Molecular Oncology: *Principles and Recent Advances*

Editor

Javier Camacho

Centro de Investigación y de Estudios Avanzados, CINVESTAV
Department of Pharmacology
Avenida Instituto Politécnico Nacional
Mexico

CONTENTS

Foreword   *i*

Preface   *ii*

List of Contributors   *iii*

CHAPTERS

1. **Cell Proliferation, Differentiation and Apoptosis**   3
   Miriam Huerta, Carla Angulo and Esther López-Bayghen

2. **Causes of Cancer**
   I) The Influence of the Environment   18
   Andrea De Vizcaya-Ruiz and Araceli Hernández-Zavala

   II) Obesity and Cancer   28
   Ranier Gutiérrez

   III) Estrogens and Cancer   33
   Jesús Adrián Rodríguez-Rasgado, Flavia Morales-Vásquez, Luz María Hinojosa and Javier Camacho

   IV) Example 1: Hepatocellular Carcinoma   44
   Pablo Muriel

   V) Example 2: Estrogens, Retinoids and Cervical Cancer Development   48
   Jorge Gutiérrez, Enoc M. Cortés, José J. Vázquez and Patricio Gariglio

3. **Oncogenes and Tumor Suppressor Genes**   64
   Patricio Gariglio

4. **Epigenetics of Cancer**   83
   Claudia M. García-Cuellar and Alfonso Dueñas-González

5. **Signal Transduction Pathways in Cancer**   98
   Lucrecia Marquez-Rosado

6. **Metastasis**   112
   Lucrecia Márquez-Rosado

7. **Cancer Immunology and Novel Strategies for Immunotherapy**   130
   Alberto Monroy-García, María de Lourdes Mora-García and Jorge Hernández-Montes

8. ***In Vitro* and *In Vivo* Models for Cancer Research**   148
   Julio I. Pérez Carreón and Jorge M. Zajgla

9. **Molecular Diagnosis and Prognosis**   163
   M. Verónica Ponce-Castañeda and Lourdes Cabrera-Muñoz

10. **Chemotherapy and Design of New Antineoplasic Compounds** 172

   Claudia Rivera-Guevara, María E. Bravo-Gómez and Lena Ruiz-Azuara

11. **Mechanisms of Therapy Resistance in Cancer** 192

   Iván Restrepo, Cindy S. Ortiz and Javier Camacho

12. **Antisense Oligodeoxyribonucleotides (AS-ODNs) for Cancer Gene Therapy: A Clinical Perspective** 198

   María L. Benítez-Hess and Luis M. Alvarez-Salas

13. **Directions of Future Cancer Research** 219

   Javier Camacho

   Author Index 223

   Subject Index 224

FOREWORD

The presentation of basic concepts and recent scientific advances is a demanding task to achieve in a single literary resource. This particular and timely combination is excellently accomplished in this book.

Given the broad spectrum of readership that will benefit from this book, it was imperative that the book was prepared by oncologists and scientists not only having demonstrated fundamental expertise in specific fields but who also have general presentation skills. In this manner, the present book reflects the knowledge necessary to communicate molecular aspects of oncology to Graduates and PhD candidates, physicians, oncologists and a broad variety of scientists, among more general readers. It is my pleasure to encourage readers to go through all of the chapters of this well-organized book.

This work represents an extraordinary effort of both, the Editor - Dr. Javier Camacho - and the other authors in order to offer a state-of-the-art scenario and a reliable and extremely valuable information source about basic concepts in molecular oncology.

With no doubt, this book perfectly meets the key features that people interested in molecular oncology books are seeking to find.

Manfred Schwab, Dr. rer. nat.
Professor for Genetics
Director, Division of Tumor Genetics
German Cancer Research Center (DKFZ)
Heidelberg, Germany
Editor-in-Chief:
Encyclopedia of Cancer (Springer), Cancer Letters

PREFACE

Cancer is one of the major causes of death worldwide. Despite hundreds of clinical trials are currently running for cancer patients, the successful rate is still very low. Therefore, early markers for cancer as well as novel therapeutic targets and drugs are needed. Understanding of the molecular aspects of cancer development, the discovery of new molecular targets and the rational drug design on a molecular basis, with no doubt should help to decrease cancer mortality.

In consideration to these demands, and in view of cancer as a multi-factorial disease, this book describes some of the most important topics related to cancer on a molecular basis. From describing causes of cancer to rational drug design, including molecular diagnosis and prognosis, the book covers many areas of interest to many potential readers. Instead of describing very particular processes at the very fine level, this book integrates information on different cancer topics.

This approach allows the reader to find in a single book the close relationship between causes of cancer, cell and molecular biology of cancer cells and drug design, among other subjects. This book pretends to cover a broad area of interest for people in the cancer field including students, physicians, researchers, policy makers, and people from the pharmaceutical industry.

We sincerely hope this source to be useful in the understanding of cancer and in the design of new strategies to fight against this terrible disease.

Javier Camacho
Centro de Investigación y de Estudios Avanzados, CINVESTAV
Department of Pharmacology
Avenida Instituto Politécnico Nacional
Mexico

List of Contributors

Luis M. Alvarez-Salas
Department of Genetics and Molecular Biology
Centro de Investigación y de Estudios Avanzados del I.P.N.
Avenida Instituto Politécnico Nacional 2508
07360 Mexico City
Mexico

Carla Angulo
Department of Molecular Biomedicine
Centro de Investigación y de Estudios Avanzados del I.P.N.
Avenida Instituto Politécnico Nacional 2508
07360 Mexico City
Mexico

María L. Benítez-Hess
Department of Genetics and Molecular Biology
Centro de Investigación y de Estudios Avanzados del I.P.N.
Avenida Instituto Politécnico Nacional 2508
07360 Mexico City
Mexico

María E. Bravo-Gómez
Departamento de Química Inorgánica y Nuclear
Laboratorio de Química Inorgánica Medicinal
Facultad de Química
Universidad Nacional Autónoma de México, Av. Universidad 3000
Ciudad Universitaria, México D.F. 04510
Mexico

Lourdes C. Muñoz
Departamento de Patología
Hospital Infantil de México Federico Gómez
Dr. Márquez 162
México D.F. 06720
Mexico

Javier Camacho
Department of Pharmacology
Centro de Investigación y de Estudios Avanzados del I.P.N.
Avenida Instituto Politécnico Nacional 2508
07360 Mexico City
Mexico

Enoc M. Cortés
Department of Genetics and Molecular Biology
Centro de Investigación y de Estudios Avanzados del I.P.N.
Avenida Instituto Politécnico Nacional 2508
07360 Mexico City
Mexico

Andrea De Vizcaya-Ruiz
Department of Toxicology

Centro de Investigación y de Estudios Avanzados del I.P.N.
Avenida Instituto Politécnico Nacional 2508
07360 Mexico City
Mexico

Alfonso Dueñas-González
Instituto Nacional de Cancerología
San Fernando No. 22, Tlalpan, 14080 Mexico City
Mexico and Instituto de Investigaciones Biomédicas Universidad Nacional Autónoma de México (UNAM)
Mexico

Claudia García-Cuellar
Instituto Nacional de Cancerología
San Fernando No. 22, Tlalpan,
14080 Mexico City
Mexico

Patricio Gariglio
Department of Genetics and Molecular Biology
Centro de Investigación y de Estudios Avanzados del I.P.N.
Avenida Instituto Politécnico Nacional 2508
07360 Mexico City
Mexico

Ranier Gutiérrez
Department of Pharmacology
Centro de Investigación y de Estudios Avanzados del I.P.N.
Avenida Instituto Politécnico Nacional 2508
07360 Mexico City
Mexico

Jorge Gutiérrez
Department of Genetics and Molecular Biology
Centro de Investigación y de Estudios Avanzados del I.P.N.
Avenida Instituto Politécnico Nacional 2508
07360 Mexico City
Mexico

Jorge Hernández-Montes
FES-Zaragoza, National University of México (UNAM)
Avenida Guelatao 66. Iztapalapa
09230 Mexico City
Mexico

Araceli Hernández-Zavala
Department of Toxicology
Centro de Investigación y de Estudios Avanzados del I.P.N.
Avenida Instituto Politécnico Nacional 2508
07360 Mexico City
Mexico

Luz M. Hinojosa
Hospital General "Dr. Manuel Gea González"
Avenida Calzada de Tlalpan 4800

14080 Mexico City
México

Miriam Huerta
Department of Genetics and Molecular Biology
Centro de Investigación y de Estudios Avanzados del I.P.N.
Avenida Instituto Politécnico Nacional 2508
07360 Mexico City
Mexico

Esther López-Bayghen
Department of Genetics and Molecular Biology
Centro de Investigación y de Estudios Avanzados del I.P.N.
Avenida Instituto Politécnico Nacional 2508
07360 Mexico City
Mexico

Lucrecia Márquez-Rosado
Public Health Sciences Division
Fred Hutchinson Cancer Research Center
1100 Fairview Avenue North
Seattle, WA 98109,
USA

Jorge M. Zajgla
Instituto Nacional de Medicina Genómica (INMEGEN)
México. Periférico Sur 4124
Torre Zafiro II, piso 5. Mexico D.F. 011900
Mexico

Alberto Monroy-García
Oncology Hospital, National Medical Centre, IMSS and
FES-Zaragoza, National University of México (UNAM)
Avenida Guelatao 66. Iztapalapa
09230 Mexico City
Mexico

María de L. Mora-García
FES-Zaragoza, National University of México (UNAM)
Avenida Guelatao 66. Iztapalapa
09230 Mexico City
Mexico

Flavia Morales-Vásquez
Instituto Nacional de Cancerología
San Fernando No. 22, Tlalpan,
14080 Mexico City
Mexico

Pablo Muriel
Department of Pharmacology
Centro de Investigación y de Estudios Avanzados del I.P.N.
Avenida Instituto Politécnico Nacional 2508

07360 Mexico City
Mexico

Cindy S. Ortiz
Department of Pharmacology
Centro de Investigación y de Estudios Avanzados del I.P.N.
Avenida Instituto Politécnico Nacional 2508
07360 Mexico City
Mexico

Julio I. Pérez-Carreon
Instituto Nacional de Medicina Genómica (INMEGEN)
México. Periférico Sur 4124
Torre Zafiro II, piso 5. Mexico D.F. 011900
Mexico

M. Verónica P. Castañeda
Unidad de Investigación Médica en Enfermedades Infecciosas,
Hospital de Pediatría, CMN SXXI, IMSS,
Av. Cuauhtémoc 330
México D.F.
Mexico

Iván Restrepo
Department of Pharmacology
Centro de Investigación y de Estudios Avanzados del I.P.N.
Avenida Instituto Politécnico Nacional 2508
07360 Mexico City
Mexico

Claudia R. Guevara
Departamento de Química Inorgánica y Nuclear
Laboratorio de Química Inorgánica Medicinal
Facultad de Química, Universidad Nacional Autónoma de México
Av. Universidad 3000, Ciudad Universitaria
México D.F. 04510
Mexico

Jesús A. Rodríguez-Rasgado
Department of Pharmacology
Centro de Investigación y de Estudios Avanzados del I.P.N.
Avenida Instituto Politécnico Nacional 2508
07360 Mexico City
Mexico

Lena Ruiz-Azuara
Departamento de Química Inorgánica y Nuclear
Laboratorio de Química Inorgánica Medicinal
Facultad de Química
Universidad Nacional Autónoma de México
Av. Universidad 3000
Ciudad Universitaria
México D.F. 04510
Mexico

José J. Vázquez
Department of Genetics and Molecular Biology
Centro de Investigación y de Estudios Avanzados del I.P.N.
Avenida Instituto Politécnico Nacional 2508
07360 Mexico City
Mexico

2

CHAPTER 1

Cell Proliferation, Differentiation and Apoptosis

Miriam Huerta[1], Carla Angulo[2] and Esther López-Bayghen[1,*]

[1]Departmento de Genética y Biología Molecular and [2]Departmento de Biomedicina Molecular, Centro de Investigación y de Estudios Avanzados del IPN., Avenida Instituto Politécnico Nacional 2508, 07360 Mexico City, Mexico

Abstract: Tight control of the cell cycle in eukaryotic cells exists to control proliferation, differentiation or apoptosis. These processes model and shape tissue and organ relationships in multicellular organisms. Two biochemical processes, protein phosphorylation/dephosphorylation and ubiquitin-mediated degradation drive cell cycle control. A multitude of pathways control cyclin-dependent kinase activities as the major event for cell cycle progression. Differentiation and apoptosis have cell cycle withdraw in common, while cancer and degenerative processes both show altered control of the cell cycle.

Keywords: Cell cycle, cancer, cyclins, apoptosis, check points, caspase, senescence, Bcl-2, cell differentiation, cyclin-dependent kinase.

INTRODUCTION

Eukaryotic cells live under tight control of cell division. Continuous proliferation is achieved under specific conditions; most of the cells in an adult organism are committed to a highly-specialized function, acquired and accomplished by the differentiation process. Programmed cell death or apoptosis is a naturally occurring process based on genetic and epigenetic programs and an indispensable part of the development and function of a multicellular organism. Cells that are no longer needed or that will be detrimental to an organism or tissue are disposed of in a neat and orderly manner. This prevents the development of an inflammatory response, which is often associated with necrotic cell death. While cell proliferation depends on the continuity of S, G2, M and G1 cell cycle phases, differentiation and apoptosis imply a withdrawal from the cell cycle. However, the decision to cycle or withdraw depends on the behavior and activity of diverse factors, which are controlled by external and internal signals. In this introductory chapter, we analyze those factors in normal cells. The following chapters will provide further discussion about how cell cycle factors change under pathological conditions such as cancer.

Life in Cycles

The two most unique characteristics of eukaryotic cells are the presence of a nucleus and the ability to reproduce only once by going through the cell cycle. Progress through the eukaryotic cell cycle is driven by a continuum of two biochemical processes: protein-phosphorylation-dephosphorylation and ubiquitin-mediated degradations carried out by specialized degradosome complexes (Table **1**). Control of the start point is mostly based in the correct assembly of a committed DNA replication origin. However, this is a process so extended and connected that even takes into account nuclear structure as a control element. For the eukaryotic cell, withdrawal from continuous cell cycling means commitment into differentiation, or senescence and apoptosis.

Cyclins and Kinases in Cell Cycle Control

Activities of CDKs (Cyclin-Dependent Kinases) oscillate because their kinase activity is controlled by the periodic synthesis and degradation of positive regulatory subunits, the cyclins. CDKs are a family of small serine/threonine protein kinases (~34-40 kDa), composed of little more than the catalytic core shared by all protein kinases, and undergo phosphorylation and dephosphorylation themselves. By definition, all CDKs require the binding of a regulatory cyclin subunit to achieve enzymatic activation. In most cases, full activation also requires phosphorylation of a threonine residue near the kinase active site. Animal cells contain nine CDKs [1-3] (Table **2**). Cyclins

*Address Correspondence to Esther López-Bayghen: Department of Genetics and Molecular Biology, Centro de Investigación y de Estudios Avanzados del I.P.N., Avenida Instituto Politécnico Nacional 2508, 07360 Mexico City, Mexico; Email: ebayghen@cinvestav.mx

Javier Camacho (Ed)

accumulate and activate CDKs at the appropriate times during the cell cycle and then are degraded, causing kinase inactivation [4]. They also are synthesized for the G1, S, or M-phases of the cell cycle. Particular cyclin/CDK complexes are involved in regulating cell cycle transitions at specific checkpoints (Table **2**). Disruption of cyclin action leads to either cell cycle arrest, or to uncontrolled cell proliferation.

Table 1: Major players in cell cycle control

Players	Biochemical process	Targeted proteins
Cyclins D, E, A and B (by appearing order)		CDKs
CDKs (Cyclin-Dependent Kinases)	Phosphorylation	Cyclins, CDKs, CKIs
Cell cycle phosphatases	Dephosphorylation	CDKs, CKIs
CKIs (Cyclin-dependent Kinase Inhibitors)	Blockage of Phospho/dephosphorylation processes	Cyclins/CDK complexes
Ubiquitin E3-ligase complexes (degradosomes): APC/C (Anaphase Promoting Complex/Cyclosome) SCF (Skp1-Cul1-F-box protein + oc1/Rbx1)	Ubiquitin-mediated degradation	Cyclins, CDKs, CKIs

Table 2: Cyclin-CDK complexes in cell cycle control

Cyclin-CDK complexes in cell cycle control	
Cyclin-D-CDK4/6	G1 progression
Cyclin-E-CDK2	G1-S transition
Cyclin-A-CDK2	S-phase progression
Cyclin-A/B-CDK1	Entry into M-phase
Cyclin-F	Refers to F-protein in SCF degradosome complex (see Table **1**)
Cyclin-CDK complexes involved in processes not directly related to the cell cycle	
Cyclin-H -CDK7	Component of both, the CDK-activating kinase and the basal transcription factor TFIIH, can phosphorylate CDKs
Cyclin-C-CDK8	Also associated with RNA Polymerase-II in Mediator complex; this complex phosphorylates the carboxyl-terminal repeat domain (CTD)
Cyclin-T-CDK9	Known as pTEFb (positive transcriptional elongation factor b), associates with RNA polymerase-II to bypass abortive transcription
Cyclin-K- CDK9	Phosphorylates the C-terminal domain (CTD) of RNA Polymerase-II

CDK Inhibitors

A cyclin-dependent kinase inhibitor protein (CKI) or cyclin-dependent kinase inhibitor (CIP/KIP) is a protein that inhibits both cyclin and CDK subunits, modulating the activities of Cyclins D-, E-, A-, and B/CDK complexes and preventing cell cycle progression. Levels of some CKIs, which specifically inhibit certain cyclin/CDK complexes, also rise and fall at specific times during the cell cycle [2]. Two major families of genes have been defined based on their evolutionary origins, structure, and CDK specificities: the CIP/KIP family and the INK4 (inhibitor of kinase 4) [5]. The CIP/KIP family includes $p21^{KIP}$, $p27^{KIP1}$ and $p57^{KIP}$. These three CKIs contain a conserved region of sequence at the NH_2 terminus that is required and sufficient for the inhibition of cyclin/CDK complexes, whereas the COOH terminal regions are variable in length and function. They can bind and inhibit a broad range of cyclin/CDK complexes, with a preference for those containing CDK2. For example, $p21^{KIP}$ (also called WAF1, CAP20, Cip1, and Sdi1) plays an essential role in growth arrest after DNA damage, and overexpression leads to G_1 and G_2 or S-phase arrest [6]. The INK4 gene family encodes $p16^{INK4a}$, $p15^{INK4b}$, $p18^{INK4c}$, and $p19^{INK4d}$, all of which bind to CDK4 and CDK6 and inhibit their kinase activities by interfering with their association with D-type cyclins [5,6]. A complex phosphorylation network modulates CIP/KIP protein functions by altering their subcellular localization, stability, protein-protein interactions and affinity for specific cyclin-CDK complexes and other proteins. Phosphorylation of various amino acids controls many aspects of CIP/KIP protein biology, but also their stability and subcellular localization [7, 8]. In fact, they are multifunctional proteins with functions beyond cell cycle regulation, including roles in apoptosis, transcriptional regulation, cell fate determination, cell migration, cell survival, cytoskeletal dynamics and probably other undiscovered functions [6].

From the cancer biology perspective, CKIs play a dual role during tumorigenesis, acting as both tumor suppressors and oncogenes. In tumors, the deregulation of various signaling pathways such as PKB/Akt inactivates the tumor-suppressor functions of these proteins, but maintains or even exacerbates the oncogenic potential. Thus, for therapeutic purposes, simply increasing the expression of these CKIs may not be beneficial and could have consequences opposite to those intended. A major challenge is now to gain the knowledge that will permit specific targeting of the oncogenic functions of CKIs while maintaining or restoring the tumor suppressor functions [9, 10].

Cell Cycle Phosphatases

Activation of cyclin-dependent kinases in higher eukaryotic cells can be achieved at specific stages of the cell cycle through dephosphorylation by members of the Cdc25 (Cell Division Cycle 25) phosphatase family (Cdc25A, Cdc25B and Cdc25C). Cdc25A plays an important role at the G1/S-phase transition. Cdc25B undergoes activation during S-phase and plays a role in activating the mitotic kinase Cyclin B/CDK1 in the cytoplasm. Active Cyclin B/CDK1 complex then phosphorylates and activates Cdc25C, leading to a positive feedback mechanism and entry into mitosis. In addition, human Cdc25A, Cdc25B and Cdc25C are the main players of the G2 arrest caused by DNA damage or by the presence of unreplicated DNA [11]. The expression and activity of these enzymes are finely regulated by multiple mechanisms including post-translational modifications, interactions with regulatory partners, intracellular localization, and cell cycle-regulated degradation. Altered expression of these phosphatases is associated with checkpoint bypass and genetic instability. Accordingly, increased expression of Cdc25A and Cdc25B is found in many high-grade tumors and is correlated with poor prognosis in human cancers [12].

Cdc25B phosphatase plays an essential role in controlling the activity of Cyclin B/CDK1 complexes at the entry into mitosis, and together with Polo-Like Kinase 1 (PLK1) in regulating the resumption of cell cycle progression after DNA damage-dependent checkpoint arrest in G2. PLK1 activity is essential for the relocation of Cdc25B from the cytoplasm to the nucleus. By gain- and loss-of-function analyses, it has been shown that PLK1 stimulates Cdc25B-induced mitotic entry under both normal conditions and after DNA damage-induced G2/M arrest. A model in which PLK1 regulates mitosis-inducing activity at the G2-M transition by relocalization of Cdc25B to the nucleus has been proposed [13].

Cell Cycle Step 1: Transcribe Cyclin D1 Gene

A main event in G1-phase is to raise Cyclin D1 levels, mostly through transcriptional and post-transcriptional mechanisms [3]. Between other activities, Cyclin D1/CDK4/CDK6 complexes control two major events in G1: the release of negative control exerted by the tumor suppressor Rb (Retinoblastoma susceptibility protein) over the E2F transcription factors and over the Cyclin E gene transcriptional activation. Cyclin D1/CDK4/CDK6 complexes are responsible for the first phosphorylation of Rb in G1-phase [2]. During G1, the Rb-HDACs (Histone Deacetylases) repressor complex binds to the E2F-DP1 transcription factors, inhibiting downstream transcription.

The mitogenic signals that encourage the cell to commence cell division activate signal transduction pathways in which Mitogen-Activated Protein Kinases (MAPKs) lead to mitosis. Signals received by growth factor cell surface receptors communicate to the nuclear cell cycle machinery to induce cell division and mediate the exit from G0 into G1 and S-phases of the cell cycle. In normal cells, the Cyclin D1 gene receives these transduced signals about the mitogenic potential of the microenvironment and begins the shift from quiescence to cell cycle entry. Cyclin D1 induction requires coordinated signaling from the extracellular matrix (ECM), soluble growth factors, and developmental signals [14]. Many binding sites/transcription factors are final effectors in multiple pathways, each of which has its own and frequently numerous, upstream signaling molecules. Since the Cyclin D1 promoter was first described [15, 16], many different individual transcription factor sequences have been identified that are involved in the regulation of Cyclin D1 transcription (determined by luciferase reporter assays, chromatin immunoprecipitation (ChIP) and *in vitro* studies using electrophoretic mobility shift assays) [17]. A major family of Cyclin D1 inducers are the MAPKs. Ras-Raf-MEK (MAPK and extracellular signal-regulated kinase (ERK))-ERK pathways play a major role through stimulating the expression of AP-1 transcription factors dimers of Fos, Jun and Activating

Transcription Factor (ATF) families [18-20]. The most common pathway is Ras, involved in a number of cytoplasmic signaling cascades such as PI3K (Phosphatidylinositiol-3 Kinase), Raf and Rho. Ras activation leads to transcriptional induction of Cyclin D1 in early G1 through a Ras-responsive element in the Cyclin D1 gene promoter. In addition to soluble mitogens, Cyclin D1 transcription is also regulated by ECM signaling through FAK and by developmental paths such as Wnt and Notch. An extensive number of transcription factors positively or negatively modulate Cyclin D1 transcription either in a tissue-specific manner or *via* specialized stimulation [21]. During cellular transformation, Cyclin D1 is frequently altered, found in many breast, liver, lung and brain cancers. Although Cyclin D1 overexpression is clearly implicated in cancers, overexpression of Cyclin D1 is not sufficient to drive oncogenic transformation. Rather, emerging evidence suggests that nuclear retention of Cyclin D1 resulting from altered nuclear trafficking and proteolysis is critical for the manifestation of its oncogenic potential [22]. This review provides a brief overview of current data documenting various mechanisms underlying aberrant Cyclin D1 regulation in human cancers and their impact on neoplastic transformation. Conversely, repression of Cyclin D1 gene expression is a hallmark of cell differentiation [1].

Step 2: Begin DNA Synthesis in S-phase

With rising levels of activated Cyclin D1, Cyclin E is synthesized. When Cyclin E is abundant, it interacts with CDK2 and allows progression of the cell cycle from G1 to S-phase. This is the first cell cycle checkpoint. The decision to either to remain in G1 or progress into S-phase is influenced by the balance between Cyclin E production and proteolytic degradation in the proteosome. Cyclin E is targeted for destruction by the proteosome through ubiquitination when associated with a complex of proteins called the SCF or F box complex.

Rb is one of the key targets of activated Cyclin E/CDK2. When Rb is dephosphorylated in the beginning of G1, it forms complexes with and blocks the transcriptional activation of the E2F family of transcription factors. However, when Cyclin E/CDK2 phosphorylates Rb, this regulator dissociates from E2F, allowing transcription of genes required for S-phase. Active E2F consists of a heterodimeric complex of an E2F polypeptide and a DP1 protein [23]. One of the genes activated by E2F is Cyclin E itself, leading to a positive feedback cycle as Cyclin E accumulates.

Cyclin A can activate two different cyclin-dependent kinases (CDK1 and CDK2) and functions in both S-phase and mitosis. In S-phase, Cyclin A levels rise, allowing the formation of Cyclin A/CDK2 complexes, which further phosphorylates Rb. Phosphorylation of DNA replication machinery components such as CDC6 (Cell Cycle Control Protein) is important for DNA replication initiation and to restrict it to only once per cell cycle. Cyclin A synthesis is mainly controlled at the transcriptional level, involving E2F and other transcription factors. Cyclin A starts to accumulate during S-phase and is abruptly degraded before metaphase. Removal of Cyclin A (and also Cyclin B) is carried out by ubiquitin-mediated proteolysis, by the APC/C degradosome [24].

Table 3: Cyclin B/CDK1 (MPF) main activities

MPF...			
Controls nuclear dissemble; breakdown and degradation of the nuclear envelope	Controls chromosome cohesion condensation process	Prevents cytokinesis	Controls mitotic spindle formation
By phosphorylation of...			
specific lamin serines; causes depolymerization of lamin filaments, leading to of the nuclear envelope (early in mitosis)	condensins (which enable chromatin condensation (prophase), which enable chromatin condensation (prophase)	inhibitory sites on myosin early in mitosis	microtubule-associated proteins
When MPF activity falls at anaphase, the inhibitory sites are dephosphorylated and cytokinesis proceeds			

Step 3: Toward Mitosis- Cyclin B/CDK1 Checking for Correct DNA Distribution

As Cyclin-B levels rise in G2 and M-phases, [25], it combines with CDK1 to form the major mitotic kinase M-phase promoting factor (MPF). During G2, the Cyclin B/CDK1 complex is maintained in an inactive state by the dual-specificity tyrosine kinase Wee1 and by Myt1 (Myelin Transcription Factor 1). As cells approach M-phase, the phosphatase Cdc25 is activated by Polo-Like Kinase (PLK). Cdc25 then activates CDK1, establishing a feedback amplification loop that efficiently drives the cell into mitosis. MPF performs a variety of activities necessary to generate the massive changes occurring in mitosis (Table **3**). Once MPF causes entry of cells into mitosis, it activates the degradation of its own cyclin subunit (Cyclin B) *via* the APC/C degradosome complex. MPF inactivation, caused by the degradation of Cyclin B, is required to exit mitosis. The 14-3-3 proteins bind phosphorylated Cyclin B/CDK1 kinase and export it from the nucleus [26].

Ubiquitin Proteosome System: Degradation Control of the Cell Cycle

A major mechanism underlying control of cell division is regulation of protein stability through the Ubiquitin Proteasome System (UPS). Degradation *via* UPS occurs by a two-step process: the target protein is first tagged by covalent attachment of ubiquitin and subsequently degraded by a multicatalytic protease complex called the 26S proteasome. Conjugation of ubiquitin to the protein involves a cascade of three enzymes: E1, E2 and E3. Ubiquitin-Activating Enzyme (E1) forms a high-energy thioester intermediate, E1-S~Ubi, which is then trans-esterified to one of the several Ubiquitin Conjugating Enzymes (E2s). The transfer of ubiquitin from the E2-S~Ubi to an ε-NH$_2$ group of an internal lysine residue in the target protein requires an Ubiquitin Protein-Ligase (E3). Because E3 enzymes determine the substrate specificity, they play the most important role in the ubiquitination reaction [27]. Among the different classes of E3s, the SCF (or F box complex, also known as Skp1-Cullin1-F-box Protein-Roc1 ubiquitin ligase complex) and the Anaphase Promoting Complex/Cyclosome (APC/C), dominate control over DNA replication and cell cycle regulation. The SCF ubiquitin ligase complex degrades negative regulators such as CKIs at the G1-to-S-phase checkpoint, and APC/C permits progression and exit from mitosis by inducing proteolysis of different cell cycle regulators [27].

Both synthesis and destruction of cyclins are important for cell cycle progression. All cyclins are degraded by ubiquitin-mediated processes, and the modes by which these systems are connected to the cell-cycle regulatory phosphorylation network are different for mitotic (A and B) and for G1 cyclins (D and E) [4]. The cellular decision to either remain in G1 or to progress into S-phase is partly a result of the balance between Cyclin E production and its proteolytic degradation. The ubiquitin-mediated proteolysis of Cyclin E plays a central role in cell cycle progression and is triggered by multisite phosphorylation, inducing targeting for destruction, when it is associated with SCF. Cyclin E accumulation is a common event in cancer. An F-box protein, Fbx2, recognizes high-mannose oligosaccharides in Cyclin E. Skp2 and its cofactor Cks1 are substrate-targeting subunits, and structures within the Skp2 complex bound to Cyclin E peptides identify a doubly phosphorylated pThr380/pSer384 Cyclin E motif as an optimal, high-affinity degron and a singly phosphorylated pThr62 motif as a low-affinity degron [27, 28]. The budding yeast SCF^{CDC4} and the mammalian SCF^{SKP2} (with the name of the F-box protein being indicated in uppercase) are required to destroy SIC1 and p27^{KIP1}, respectively, promoting entry into S-phase [27]. The human SCF^{SKP2} E3 targets other essential regulators of S-phase progression [29], including E2F1 [30], the Rb-like p130 protein [31] and the licensing factor for DNA replication, CDT1 [32].

Final Step: Leaving Mitosis

Anaphase-Promoting Complex/Cyclosome (APC/C) is the second multi-subunit E3 ubiquitin ligase. The complex is a 1.5 MDa complex composed of a dozen different subunits and permits progression and exit from mitosis by inducing proteolysis of different cell cycle regulators. Cyclin B destruction by APC/C is essential for metaphase-anaphase transition; expression of an indestructible Cyclin B traps cells in mitosis (reviewed in [33, 34]). APC/C is conserved from yeast to human and relies on two adaptor proteins, Cdc20 and Cdh1, to bring in substrates. Both APCCdc20 and APCCdh1 control mitosis through ubiquitination and degradation of mitotic regulators such as Securin and Plk1. APCCdh1 is thought to prevent premature S-phase entry by limiting the accumulation of mitotic cyclins in G1-phase, and also to regulates processes unrelated to cell cycle [26]. Anaphase induction is regulated by cohesin complexes. Cohesin complexes connect chromosomes within their centromeric regions and also along the arms of sister chromatids. The dissolution of sister chromatid cohesion is catalyzed by the Separase protease after the destruction of its inhibitor Securin, which is polyubiquitinated by the APC/C during early anaphase [26].

Cell Cycle Checkpoints

High fidelity genome transmission for the maintenance of genome integrity depends on the existence of specific cell cycle checkpoints. Many different stimuli exert stop signals at different checkpoints within the cell cycle. Checkpoint pathways suppress initiation of the next event by inhibiting cell cycle regulators until completion of previous events or correction of anomalies such as DNA damage.

The G1/S-phase border is mainly controlled by interpreting growth factor withdrawal or mitogenic signals to determine if the cell's environment is favorable. DNA damage from irradiation or chemical modification also prevents cells from entering the S-phase mainly by blocking the activation of cyclin E-CDK2 until enough pre-replicative complexes are formed. This checkpoint has two functions. The first is to inhibit DNA replication initiation from hitherto unfired origins through targeting the Cyclin E/CDK2 and CDC7-DBF4 kinases that regulate the assembly and firing of replication-competent origins. The second function is to protect replication fork integrity and allow the recovery of cell-cycle progression after DNA repair and/or restoration of the dNTP pools. Many proteins influence the intra-S-phase DNA damage checkpoint. Parallel to implementing a cell cycle arrest, checkpoint signaling also mediates the recruitment of DNA repair systems. If the extent of damage exceeds repair capacity, additional signaling cascades are activated to ensure elimination of these damaged cells (see Apoptosis). DNA damage activates the DNA-PK/ATM/CHK2-ATR/CHK1 kinases that control phosphatase Cdc25 (see Mitosis) a positive regulator of cell cycle progression that is inhibited by CHK1-mediated or CHK2-mediated phosphorylation [35, 36].

The G2/M checkpoint ensures that only completely replicated, undamaged DNA is present, preventing cells in G_2 from entering mitosis. Moderate DNA damage activates p53, a transcription factor that stimulates expression of $p21^{KIP}$, and with inactivation of Cyclins E and D, inhibits all CDK-cyclin complexes causing arrest in G_1 and G_2. In response to extensive DNA damage, p53 activates genes that induce apoptosis. Loss of the important regulator p53 leads to genome instability [37].

The metaphase checkpoint, occurring almost at the end of M-phase, can be overcome when all chromosomes are attached to the spindle. A stop occurs by blocking APC/C activation. Cells do not enter anaphase until all kinetochores are bound to spindle microtubules. Consequently, defects in mitotic spindle assembly or in the attachment of kinetochores to spindle microtubules prevent APC/C activation. DNA damage activates the sensor systems (DNA-PK/ATM/ATR kinases, the transducers as Cds1), initiating cascades to implement cell cycle arrest by inactivation of Cyclin B/CDK1, in turn blocking degradosome APC/C activation. Cdc25 (prevent activation of Cyclin B/CDK1 (MPF) [12, 37].

TGF-Beta, DNA damage, contact inhibition and replicative senescence occur through induction of INK4A family or KIP/CIP families of cell cycle kinase inhibitors. TGF-Beta additionally inhibits the transcription of Cdc25A. Defects in many of the molecules that regulate the cell cycle checkpoints also lead to tumor progression. Key among these are p53, the CKIs p15 (INK4B), p16 (INK4A), p18 (INK4C), p19 (INK4D), $p21^{KIP}$, $p27^{KIP1}$ and Rb, which act to halt cell cycle progression until DNA repair has been completed [38].

Cell Cycle and Cell Differentiation

All cellular processes that confer new abilities, allowing that cell to perform specialized functions are globally referred to as cell differentiation. Unlike the cell cycle where molecular events are highly conserved across all cells, signals, cascades, and gene expression patterns during differentiation are specific for a defined cell type and for that development timing. Differentiation is induced by specific signals, recruiting transcription factors as effectors that accomplish new gene expression patterns by turning on and off certain genes. Differentiation dramatically changes a cell's size, shape, membrane potential, metabolic activity and responsiveness to signals. As multicellular organisms develop from the fertilized egg to the complete body, differentiation occurs often to produce a vast number of specialized cell types and tissues.

Of particular recent interest is the process by which the descendants of a single cell undergo specialization and organize into a complex organism. Adult stem cells divide and create fully-differentiated daughter cells during tissue repair and during normal cell turnover. A cell that is able to differentiate into any cell type is known as totipotent, and a pluripotent cell is a stem cell that is able to differentiate into many cell types. In mammals, only the zygote and early embryonic cells are totipotent [39]. De-differentiation is a cellular process often seen as an aberration of the normal development cycle that often results in cancer. In cytopathology, the differentiation grade of tumors is frequently used as a marker to measure cancer progression.

The phenomenon of nuclear reprogramming was first demonstrated in the context of somatic cell nuclear transfer experiments. These experiments showed that the nucleus from an adult somatic cell can be reprogrammed to an earlier developmental state upon transfer into an unfertilized oocyte. This strategy resulted in the generation of cloned embryos with the potential to develop into an identical animal, the first of which was Dolly the sheep [40]. Embryonic Stem (ES) cells are embryo-derived cell lines that retain pluripotency and represent invaluable tools for research into the mechanisms of tissue formation [39]. Takahashi and Yamanaka (2006) [41] took a significant step toward delineating the minimal set of factors required to confer the developmental potential of an ES cell onto a terminally-differentiated somatic cell. As ES cells have reprogramming capabilities, the authors performed retroviral transduction of ES cell-specific genes, particularly transcription factors, into somatic cells to induce them to take on a more embryonic character. More recently, fibroblasts have been directly reprogrammed back to pluripotency by ectopic expression of four transcription factors (Oct4, Sox2, Klf4 and Myc), yielding induced pluripotent stem (iPS) cells [42, 43]. The surprising fact that pluripotency could be achieved by introducing embryonic transcription factors into fully-differentiated somatic cells provides an additional perspective on the regulation of a cell's developmental identity. Extensive reprogramming of adult human somatic cells is a dream for tissue regeneration, aging, and disease therapies that is ever closer to becoming reality.

What is Apoptosis?

Cell death occurs by one of three events: necrosis, autophagy, or apoptosis. Apoptosis (Greek: *apo* - from, *ptosis* - falling) or programmed cellular death, is a normal cellular process that is essential for the proper development and maintenance of all multicellular organisms. Apoptosis is also necessary for the destruction of cells considered a threat, such as cells infected with viruses, cells with DNA damage, cancerous cells, and cells of the immune system after they have fulfilled their function. Apoptosis is a highly organized process characterized by nuclear changes, chromatin shrinkage, DNA fragmentation, membrane blebbing, and the formation of apoptotic bodies. Programmed cell death occurs through rapid ingestion and degradation of apoptotic bodies by the surrounding surviving cells without the participation of professional phagocytic cells, and in the absence of subsequent inflammatory reaction [44, 45]. Although apoptosis has been described since 1842, many molecular mechanisms of this process are still under analysis. A number of key genes have been characterized in several species, along with their human counterparts (Table **4**) [46-48]. Scores of new proteins have been found to play a role in apoptosis, and many proteins that have defined roles in other cellular events are able to modulate the process [49-51].

Table 4: Comparison of apoptosis proteins in different species

Human, Mouse and *X. laevis*	*C. elegans*	*D. melanogaster*
Bcl-2	Ced-9	Buffy and Debcl
BH3-only proteins	Egl1	ND
Apaf-1	Ced-4	ARK
Caspase-9	Ced-3	DRONC
Caspase-3	ND	DRICE/DCP-1
IAP	ND	DIAP1

Two Ways into Apoptosis

In mammals, two alternative pathways into apoptosis involve activation of executioner proteases. The first pathway is extrinsic, carried out by proteins as transmembrane death receptors, scaffold proteins and non-active forms of cysteine-dependent aspartate-specific proteases, the caspases. The death receptors belong to the Tumor Necrosis Factor (TNF) receptor gene superfamily, consisting of more than 20 proteins with a wide range of biological functions including cell death regulation, survival, differentiation, and immune responses (Table **5**) [52, 53].

These receptors contain a conserved 80 amino acid sequence called the "death domain" in the cytosolic tail that is responsible for transduction of cytotoxic signals [54]. Two scaffold proteins bind to death domains: FAS-associated death domain protein (FADD) and TNFR-1 associated death domain protein (TRADD) [55, 56]. The non-active forms of mammalian caspases can be classified in two groups: those involved in inflammatory responses and innate immunity as caspases 1, 4, and 5; and those that regulate programmed cell death such as caspases 2, 3, 6, 7, 8, and 9

[57]. All of these proteins constitute the death-inducing signaling complex (DISC) [58]. The extrinsic pathway starts with ligand binding to the death receptor followed by receptor trimerization. For TNFR-1, interaction of the cytosolic receptor domains with TRADD occurs first, followed by FADD [56]. Next a pro-caspase (8, 10, or 2) binds to FADD and becomes activated. The so-called "initiator" caspases 8, 10, or 2 activate pro-caspases 3, 6, and 7. In turn, caspase 3 also activates caspase 6 [59]. Executor caspases translocate into the cell nucleus and activate the DNA fragmentation factor (DFF), a heterodimeric protein (40/50 kDa) that triggers chromatin condensation and acts as a DNase [60]. Cleavage of many structural, functional, or housekeeping proteins including nuclear lamins, actin, α-fodrin, α II-spectrin, β II-spectrin, nuclear replication factor MCM3, the large subunit of DNA replication factor C, Rad51, (ADP-ribose) polymerase (PARP), U1-ribonucleoprotein (U1-70 kDa), the catalytic subunit of the DNA-dependent protein kinase (DNA-PKcs), the protein β NAC involved in binding to nascent chains as they emerge from the ribosome, and others, facilitate the structural disassembly of the cell undergoing apoptosis [61-63] (Fig. **1**).

Table 5: Tumor Necrosis Factor (TNF) Receptor family members associated with apoptosis

Receptor	Also known as	Ligand	Also known as
TNFRSF1B	CD120, p75, **TNF-R**, TNF-R-II, TNFR80, TNFR2, TNF-R75, TNFBR, p75 TNFR	TNFSF2	**TNFα**, TNF, DIF
TNFRSF6	**CD95, Fas**, APO-1, APT1	TNFSF6 TNF	**FasL**, APO-1L, APT1LG1
TNFRSF10A	**TRAIL-R1**, DR4, APO-2	TNFSF10	**TRAIL**, APO-2L. TL2
TNFRSF10B	**TRAIL-R2**, DR5, Killer, Trick2A, Trick2B	TNFSF10	**TRAIL**, APO-2L. TL2
TNFRSF10C	**TRAIL-R3**, DcR1, LIT, TRID	TNFSF10	**TRAIL**, APO-2L. TL2
TNFRSF10D	**TRAIL-R4**, DcR2, TRUNDD	TNFSF10	**TRAIL**, APO-2L. TL2
Adapted from http://www.gene.ucl.ac.uk/nomenclature/genefamily/tnftop.html. TRAIL: tumor necrosis factor (TNF)-related apoptosis-inducing ligand.			

The second pathway is the intrinsic or mitochondria-associated apoptosis pathway. After an apoptotic stimulus, such as UV light or radiation, there is an imbalance of pro- and anti- apoptotic proteins from the Bcl-2 family (Table **6**), leading to the activation of Bax and/or Bak proteins [64]. The mitochondrial inner membrane is disassembled through the permeability transition pore (PTP) complex [65]. As a consequence, cytochrome C translocates into the cytoplasm [66], where it binds to Apaf-1 in the presence of dATP, to form the apoptosome, a ring-shaped heptamer complex [67-69]. The apoptosome formation is important for creating a scaffold for procaspase-9 activation [70-72], leading to activation of caspases 3, 6, and 7 [71] (Fig. **1**). Some cells undergo amplified feedback mechanisms to enhance the apoptosis pathways. Cross-talk between the extrinsic and intrinsic pathways is established through BID, a specific substrate of caspase 8. Cytosolic BID translocates into mitochondria after being cleaved by caspase 8. Truncated BID (tBID) promotes clustering of mitochondria around the nuclei and caspase-independent release of cytochrome c by inducing MAC (mitochondrial apoptosis-induced channel) [73, 74] (Fig. **1**). Another enhanced apoptosis mechanism requires that activated caspase 3 cleaves procaspases 2, 6, 8, and 10 prior to procaspase 9 processing [75] (Fig. **1**).

Table 6: Proteins that participate in the intrinsic apoptotic pathway

Bcl-2 Family		
Anti-apoptotic	**Pro-Apoptotic**	
	Bax-like roup	**BH3-only proteins**
Bcl-2	Bax	Bad, Bik, BID,
Bcl-X$_L$	Bak	Bim (EL, L, S),
Mcl-1	Bok	Bmf, Hrk
Diva		Noxa, Puma
Bcl-w		
A1		

Reviewed in [76, 82, 83].

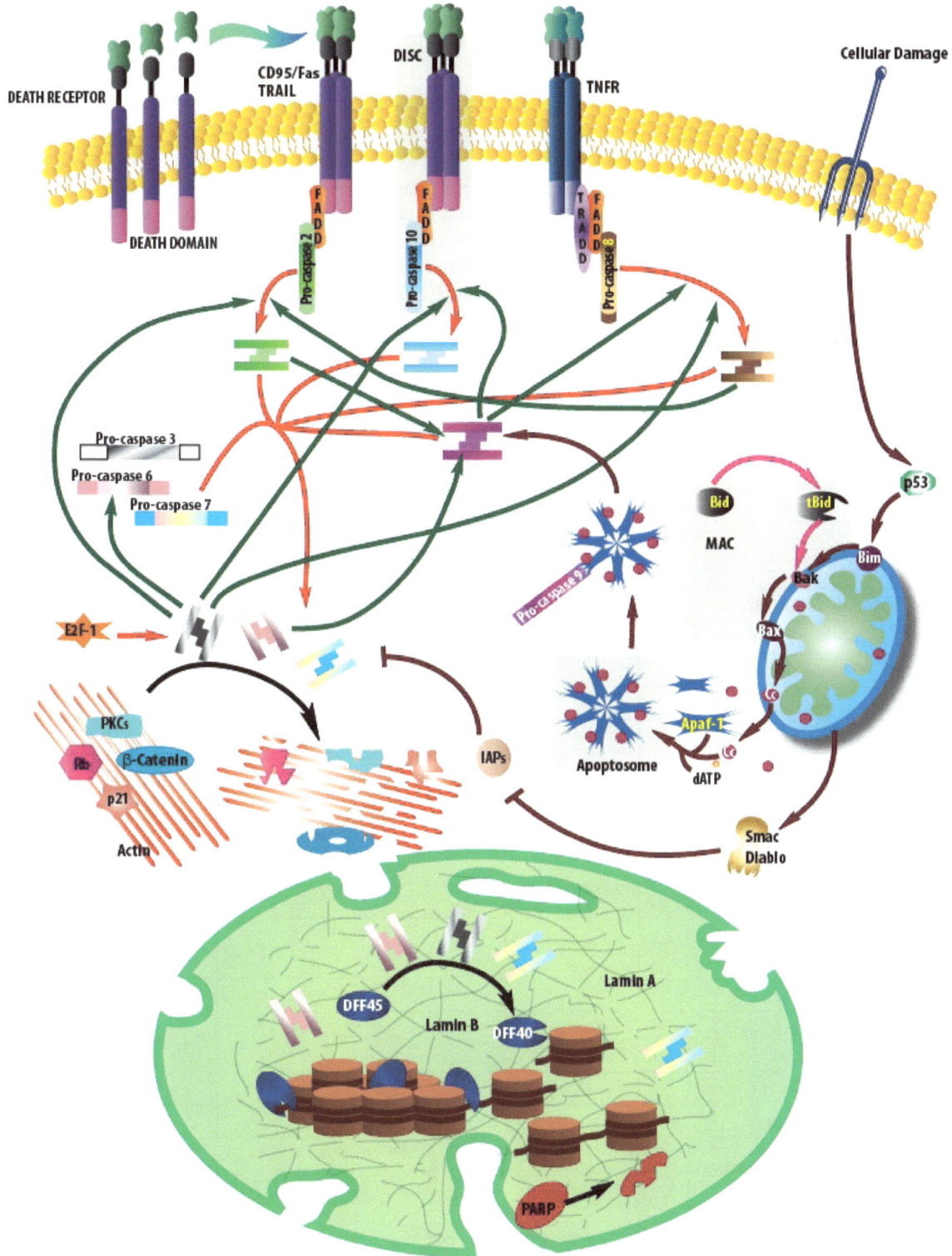

Figure 1: Schematic representation of apoptosis pathways in mammalian cells. Red arrows represent the extrinsic pathway, the brown ones correspond to the intrinsic pathway, the pink ones indicate the cross-talk between extrinsic and intrinsic pathways, the black ones point to the common mechanism, and the green ones symbolize the feedback mechanisms. The light gray boxes indicate the main complexes form in each pathway. For the description of each pathway see the text.

Since the caspases are the main effectors of apoptosis, their expression and function are tightly regulated by a family of antiapoptotic proteins that bind and inhibit caspases (IAP, Inhibitors of Apoptosis Proteins) including cIAP1, cIAP2, XIAP, NAIP, ML-IAP, ILP2, Livin, Apolon, and Survivin [76]. IAPs themselves are subject to inhibition by the mitochondrial proteins Smac/Diablo and Omi/HtrA2 [77-81].

Apoptosis Serves Several Purposes

Apoptosis plays a critical role in development and homeostasis. To maintain cell division integrity, the exit to programmed cell death occurs at two specific points during the cell cycle: entry into DNA division and the exit from mitosis. When irreversible DNA damage occurs, or the replicated chromosomes have not properly aligned on the mitotic spindle, the cell undergoes apoptosis. Hence, the cell cycle and apoptosis share some common participants such as Rb, E2F, and p53 proteins [84, 85] (Fig. **1**). Moreover, altered expression of some apoptosis proteins is associated with some diseases where cell proliferation is misregulated. For example, decreased expression or mutation of CD95/Fas has been reported in T cell leukemia [86], non-small cell lung cancer [87], and urinary bladder carcinomas [88]. In many allergic diseases, eosinophil apoptosis is delayed due to overexpression of Bim and Bcl-xL proteins [89].

Table 7: Most common cancers

Cancer type	Am	Eu	SEAs	Af	WP
Bladder		■			
Bone					
Brain and nervous system					
Colon and Rectum	■	■			■
Endometrial					
Female Breast	■	■	■	■	■
Hodgkin lymphoma					
Kidney					
Leukaemia					
Liver			■	■	■
Lung and Bronchus	■	■	■	■	■
Melanoma of the skin					
Multiple myeloma	■		■	■	
Non-Hodgkin Lymphoma					
Oesophagus			■	■	■
Oral cavity/ pharynx					
Ovary					
Pancreas					
Prostate	■	■		■	
Stomach	■	■	■	■	■
Testis					
Thyroid					
Urinary bladder					
Uterine cervix	■	■	■	■	

Modified from [100]. Am, Americas; Eu, Europe; SEAs, South East Asia; Af, Africa; WP, Western Pacific. Color stands for an extraordinary incidence of the particular cancer type in the geographical region.

During embryogenesis, apoptosis plays an important role in modulating normal tissue development. In the limb formation, programmed cell death occurs in the interdigital region to eliminate the membrane between each finger

[90]. Even after birth, some tissues are remodeled by apoptosis, such as the mouse vaginal opening [91]. In lymphoid cell development where the aim is to keep only the cells that do not recognize auto-antigens, selection of negative T and B cells and fail-positive selection results in apoptosis. Moreover, apoptosis is involved in control of T and B cell numbers at the peripheral lymphoid organs, *via* receptor-induced apoptosis or the loss of extracellular survival signals [83, 92, 93]. Apoptosis is also particularly important in nervous system development, whereby a large number of newly-generated neurons die by apoptosis. Apoptosis occurs in cells that are damaged by a variety of xenobiotic stimuli, including many toxic metals such as arsenic. This poisonous metalloid induces apoptosis by several mechanisms, including increased intracellular calcium, which in turn activates mitochondrial PTP, depletion of intracellular glutathione, cytochrome C release, and DNA strand breakage; all stimuli for starting the intrinsic apoptosis pathway [94-97].

Cellular antiproliferation is also mediated through apoptosis. When the liver suffers an acute damage, the hepatic stellate cells activate myofibroblastic cells to proliferate and repair the organ by the synthesis of matrix proteins. After this process, hepatic stellate cells self-activate programmed cell death *via* the CD95/Fas pathway [98]. Apoptosis also plays a role in regulating and limiting numbers of Hematopoietic Stem Cells (HSC), which need to be maintained at an adequate number throughout life. In transgenic mice overexpressing the anti-apoptotic protein Bcl-2, the population of HSC increases, potentially giving rise to certain proliferative diseases [99].

APOPTOSIS IN CANCER THERAPEUTICS

Apoptosis is an essential anti-neoplastic mechanism that functions in normal individuals to prevent tumorigenesis. Apoptosis induction is a goal in some cancer therapies, due to tumor cells that express low levels or non-functional pro-apoptotic proteins as CD95, TNFR, Bcl-x, and others. In pancreatic ductal adenocarcinoma cells that are CD95/TRAIL-resistant, the survival rate depends on many mechanisms, including activation of Decoy receptor 3 (DcR) that competes with CD95 for CD95L binding and interferes with FAS-triggered apoptosis [101], the increase of IAPs proteins that block caspase function [102], and over-expression of the anti-apoptotic Bcl-XL and Mcl-1 proteins [103, 104]. In other cancers such as neuroblastoma, the caspase 8 gene is silenced [105]. Apaf-1 is mutated and transcriptionally silenced in melanomas and leukemias [106], and TRAIL R1/R2 is mutated in breast cancer [107]. The altered mechanisms of apoptosis in these and other examples have been used to develop new strategies for treating certain diseases. For example, small molecules that inhibit the XIAP Protein Function (XIAP antagonists or Xantags) may show promise [108-110].

REMARKS

Changes in cell cycle factors under pathological conditions are associated with cancer development. There are as many cancer types as the number of different cell types in the human body...and more, as many tissues can give rise to several cancer types. For example, brain tumors include astrocytomas and glioblastomas, both derived from glial cells but with different pathologies. Table **7** lists the most frequently-diagnosed cancer types. The study of cell cycle control elements has shown remarkable progress. In-depth pursuit of specific factors and pathways reveals key targets that may be pharmacologically modified in order to regain normality or to induce apoptosis when cellular damage is beyond repair.

REFERENCES

[1]   Fu M, Wang C, Li Z, Sakamaki T, Pestell RG. Minireview: Cyclin D1: normal and abnormal functions. Endocrinology 2004; 145(12): 5439-47.

[2]   Coqueret O. Linking cyclins to transcriptional control. Gene 2002; 299(1-2): 35-55.

[3]   Musgrove EA. Cyclins: roles in mitogenic signaling and oncogenic transformation. Growth Factors 2006; 24(1): 13-19.

[4]   Tenderenda M. A study on the prognostic value of cyclins D1 and E expression levels in resectable gastric cancer and on some correlations between cyclins expression, histoclinical parameters and selected protein products of cell-cycle regulatory genes. J Exp Clin Cancer Res 2005; 24(3): 405-14.

[5]   Sherr CJ, Roberts JM. CDK inhibitors: positive and negative regulators of G1-phase progression. Genes Dev 1999; 13(12): 1501-12.

[6]   Besson A, Dowdy SF, Roberts JM. CDK inhibitors: cell cycle regulators and beyond. Dev Cell 2008; 14(2): 159-69.

[7]   Child ES, Mann DJ. The intricacies of p21 phosphorylation: protein/protein interactions, subcellular localization and stability. Cell Cycle 2006; 5(12): 1313-9.

[8]   Borriello A, Cucciolla V, Oliva A, Zappia V, Della Ragione F. p27Kip1 metabolism: a fascinating labyrinth. Cell Cycle 2007; 6(9): 1053-61.

[9]   Boyer MJ, Cheng T. The CDK inhibitors: potential targets for therapeutic stem cell manipulations? Gene Ther 2008; 15(2): 117-25.

[10]   Diaz-Padilla I, Siu LL, Duran I. Cyclin-dependent kinase inhibitors as potential targeted anticancer agents. Invest New Drugs 2009; 27(6): 5862-94.

[11]   Nilsson I, Hoffmann I. Cell cycle regulation by the Cdc25 phosphatase family. Prog Cell Cycle Res 2000; 4107-114.

[12]   Aressy B, Ducommun B. Cell cycle control by the CDC25 phosphatases. Anticancer Agents Med Chem 2008; 8(8): 818-24.

[13]   Lobjois V, Jullien D, Bouche JP, Ducommun B. The polo-like kinase 1 regulates CDC25B-dependent mitosis entry. Biochim Biophys Acta 2009; 1793(3): 462-8.

[14]   Assoian RK, Klein EA. Growth control by intracellular tension and extracellular stiffness. Trends Cell Biol 2008; 18(7): 347-52.

[15]   Herber B, Truss M, Beato M, Muller R. Inducible regulatory elements in the human cyclin D1 promoter. Oncogene 1994; 9(7): 2105-7.

[16]   Motokura T, Arnold A. Cyclins and oncogenesis. Biochim Biophys Acta 1993; 1155(1): 63-78.

[17]   Klein EA, Assoian RK. Transcriptional regulation of the cyclin D1 gene at a glance. J Cell Sci 2008; 121(23): 3853-7.

[18]   Balmanno K, Cook SJ. Sustained MAP kinase activation is required for the expression of cyclin D1, p21Cip1 and a subset of AP-1 proteins in CCL39 cells. Oncogene 1999; 18(20): 3085-97.

[19]   Karin M, Shaulian E. AP-1: linking hydrogen peroxide and oxidative stress to the control of cell proliferation and death. IUBMB Life 2001; 52(1-2): 17-24.

[20]   Shaulian E, Karin M. AP-1 in cell proliferation and survival. Oncogene 2001; 20(19): 2390-400.

[21]   Joung YH, Lim EJ, Lee MY, *et al.* Hypoxia activates the cyclin D1 promoter *via* the Jak2/STAT5b pathway in breast cancer cells. Exp Mol Med 2005; 37(4): 353-64.

[22]   Kim JK, Diehl JA. Nuclear cyclin D1: An oncogenic driver in human cancer. Journal of cellular physiology 2009; 220(2): 292-6.

[23]   Mundle SD, Saberwal G. Evolving intricacies and implications of E2F1 regulation. Faseb J 2003; 17(6): 569-74.

[24]   King RW, Peters JM, Tugendreich S, *et al.* A 20S complex containing CDC27 and CDC16 catalyzes the mitosis-specific conjugation of ubiquitin to cyclin B. Cell 1995; 81(2): 279-88.

[25]   Coverley D, Laman H, Laskey RA. Distinct roles for cyclins E and A during DNA replication complex assembly and activation. Nat Cell Biol 2002; 4(7): 523-8.

[26]   Li M, Zhang P. The function of APC/CCdh1 in cell cycle and beyond. Cell Div 2009; 42.

[27]   Pagano M. Control of DNA synthesis and mitosis by the Skp2-p27-Cdk1/2 axis. Mol Cell 2004; 14(4): 414-6.

[28]   Hao B, Oehlmann S, Sowa ME, Harper JW, Pavletich NP. Structure of a Fbw7-Skp1-cyclin E complex: multisite-phosphorylated substrate recognition by SCF ubiquitin ligases. Mol Cell 2007; 26(1): 131-43.

[29]   Nakayama K, Nagahama H, Minamishima YA, *et al.* Targeted disruption of Skp2 results in accumulation of cyclin E and p27(Kip1), polyploidy and centrosome overduplication. EMBO J 2000; 19(9): 2069-81.

[30]   Marti A, Wirbelauer C, Scheffner M, Krek W. Interaction between ubiquitin-protein ligase SCFSKP2 and E2F-1 underlies the regulation of E2F-1 degradation. Nat Cell Biol 1999; 1(1): 14-19.

[31]   Tedesco D, Lukas J, Reed SI. The pRb-related protein p130 is regulated by phosphorylation-dependent proteolysis *via* the protein-ubiquitin ligase SCF(Skp2). Genes Dev 2002; 16(22):2946-57.

[32]   Li X, Zhao Q, Liao R, Sun P, Wu X. The SCF(Skp2) ubiquitin ligase complex interacts with the human replication licensing factor Cdt1 and regulates Cdt1 degradation. J Biol Chem 2003; 278(33): 30854-8.

[33]   Peters JM. The anaphase promoting complex/cyclosome: a machine designed to destroy. Nat Rev Mol Cell Biol 2006; 7(9):644-56.

[34]   Fung TK, Siu WY, Yam CH, Lau A, Poon RY. Cyclin F is degraded during G2-M by mechanisms fundamentally different from other cyclins. J Biol Chem 2002; 277(38): 35140-9.

[35]   Misri S, Pandita S, Pandita TK. Detecting ATM-dependent chromatin modification in DNA damage and heat shock response. Methods Mol Biol 2009; 523395-410.

[36]   Reinhardt HC, Yaffe MB. Kinases that control the cell cycle in response to DNA damage: Chk1, Chk2, and MK2. Curr Opin Cell Biol 2009; 21(2): 245-55.

[37]   Decordier I, Cundari E, Kirsch-Volders M. Mitotic checkpoints and the maintenance of the chromosome karyotype. Mutat Res 2008; 651(1-2): 3-13.

[38]   Chesnokova V, Pechnick RN. Antidepressants and Cdk inhibitors: releasing the brake on neurogenesis? Cell Cycle 2008; 7(15): 2321-6.

[39]   Dick JE. Stem cell concepts renew cancer research. Blood 2008; 112(13): 4793-807.

[40]   Wilmut I, Schnieke AE, McWhir J, Kind AJ, Campbell KH. Viable offspring derived from fetal and adult mammalian cells. Nature 1997; 385(6619): 810-3.

[41]   Takahashi K, Yamanaka S. Induction of pluripotent stem cells from mouse embryonic and adult fibroblast cultures by defined factors. Cell 2006; 126(4): 663-76.

[42]   Takahashi K, Okita K, Nakagawa M, Yamanaka S. Induction of pluripotent stem cells from fibroblast cultures. Nat Protoc 2007; 2(12): 3081-9.

[43]   Nakagawa M, Koyanagi M, Tanabe K, *et al.* Generation of induced pluripotent stem cells without Myc from mouse and human fibroblasts. Nat Biotechnol 2008; 26(1): 101-6.

[44]   Pipan N, Sterle M. Cytochemical analysis of organelle degradation in phagosomes and apoptotic cells of the mucoid epithelium of mice. Histochemistry 1979; 59(3): 225-32.

[45]   Edinger AL, Thompson CB. Death by design: apoptosis, necrosis and autophagy. Curr Opin Cell Biol 2004; 16(6): 663-9.

[46]   Brenner S. The genetics of Caenorhabditis elegans. Genetics 1974; 77(1): 71-94.

[47]   Avery L, Horvitz HR. A cell that dies during wild-type C. elegans development can function as a neuron in a ced-3 mutant. Cell 1987; 51(6): 1071-8.

[48]   Sulston JE. Post-embryonic development in the ventral cord of Caenorhabditis elegans. Philos Trans R Soc Lond B Biol Sci 1976; 275(938): 287-97.

[49]   Chan CM, Tsoi H, Chan WM, *et al.* The ion channel activity of the SARS-Coronavirus 3a protein is linked to its pro-apoptotic function. Int J Biochem Cell Biol 2009;.

[50]   Kong M, Fox CJ, Mu J, *et al.* The PP2A-associated protein alpha4 is an essential inhibitor of apoptosis. Science 2004; 306(5696): 695-8.

[51]   Cook PJ, Ju BG, Telese F, *et al.* Tyrosine dephosphorylation of H2AX modulates apoptosis and survival decisions. Nature 2009; 458(7238): 591-6.

[52]   Ashkenazi A. Targeting the extrinsic apoptosis pathway in cancer. Cytokine Growth Factor Rev 2008; 19(3-4): 325-31.

[53]   Lavrik I, Golks A, Krammer PH. Death receptor signaling. J Cell Sci 2005; 118(Pt 2): 265-7.

[54]   Tartaglia LA, Ayres TM, Wong GH, Goeddel DV. A novel domain within the 55 kd TNF receptor signals cell death. Cell 1993; 74(5): 845-53.

[55]   Boldin MP, Varfolomeev EE, Pancer Z, *et al.* A novel protein that interacts with the death domain of Fas/APO1 contains a sequence motif related to the death domain. J Biol Chem 1995; 270(14): 7795-8.

[56]   Hsu H, Xiong J, Goeddel DV. The TNF receptor 1-associated protein TRADD signals cell death and NF-kappa B activation. Cell 1995; 81(4): 495-504.

[57]   Chowdhury I, Tharakan B, Bhat GK. Caspases - an update. Comp Biochem Physiol B Biochem Mol Biol 2008; 151(1): 10-27.

[58]   Kischkel FC, Hellbardt S, Behrmann I, *et al.* Cytotoxicity-dependent APO-1 (Fas/CD95)-associated proteins form a death-inducing signaling complex (DISC) with the receptor. EMBO J 1995; 14(22): 5579-88.

[59]   Hirata H, Takahashi A, Kobayashi S, *et al.* Caspases are activated in a branched protease cascade and control distinct downstream processes in Fas-induced apoptosis. J Exp Med 1998; 187(4): 587-600.

[60]   Liu X, Li P, Widlak P, *et al.* The 40-kDa subunit of DNA fragmentation factor induces DNA fragmentation and chromatin condensation during apoptosis. Proc Natl Acad Sci U S A 1998; 95(15): 8461-6.

[61]   Nunez G, Benedict MA, Hu Y, Inohara N. Caspases: the proteases of the apoptotic pathway. Oncogene 1998; 17(25): 3237-45.

[62]   Casciola-Rosen L, Nicholson DW, Chong T, *et al.* Apopain/CPP32 cleaves proteins that are essential for cellular repair: a fundamental principle of apoptotic death. J Exp Med 1996; 183(5): 1957-64.

[63]   Creagh EM, Brumatti G, Sheridan C, *et al.* Bicaudal is a conserved substrate for Drosophila and mammalian caspases and is essential for cell survival. PLoS ONE 2009; 4(3): e5055.

[64]   Oltvai ZN, Milliman CL, Korsmeyer SJ. Bcl-2 heterodimerizes *in vivo* with a conserved homolog, Bax, that accelerates programmed cell death. Cell 1993; 74(4): 609-19.

[65]   Kinnally KW, Antonsson B. A tale of two mitochondrial channels, MAC and PTP, in apoptosis. Apoptosis 2007; 12(5): 857-68.

[66]   Kluck RM, Bossy-Wetzel E, Green DR, Newmeyer DD. The release of cytochrome c from mitochondria: a primary site for Bcl-2 regulation of apoptosis. Science 1997; 275(5303): 1132-6.

[67]   Zou H, Henzel WJ, Liu X, Lutschg A, Wang X. Apaf-1, a human protein homologous to C. elegans CED-4, participates in cytochrome c-dependent activation of caspase-3. Cell 1997; 90(3): 405-13.

[68]   Pan G, O'Rourke K, Dixit VM. Caspase-9, Bcl-XL, and Apaf-1 form a ternary complex. J Biol Chem 1998; 273(10): 5841-5.

[69]   Yu X, Acehan D, Menetret JF, *et al.* A structure of the human apoptosome at 12.8 A resolution provides insights into this cell death platform. Structure 2005; 13(11): 1725-35.

[70]   Li P, Nijhawan D, Budihardjo I, *et al.* Cytochrome c and dATP-dependent formation of Apaf-1/caspase-9 complex initiates an apoptotic protease cascade. Cell 1997; 91(4): 479-89.

[71]   Pan G, Humke EW, Dixit VM. Activation of caspases triggered by cytochrome c *in vitro*. FEBS Lett 1998; 426(1): 151-54.

[72]   Tsujimoto Y. Role of Bcl-2 family proteins in apoptosis: apoptosomes or mitochondria? Genes Cells 1998; 3(11): 697-707.

[73]   Li H, Zhu H, Xu CJ, Yuan J. Cleavage of BID by caspase 8 mediates the mitochondrial damage in the Fas pathway of apoptosis. Cell 1998; 94(4): 491-501.

[74]   Harrington HA, Ho KL, Ghosh S, Tung KC. Construction and analysis of a modular model of caspase activation in apoptosis. Theor Biol Med Model 2008; 526.

[75]   Slee EA, Harte MT, Kluck RM, *et al.* Ordering the cytochrome c-initiated caspase cascade: hierarchical activation of caspases-2, -3, -6, -7, -8, and -10 in a caspase-9-dependent manner. J Cell Biol 1999; 144(2): 281-92.

[76]   Hamacher R, Schmid RM, Saur D, Schneider G. Apoptotic pathways in pancreatic ductal adenocarcinoma. Mol Cancer 2008; 764.

[77]   Srinivasula SM, Datta P, Fan XJ, *et al.* Molecular determinants of the caspase-promoting activity of Smac/DIABLO and its role in the death receptor pathway. J Biol Chem 2000; 275(46): 36152-7.

[78]   Chai J, Du C, Wu JW, *et al.* Structural and biochemical basis of apoptotic activation by Smac/DIABLO. Nature 2000; 406(6798): 855-62.

[79]   Wu G, Chai J, Suber TL, *et al.* Structural basis of IAP recognition by Smac/DIABLO. Nature 2000; 408(6815): 1008-12.

[80]   Liu Z, Sun C, Olejniczak ET, *et al.* Structural basis for binding of Smac/DIABLO to the XIAP BIR3 domain. Nature 2000; 408(6815): 1004-8.

[81]   Suzuki Y, Imai Y, Nakayama H, *et al.* A serine protease, HtrA2, is released from the mitochondria and interacts with XIAP, inducing cell death. Mol Cell 2001; 8(3): 613-21.

[82]   Colin J, Gaumer S, Guenal I, Mignotte B. Mitochondria, Bcl-2 family proteins and apoptosomes: of worms, flies and men. Front Biosci 2009; 144127-37.

[83]   Rathmell JC, Thompson CB. Pathways of apoptosis in lymphocyte development, homeostasis, and disease. Cell 2002; 109 SupplS97-107.

[84]   Tyson JJ, Novak B. Temporal organization of the cell cycle. Curr Biol 2008; 18(17):R759-R768.

[85]   Liu DX, Greene LA. Neuronal apoptosis at the G1/S cell cycle checkpoint. Cell Tissue Res 2001; 305(2): 217-28.

[86]   Maeda T, Yamada Y, Moriuchi R, *et al.* Fas gene mutation in the progression of adult T cell leukemia. J Exp Med 1999; 189(7): 1063-71.

[87]   Lee SH, Shin MS, Park WS, *et al.* Alterations of Fas (Apo-1/CD95) gene in non-small cell lung cancer. Oncogene 1999; 18(25): 3754-60.

[88]   Lee SH, Shin MS, Park WS, *et al.* Alterations of Fas (APO-1/CD95) gene in transitional cell carcinomas of urinary bladder. Cancer Res 1999; 59(13): 3068-72.

[89]   Alfredsson J, Puthalakath H, Martin H, Strasser A, Nilsson G. Proapoptotic Bcl-2 family member Bim is involved in the control of mast cell survival and is induced together with Bcl-XL upon IgE-receptor activation. Cell Death Differ 2005; 12(2): 136-44.

[90]   Zakeri Z, Quaglino D, Ahuja HS. Apoptotic cell death in the mouse limb and its suppression in the hammertoe mutant. Dev Biol 1994; 165(1): 294-7.

[91]   Rodriguez I, Araki K, Khatib K, Martinou JC, Vassalli P. Mouse vaginal opening is an apoptosis-dependent process which can be prevented by the overexpression of Bcl2. Dev Biol 1997; 184(1): 115-21.

[92]   Jenkinson EJ, Kingston R, Smith CA, Williams GT, Owen JJ. Antigen-induced apoptosis in developing T cells: a mechanism for negative selection of the T cell receptor repertoire. Eur J Immunol 1989; 19(11): 2175-7.

[93]   Carsetti R, Kohler G, Lamers MC. Transitional B cells are the target of negative selection in the B cell compartment. J Exp Med 1995; 181(6): 2129-40.

[94]   Larochette N, Decaudin D, Jacotot E, *et al.* Arsenite induces apoptosis *via* a direct effect on the mitochondrial permeability transition pore. Exp Cell Res 1999; 249(2): 413-21.

[95]   Li JJ, Tang Q, Li Y, *et al.* Role of oxidative stress in the apoptosis of hepatocellular carcinoma induced by combination of arsenic trioxide and ascorbic acid. Acta Pharmacol Sin 2006; 27(8): 1078-84.

[96]   Bustamante J, Nutt L, Orrenius S, Gogvadze V. Arsenic stimulates release of cytochrome c from isolated mitochondria *via* induction of mitochondrial permeability transition. Toxicol Appl Pharmacol 2005; 207(2 Suppl): 110-16.

[97]   Yih LH, Lee TC. Arsenite induces p53 accumulation through an ATM-dependent pathway in human fibroblasts. Cancer Res 2000; 60(22): 6346-52.

[98]   Saile B, Knittel T, Matthes N, Schott P, Ramadori G. CD95/CD95L-mediated apoptosis of the hepatic stellate cell. A mechanism terminating uncontrolled hepatic stellate cell proliferation during hepatic tissue repair. Am J Pathol 1997; 151(5): 1265-72.

[99]   Domen J, Cheshier SH, Weissman IL. The role of apoptosis in the regulation of hematopoietic stem cells: Overexpression of Bcl-2 increases both their number and repopulation potential. J Exp Med 2000; 191(2): 253-64.

[100]   World Health Organization W. The global burden of disease: 2004 update. In. Geneva, Switzerland.: http://www.who.int/healthinfo/global_burden_disease/GBD_report_2004update_full.pdf; 2008.

[101]   Elnemr A, Ohta T, Yachie A, *et al.* Human pancreatic cancer cells disable function of Fas receptors at several levels in Fas signal transduction pathway. Int J Oncol 2001; 18(2): 311-6.

[102]   Trauzold A, Schmiedel S, Roder C, *et al.* Multiple and synergistic deregulations of apoptosis-controlling genes in pancreatic carcinoma cells. Br J Cancer 2003; 89(9): 1714-21.

[103]   Hinz S, Trauzold A, Boenicke L, *et al.* Bcl-XL protects pancreatic adenocarcinoma cells against CD95- and TRAIL-receptor-mediated apoptosis. Oncogene 2000; 19(48): 5477-86.

[104]   Boucher MJ, Morisset J, Vachon PH, *et al.* MEK/ERK signaling pathway regulates the expression of Bcl-2, Bcl-X(L), and Mcl-1 and promotes survival of human pancreatic cancer cells. J Cell Biochem 2000; 79(3): 355-69.

[105]   Teitz T, Wei T, Valentine MB, *et al.* Caspase 8 is deleted or silenced preferentially in childhood neuroblastomas with amplification of MYCN. Nat Med 2000; 6(5): 529-35.

[106]   Soengas MS, Capodieci P, Polsky D, *et al.* Inactivation of the apoptosis effector Apaf-1 in malignant melanoma. Nature 2001; 409(6817): 207-11.

[107]   Shin MS, Kim HS, Lee SH, *et al.* Mutations of tumor necrosis factor-related apoptosis-inducing ligand receptor 1 (TRAIL-R1) and receptor 2 (TRAIL-R2) genes in metastatic breast cancers. Cancer Res 2001; 61(13): 4942-6.

[108]   Mori T, Doi R, Kida A, *et al.* Effect of the XIAP inhibitor Embelin on TRAIL-induced apoptosis of pancreatic cancer cells. J Surg Res 2007; 142(2): 281-6.

[109]   Karikari CA, Roy I, Tryggestad E, *et al.* Targeting the apoptotic machinery in pancreatic cancers using small-molecule antagonists of the X-linked inhibitor of apoptosis protein. Mol Cancer Ther 2007; 6(3): 957-66.

[110]   Oost TK, Sun C, Armstrong RC, *et al.* Discovery of potent antagonists of the antiapoptotic protein XIAP for the treatment of cancer. J Med Chem 2004; 47(18): 4417-26.

Causes of Cancer

I. The Influence of the Environment

Andrea De Vizcaya-Ruiz[*] and Araceli Hernández-Zavala

Department of Toxicology, Centro de Investigación y de Estudios Avanzados del I.P.N., Avenida Instituto Politécnico Nacional 2508, 07360 Mexico City, Mexico

Abstract. There is a close and direct relationship between the magnitude of the exposure of compounds in the environment that disrupts its natural equilibrium and the development of disease. Many of these substances act as mutagens or promoters or synergistically behave as carcinogens, and thus contribute to the growing incidence of cancer worldwide. However, the underlying mechanisms involved in the induction of genomic instability, genotoxicity, mutations and consequent increased cell proliferation are still a matter of intense research. In particular, tobacco smoke, exposure to radiation, pesticides, dioxins, organic compounds, metals and metalloids, and outdoor air pollution, will be reviewed with respect to epigenetic events, genetic polymorphism susceptibility, gene expression and signal transduction modification, and oxidative stress cellular events related to carcinogenesis.

Keywords: Environment, genes, tobacco, UV radiation, pesticides, dioxins, benzene, estrogens, cancer, chromium, cadmium, arsenic, air pollution, particulate matter, reactive oxygen species.

INTRODUCTION

Modern lifestyles and increase in the world's population have increased the demand for energy, transportation, agriculture, food and health services, and as a result, a vast number of chemicals or foreign substances have been introduced into the environment. The presence of these chemicals in air, soil, sediments and water disrupts the natural equilibrium of the environment, and there is a direct relationship between the magnitude of the exposure and the development of disease. Many of these substances act as mutagens, promoters or synergistic carcinogens, and thus contribute to the growing incidence of cancer worldwide. However, the etiology of many types of cancer and/or the mechanisms and molecular aspects by which a specific exposure may cause a specific type of cancer are still under investigation. Most of the evidence linking environmental exposures and the development of cancer has been obtained from epidemiological studies that have identified environmental and lifestyle factors that influence cancer risk. In this section, the etiology of cancer caused by compounds in the environment will be described in relation to known cancer-related molecular markers of exposure or cellular damage.

GENE-ENVIRONMENT INTERACTION

Cancer is a multistage disease caused by the accumulation of mutations in stem cells [1]. Endogenous genetic markers related to cancer have been identified, including cell-cycle control or tumor suppressor, DNA repair and susceptibility, and metabolism and apoptosis genes; however, because of the presence of chemicals in the environment, these genes may or may not influence or aggravate cellular outcomes. For example, exposure to tobacco smoke or asbestos individually induces lung cancer; however, exposure to both agents in combination causes a higher risk of developing tumors than the sum of the separate risks [2]. Other examples come from epidemiological studies of twin or immigrant populations in which changes in the environment determine the occurrence or absence of cancer development. Although the heritable information is present within an individual, if there is no stimulus from the environment, no development of the disease occurs [3]. However, the same rule applies for the opposite hypothesis in which the susceptibility factor due to inherited genetic characteristics or gene allelic variation will

Address correspondence to Andrea De Vizcaya-Ruiz: Department of Toxicology, Centro de Investigación y de Estudios Avanzados del I.P.N., Avenida Instituto Politécnico Nacional 2508, 07360 Mexico City, Mexico; E-mail: avizcaya@cinvestav.mx

determine whether specific factors, in this case the involuntary exposure to chemical agents in the environment, will induce cancer development. Therefore, efforts to understand the interaction of genes and the environment should consider all factors, including the influence of different environmental scenarios, the presence of weak and moderate risk genes, the study of heterogeneous large populations, and the reproducibility of the results describing biological or molecular mechanisms, in adequately planned studies that include molecular and epidemiological components [3, 4].

The magnitude of the exposure in a given organism can be estimated with the use of markers of exposure, which are indicators present in biological fluids, and they allow the characterization of levels of exogenous factors in the organism. Chemicals in the environment such as polychlorinated biphenyls, aromatic amines, dioxins, heavy metals, Polycyclic Aromatic Hydrocarbons (PAHs) and/or products of their metabolism, and constituents of tobacco smoke can be identified in biological fluids and are used as markers of exposure.

Macromolecular adducts, such as carcinogen-protein or carcinogen-DNA adducts, are also used as markers of exposure and can be indicators of biological responses to chemical exposure; they reveal processes of carcinogenic metabolism, activation and/or detoxification, DNA damage and/or repair, and biologically effective doses [4]. The presence and persistence of carcinogen-DNA or carcinogen-protein adducts are considered early markers of carcinogenesis [5]. One of the main mechanisms by which DNA is damaged is through the generation of Reactive Oxygen Species (ROS), which originate *via* redox reactions from the intrinsic ability of transition metals, quinones and organic compounds that originate the quinones. ROS contribute to cell transformation and tumor development [6]. Site-specific damage to DNA is mainly caused by OH$^\bullet$ radicals [7]. All four DNA bases and the sugar backbone can be oxidatively modified, and thymidine is the most susceptible. The most studied DNA oxidative modification is the 8-hydroxy-2'-deoxyguanosine (8-HO-dG) [6].

The involuntary exposure to pollutants in the environment (*e.g.*, tobacco smoke, pesticides, dioxins, radiation, metals, and air pollution) can lead to carcinogenic cellular events from a gene regulation level (gene expression and transcriptional and cell cycle checkpoint activation) to epigenetic modifications and DNA damage and repair. These processes most likely occur because of cellular metabolism and consequently induce apoptosis and/or proliferation and thus contribute to increased cancer risk. Scientific research is actively searching for specific genes that can identify subtle increases in individual risk and that account for residual risk associated with family history after the exposure to pollutants in the environment (Fig. **1**).

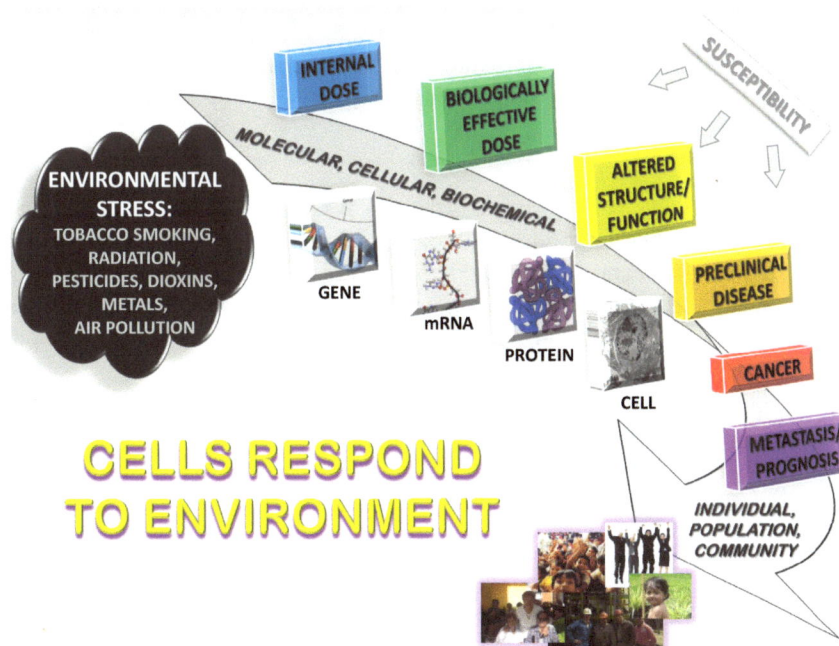

Figure 1: Cells respond to environmental stimulus, from a gene regulation level up to changes in mRNA and protein complements, influencing cell response and creating a broad pathway from exposure to disease manifestation as a consequence of the modification of our environment.

ENVIRONMENTAL CHEMICAL CARCINOGENS

Tobacco Smoking

Tobacco smoking is the single largest preventable cause of cancer [8]. Tobacco smoking accounts for the majority of lung cancer (adenocarcinomas and squamous cell carcinoma) morbidity and deaths worldwide. It has also been associated with breast, urinary bladder (transitional cell carcinomas) and head and neck cancer (tumors of the supraglottis and glottis and larynx squamous cell carcinomas) [9].

Studies performed by Zaridze [4] have identified two types of mutations in the *p53* gene in tumors of current smokers: transversions (G:C→T:A) and transitions (A:T→G:C), localized in PAH-DNA adduct sites. Transversion mutations have more often been found in tumors of never smokers at non-CpG sites, probably from the formation of promutagenic O^6-alkyl-DNA adducts induced by N-nitrosonornicotine, which is found in high concentrations in side-stream smoke. The author proposes that the type and location of mutations in *p53* can serve as markers of exposure to PAHs and tobacco-specific nitrosamines, in addition to active and passive smoking. An important increase in lung cancer incidence in never smokers has also been documented; evidence indicates that tobacco-related lung cancer and never smoker cancer are biologically different. Mutations in *KRAS, EGRF*, *p53* and methylation index are different in lung cancer patients who have never smoked compared with those with tobacco-related lung cancer [10]. This evidence is very relevant when deciding on preventive measures and therapy strategies because the target molecules may not be the same. More data comparing profile expression studies in large populations is needed to identify significant differences in the physio-pathological processes related to tobacco smoking in active and never smokers [11].

Various studies investigating the distribution and the potential gene-gene and gene-environment interaction have established a relationship of selected metabolic genetic polymorphisms with cancer risk. Polymorphisms in *GSTT1, SULT1A1* and *NAT2* were shown to modulate susceptibility to gastric cancer associated with cigarette-smoke in a case-control study of an Italian population [12]. In addition, current evidence indicates that allelic variants in cytochrome p450 (CYP) phase I metabolic enzymes involved in tobacco smoke-carcinogen bioactivation influence individual cancer development. Associations between members of the CYP family, such as CYP1A1, 1B1, 2A6, 2A13, 2B6, 2C18, 2E1, 2F1, 3A5 and 4B1, present in the lung, urinary bladder and head and neck and their involvement with tobacco smoke compound, PAH and nitrosamine metabolism and activation with various tumor types have been established, suggesting a direct interrelationship between the metabolic capacity of certain cell types and the cell type-specific susceptibility to xenobiotics. Such is the case of the polymorphic variant *CYP1B1*3/*3*, which significantly relates to the individual susceptibility of smokers to head and neck cancer, reinforcing the evidence that PAHs are metabolically activated by CYP1B1, which could be used as a biomarker of susceptibility [13].

Radiation

The flux of elementary particles, photons or electrons, is defined as radiation. How radiation is originated defines the magnitude of the effects induced when interacting with biological matter. Two categories apply: ionizing radiation (*i.e.*, radon and radon decay products) and nonionizing radiation (*i.e.*, UV rays). Cancers induced from the exposure to ionizing and nonionizing radiation are stochastic late effects, and among these cancers are the following: leukemias, lymphomas, thyroid cancers, skin cancers, some sarcomas and lung and breast carcinomas [14].

Particles in ionizing radiation (X-rays and α-particles) have sufficient energy to collide and remove an electron from an atom or molecule, generating an electrically charged ion pair, which can lead to DNA damage either by a direct interaction or by creating a chemically reactive free radical. •HO is the most abundant radical formed. This DNA damage can induce cell death or nonlethal DNA modifications that if misrepaired or unrepaired lead to cell proliferation and tumor progression. Particles in nonionizing radiation (microwaves and extremely low-frequency electric and magnetic fields (ELF-EMF)) do not have sufficient energy to break chemical bonds and thus, to produce ionization. Ultraviolet, visible and infrared radiations (also called optical radiation) have sufficient energy to generate photoelectric excitation with biological matter and consequently induce damaging effects (*e.g.*, Ultraviolet Radiation (UVR) for which associations of photochemical damage with the manifestation of skin cancer has been established) [15, 16]. Moreover, cyclobutane pyrimidine dimer DNA lesions and 6,4 pyrimidine photoproducts caused by the absorption of UVB radiation (290-320 nm) from sunlight have been implicated in skin cancer [17].

UVA radiation (320-400 nm), the predominant energy source in incident sunlight, is poorly absorbed by DNA and therefore is considered to be less harmful. However, the danger from UVA exposure is indirect because it produces thymine:thymine cyclobutane photoproducts in DNA, probably through photosensitized reactions involving non-DNA chromophores. UVA generates ROS, mainly singlet oxygen ($^1O_2$), which induces damage to the Proliferating Cell Nuclear Antigen (PCNA), the homotrimeric DNA polymerase sliding clamp, and causes covalent oxidative crosslinking between the PCNA subunits through a histidine residue in the intersubunit domain in exposed A2780 SC5 ovarian carcinoma cells and HCT116 colorectal carcinoma cells [18]. Persistent oxidative DNA damage can induce mutations and cancer progression.

Pesticides

Pesticides, from natural origin or chemically synthesized, have been extensively used in the last half-century in agriculture to eliminate or control unwanted or harmful insects, plants, fungi, animals, or microorganisms. Because of their extensive use, residues of chlorinated, organophosphate and carbamate pesticides are found in the air, soil, and water, with a concomitant presence in humans. Current evidence indicates an association between human exposure and cancer or carcinogenic events from pesticides' modes of action. Exposure to high concentrations of pesticides is linked with a high incidence of blood and lymphatic system cancers (lip, stomach, lung, brain, and prostate) as well as melanoma and other skin cancers [19]. Several pesticides are classified as probable or possible human carcinogens according to IARC and US-EPA, including organochlorines, carbamates, chlordane, and carbonyl groups, such as Dichlorodiphenyltrichloroethane (DDT), and their metabolites [20]. Pesticides have molecular structures similar to those of estrogens or androgens and have been identified as endocrine disruptors, and they can act as promoters or mutagens.

Direct observations of carcinogenicity events in animal models exposed to these chemical agents have been observed. Metabolites of *Ortho*-Phenylphenol (OPP) and Phenyl-1,4-Benzoquinone (PBQ) induce oxidative DNA damage through H_2O_2 generation in HL60 cells, and this damage that may lead to mutations and carcinogenesis [21].

Epigenetic events induced by pesticide exposure are reported as one of the main carcinogenicity mechanisms of pesticides. Pesticides are known to be hepatocarcinogenic (DDT), peroxisome proliferators (phenoxypropionic herbicides, fluazifop-butyl and haloxyfop), goitrogenic pesticides (dithiocarbamates such as mancoceb, maneb, ziram, metyram, zineb, and propylenthiourea) and inducers of sustained cell proliferation (chlorothalonil and p-dichlorobenzene). Pesticides' main mechanisms of carcinogenicity are the promotion of spontaneous initiation, cytotoxicity with sustained cell proliferation, oxidative stress and formation of activated receptors. No direct correlation between genotoxicity and carcinogenicity from exposure to pesticides has been reported. Some pesticides are genotoxic (although not strongly) but noncarcinogenic, and others are considered as nongenotoxic but are strongly carcinogenic (chlorothalonil and acetochlor). Most recently, CYP-induced formation of ROS and peroxisome proliferation have been proposed as the main promoter mechanisms of pesticide carcinogenesis [22].

Organochlorine insecticides (dieldrin, endosulfan, heptachlor and lindane) induce the formation of ROS, which activate ERK1/2, a subfamily of Mitogen-Activated Protein Kinases (MAPK), in human HaCaT keratinocytes. The deregulation of MAPK signaling pathways in epithelial cells has been associated with hyperproliferation and altered differentiation, contributing to malignant skin transformation [23].

Dioxins and Organic Compounds

2,3,7,8-Tetrachlorodibenzeno-P-Dioxin (TCDD) is the most toxic congener of a family of halogenated aromatic hydrocarbons produced from common industrial processes such as combustion, bleaching of wood pulp and chlorination of phenols [24]. TCDD and structurally related compounds are widely distributed in the environment and elicit a broad spectrum of biological responses in mammalian systems. At doses in the ng/kg range, TCDD leads to xenobiotic metabolism gene up-regulation (CYP1A1, 1A2, 1B1, UGT1A6 and members of the GST family) and endogenous hormone (estrogens) up-regulation. At doses in the μg/kg range, TCDD up-regulates xenobiotic toxic responses and causes hepatotoxicity, thymic involution, birth defects, cancer and lethality [25]. Extensive pharmacological and genetic research has demonstrated that TCDD toxicity is mediated through activation of the Aryl Hydrocarbon Receptor (AHR or Ah receptor), a ligand-activated member of the PAS (Per-ARNT-Sim) [26]. The Aryl Hydrocarbon Receptor Nuclear Translocator (ARNT) receptors were originally identified and characterized because of their central role in the vertebrate response to planar aromatic hydrocarbons. The AHR-ARNT complex binds to dioxin-responsive elements (DREs), which facilitates nuclear translocation of AHR and ARNT heterodimerization, facilitating gene-transcription [27]. In its non-bound state, the AHR is maintained in the cytosol in a complex with chaperones such as HSP90 and ARA9 (also known as AIP-1 or XAP2) [28]. Upon binding to TCDD, the AHR translocates to the nucleus where it dimerizes with another PAS protein, usually ARNT. The most potent known ligand for the AHR is TCDD, which is highly resistant to metabolic degradation and elicits numerous AHR-dependent toxic events, including late stage terata, thymic atrophy, chloracne, tumor promotion, hepatomegaly, and cachexia [29]. Although the carcinogenic mechanism of dioxin is not clear, there is a strong association between chronic exposure and an increased incidence of all cancer types, indicating the important and extensive spectrum of the carcinogenic effects of dioxin [30]. In the liver, evidence suggests that DRE-regulated gene expression within the hepatocyte is a fundamental aspect of TCDD-induced liver toxicity. For example, recombinant mouse models with mutations in the DNA binding domain for AHR, hepatocyte specific deletions of the AHR, or hypomorphic expression of ARNT are all resistant to TCDD-induced hepatotoxicity. This genetic evidence highlights the importance of AHR-ARNT-DRE interactions in TCDD-induced hepatotoxicity, although it does not identify the causally related DRE-driven genes. The number of steps between the DRE-regulated genes and any given pathological endpoint, which could be the induction of cell proliferation and/or carcinogenesis, are the subject of intense research.

Benzene

Exposure to benzene, a widespread airborne pollutant emitted from traffic exhaust fumes and cigarette smoking, has been consistently associated with acute myelogenous leukemia (AML); however, the mechanisms relating benzene to AML are still under investigation [31]. Aberrant DNA methylation patterns, including global hypomethylation, gene-specific hypermethylation or hypomethylation, and loss of imprinting, are common in AML and other cancer tissues [32]. Gene-specific hypomethylation has been reported in cancer cells. For example, MAGE-1 has been found to be hypomethylated in malignant cells and in AML showing a specific pattern, including frequent hypermethylation and p15 tumor suppressor gene inactivation [33].

Estrogens

Epidemiological studies have established a firm link between female reproductive history and increased risk of developing breast cancer and endometrius [34]. The mechanisms of estrogen carcinogenesis are not well understood. Malignant phenotypes arise as a result of a series of mutations, most likely in genes associated with tumor suppression, oncogenesis, DNA repair, or endocrine functions [35]. One major pathway considered to be important in the extensively studied hormonal pathway by which estrogen stimulates cell proliferation is the nuclear Estrogen Receptor (ER)-Mediated Signaling Pathway, which results in an increased risk of genomic mutations during DNA replication. The second pathway (a nongenomic pathway) involves membrane-associated ER and also appears to regulate other extranuclear estrogen signaling pathways. Various xenoestrogenic contaminants from natural or anthropogenic origin may act with endogenous estrogen and increase cancer risk [36]. A third pathway involves estrogen metabolism; it is mediated by Cytochrome p450, which generates reactive electrophilic estrogen *o*-quinones and ROS through redox cycling of these *o*-quinones [37].

Estrogen quinoids can directly damage cellular DNA, leading to genotoxic effects. There are some reports in MCF-7 (breast cancer cells) cells exposed to 3,4-quinone that show that the major DNA adducts produced from 4-hydroxyestradiol-*o*-quinone are depurinating N7-guanine and N3 adenine adducts [38]. Epidemiological studies have suggested a link between genetic polymorphisms in estrogen 4-hydroxylases and a risk for developing breast cancer, suggesting that estrogen metabolites are likely contributors to cancer development [39].

Metals and Metalloids

Several metals and metalloids have been rated as certain or probable carcinogens by IARC [40]. The inhalation of arsenic oxides can cause lung cancer, and if arsenic is absorbed through the gut, cancer can appear in organs such as bladder, kidney, liver and lung, yet the cancer reported with highest prevalence is skin cancer [41]. Aside from arsenic oxide exposure, lung cancer has also been reported to be associated with exposure to many metals, including lead, hexavalent Chromium (Cr(VI)) and nickel. Furthermore, exposure to Cr(VI) or nickel has been found to be associated with nasopharyngeal carcinoma, exposure to lead or mercury with brain tumors, exposure to lead or cadmium with kidney cancer and exposure to cadmium with prostate cancer [30]. The mechanism of action of metals and metalloids is not clear. They can act as co-carcinogens by activating procarcinogens in the liver [42], or they can replace natural metal-associated enzymes, thus inactivating the metabolic pathway of key enzymes. Such is the case of carcinogenic metals and metalloids, such as As, Cd, Ni and putative carcinogens including Co and Pb, which have been observed to inhibit Zn finger containing DNA repair proteins. Damage in these proteins can therefore be considered a novel mechanism in carcinogenesis [43]. Moreover, some metals and metalloids may also be mutagenic through other mechanisms, interacting with DNA. For example, compounds such as Cr(VI) are taken up by cells as chromate anion and are reduced intracellularly *via* reactive intermediates to stable Cr(III), which may directly interact with DNA, affecting DNA by terminating its replication or reducing replication fidelity and leading to mutations.

In the last two decades, there has been an explosive interest in the role of ROS in metal-induced carcinogenesis [44]. ROS, including superoxide anion, nitric oxide and hydrogen peroxide, can be produced from both endogenous and exogenous substances. Endogenous sources include mitochondria, Cytochrome p450 metabolism, peroxisomes, and inflammatory cell activation (neutrophils, eosinophils and macrophages generate ROS). ROS are also produced by exogenous processes; environmental agents including non-genotoxic carcinogens can directly generate or indirectly induce ROS in cells. The induction of oxidative stress and damage has been observed following exposure to various xenobiotics, including metals [45]. Metal-mediated formation of free radicals may cause various modifications to DNA bases, enhanced lipid peroxidation, changes in calcium and sulfhydryl homeostasis, and protein oxidation.

Chromium

Chromium (III), which is ubiquitous in nature, is an essential trace element that plays an important role in regulating blood levels of glucose. Chromium (VI) or chromate is potentially toxic and carcinogenic. Chromates can actively enter cells through channels for the transfer of isoelectric and isostructural anions, such as those for SO_4^{2-} and HPO_4^{2-}. Insoluble chromates like lead, calcium and zinc are absorbed by cells *via* phagocytosis, and the uptake of reduced Cr species is generated from extracellular redox mechanisms. Once inside the cell, chromates are able to generate free radicals [46], and in the presence of cellular reductants, Cr causes a wide variety of DNA lesions including Cr-DNA adducts, DNA-proteins crosslinks, DNA-DNA crosslinks and oxidative damage [45, 46]. Cr(VI) has been reported to cause lung cancer in humans; workers exposed to Cr(VI) in the workplace air showed higher rates of lung cancer from cell transformation than workers who were not exposed. Moreover, Cr was recently implicated as a causal agent in an increased rate of breast cancer [47].

Cadmium

Cadmium is a highly toxic metal. It is unable to generate free radicals directly; however, indirect generation of various radicals involving the superoxide radical, hydroxyl radical and nitric oxide from Cd exposure have been reported. Cadmium is a potent human carcinogen in occupational exposure scenarios and it has been associated with lung, prostate, pancreas and kidney cancers [45].

Arsenic

Arsenic is well known as a poison, and it is a carcinogen in humans. Many studies have confirmed the generation of free radicals during arsenic metabolism in cells. ROS generation can cause cell damage and death through activation of oxidative sensitive signaling pathways [48]. Arsenic-mediated generation of ROS is a complex process that involves the generation of a variety of ROS including superoxide, singlet oxygen, peroxyl radical, nitric oxide, hydrogen peroxide, dimethylarsinic peroxyl radical and dimethylarsinic radical. The exact mechanism responsible for the generation of all of these ROS is not clear, but some studies have proposed the formation of intermediary arsine species [45]. UROtsa cells exposed to methyl arsonous acid MMA^{III} (50 nM) for 52 weeks achieved hyperproliferation, anchorage-independent growth, and enhanced tumorigenicity. MMA^{III} has been shown to induce ROS, which can lead to activation of signaling cascades causing stress-related proliferation of cells and even cellular transformation [49].

Arsenic is a well-established human carcinogen. As compounds bind to SH-groups and inhibit various enzymes including glutathione reductase. Arsenic may act as a co-carcinogen, not causing cancer directly, but allowing other substances, such as cigarette smoke and UV radiation, to cause DNA mutations more effectively [50].

Air Pollution

The presence of foreign elements that are not part of the natural air composition and that can potentially cause damage to human health, is recognized as air pollution. The most important air quality indicators used in urban atmospheres are sulfur dioxide, nitric oxides, ozone, carbon monoxide and airborne particulate matter (PM). Among air pollutants, PM has been the most strongly associated with the increase in lung cancer risk in exposed populations [51, 52]. The mixture of chemical components, such as PAHs, transition metals, soluble ions, and benzene and surface physical characteristics stimulate the generation of ROS and reactive nitrogen species (RNS) that arise from cellular metabolism, NADPH-oxidase or mitochondrial stimulation, and/or inflammatory cell activation. Experimental evidence of damage to cellular macromolecules, particularly to DNA, from the exposure to PM in relation with its chemical composition has been extensively documented [53-57]. Oxidative stress is the main mechanism implicated in PM-induced DNA damage [58]. Non-regulated and/or prolonged production of reactive species have been linked with DNA strand breaks, mutations and modifications or regulation of gene expression implicated in carcinogenic processes [59]. It has been shown that exposure of A549 cells to $PM_{2.5}$ induced the generation of ROS primarily from site III of the mitochondrial electron transport chain, activating the intrinsic apoptotic pathway through ASK1, JNK and p53 [60].

Fig. 2 illustrates the potential mechanisms of PM-mediated oxidative stress induction involving cellular signal transduction pathways Nrf-2, AP-1 and NFkB, which are members of the antioxidant response, and the consequent effects on DNA and carcinogenesis in relation to emission sources that define PM physicochemical characteristics.

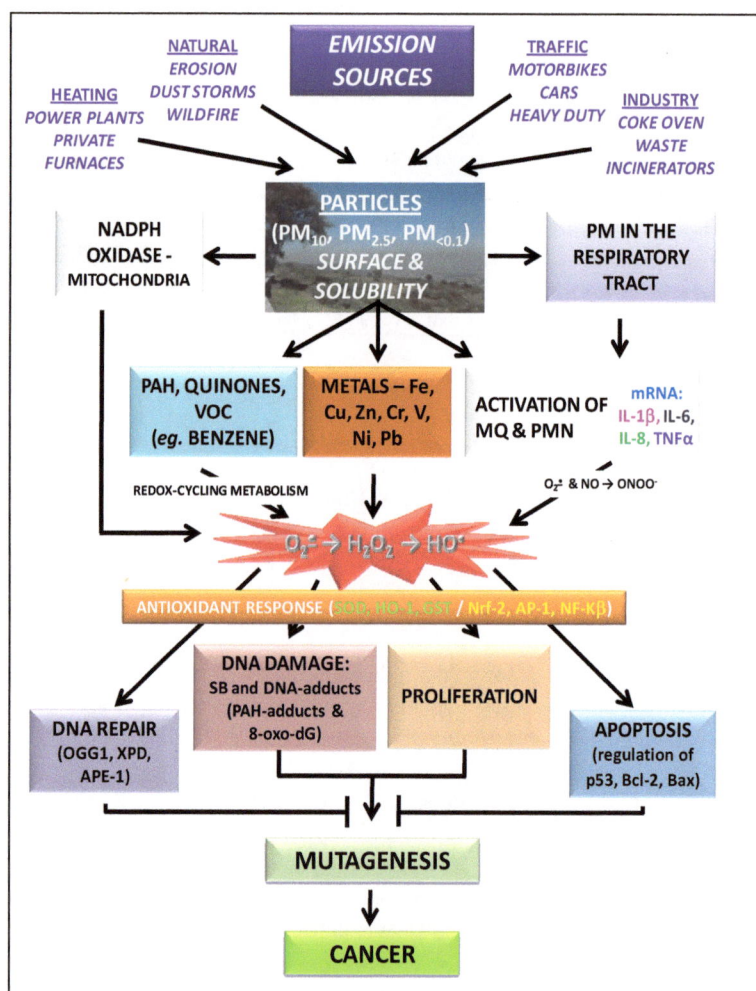

Figure 2: Potential mechanisms of oxidative stress and induction of DNA damage and carcinogenesis from exposure to airborne particulate matter.

Oxidative DNA damage has been suggested to come from PM that can traverse to the nucleus or from ROS that originate extracellularly, trigger free radical chain reactions, reach the nucleus and damage DNA. Studies in experimental animals show that elevated levels of oxidized guanines in lungs and other organs are associated with exposure to traffic-related PM, which could eventually be related to cancer development [61]. Studies in human populations exposed to different levels of air pollutants suggest a dose-response relationship in the context of increased levels of DNA adducts when air pollutant levels are higher; the 8-oxo-7,8-dihydro-2'-deoxyguanosine (8-oxo-dG) DNA adduct in lymphocytes is the most common promutagenic lesion reported [62]. In addition, the formation of PAH bulky adducts, presence of 8-oxo-dG and strand breaks, and the expression of *ERCC1* and *OGG1*, relevant DNA repair genes, in lymphocytes from exposed individuals have been associated with seasonal variations of PM, particularly $PM_{2.5}$ [63].

CONCLUSIONS

Chemicals or substances present in air, soil and water act as mutagens and/or carcinogens and may contribute to the increase in cancer incidence worldwide. Although genetic background plays an important role in the susceptibility to cancer, exposure to environmental chemical contaminants is without a doubt an elemental factor that can induce damaging effects to DNA, mainly through the ability to catalyze redox reactions.

Linking experimental studies with health outcomes related to environmental exposures in open populations requires greater advancement of knowledge. Emphasis on methodological rigor in study design, conduct and analysis and improvement in reliable and valid high-throughput biomarkers (based on exposure assessment and molecular targets) is imperatively needed in cancer epidemiology.

ACKNOWLEDGEMENTS

This work was partially supported by CONACYT 57752.

REFERENCES

[1]   Loeb KR, Loeb LA. Significance of multiple mutations in cancer. Carcinogenesis 2000; 21: 379-85.

[2]   IARC. Tobacco smoke and involuntary smoking. IARC, Lyon, 2004.

[3]   Hemminki K, Lorenzo Bermejo J, Försti A. The balance between heritable and environmental aetiology of human disease. Nat Rev Genet 2006; 7 (12): 958-65.

[4]   Zaridze D.G. Molecular epidemiology of cancer. Biochemistry (Moscow) 2008; 73 (5): 532-42.

[5]   Barr DB, Needham LL. Analytical methods for biological monitoring of exposure to pesticides: a review. J Chromatogr B Analyt Technol Biomed Life Sci 2002; 778 (1-2): 5-29.

[6]   Goetz ME, Luch A. Reactive species: a cell damaging rout assisting to chemical carcinogens. Cancer Lett 2008; 266: 73-83.

[7]   Marnett LJ. Oxyradicals and DNA damage. Carcinogenesis 2000; 21: 361-70.

[8]   World Health Organization. WHO Report on the Global Tobacco Epidemic 2008.

[9]   Centers for Disease Control and Prevention. Annual smoking attributable mortality, years of potential life lost, and productivity losses—United States, 1997-2001. Morb Mortal Wkly Rep 2005; 54: 625-8.

[10]   Subramanian J, Govindan R. Molecular genetics of lung cancer in people who have never smoked. Lancet Oncol 2008; 9: 676-82.

[11]   Subramanian J, Govindan R. Lung cancer in never smokers: a review. J Clin Oncol 2007; 25: 561-70.

[12]   Boccia S, Sayed-Tabatabaei FA, Persiani R, *et al.* Polymorphisms in metabolic genes, their combination and interaction with tobacco smoke and alcohol consumption and risk of gastric cancer: a case-control study in an Italian population. BMC Cancer 2007; 8 (7): 206 (http://www.biomedcentral.com/1471-2407/7/206).

[13]   Roos PH, Bolt HM. Cytochrome P450 interactions in human cancers: new aspects considering CYP1B1. Expert Opin Drug Metab Toxicol 2005; 1 (2): 187-202. [14] Irigaray P, Newby J.A, Clapp R, *et al.* Lifestyle-related factors and environmental agents causing cancer: an overview. Biomed Pharmacother 2007; 61 (10): 640-58.

[15]   International Commission on Radiological Protection (ICRP). 1990 Recommendations of the International Commission on Radiological Protection ICRP, Publication 60. Annals of the ICRP 1991; 21 (1-3). Pergaman: Oxford.

[16]   Wakeford R. The cancer epidemiology of radiation. Oncogene 2004; 23 (38): 6404-28.

[17] Friedberg EC, Walker GC, Siede W, Wood RD, Schultz RA, Ellenberger T. DNA Repair and Mutagenesis 2006; Washington, USA: ASM.

[18] Montaner B, O'Donovan P, Reelfs O, *et al.* Reactive oxygen-mediated damage to a human DNA replication and repair protein. EMBO Rep 2007; 8 (11): 1074-9.

[19] Cancer Trends Progress Report, 2007. National Cancer Institute, U.S. National Institutes of Health.

[20] IARC (International Agency for Research on Cancer). Occupational exposures in insecticide application, and some pesticides. In: IARC monographs on the evaluation of carcinogenic risk to humans 1991; Vol. 53. Lyon: IARC Press.

[21] Murata M, Moriya K, Inoue S, Kawanishi S. Oxidative damage to cellular and isolated DNA by metabolites of a fungicide ortho-phenylphenol. Carcinogenesis 1999; 20 (5): 851-7.

[22] Rakitsky VN, Koblyakov VA, Turusov VS. Nongenotoxic (epigenetic) carcinogens: pesticides as an example. a critical review. Teratogenesis Carcinog Mutagen 2000; 20: 229-40.

[23] Ledirac N, Antherieu S, d'Uby A.D, Caron J.C, Rahmani R. Effects of organochlorine insecticides on MAP kinase pathways in human HaCaT keratinocytes: key role of reactive oxygen species. Toxicol Sci 2005; 86 (2): 444-52.

[24] Adachi J, Mori Y, Matsui S, Matsuda T. Comparison of gene expression patterns between 2,3,7,8-tetrachlorodibenzo-p-dioxin and a natural arylhydrocarbon receptor ligand, indirubin. Toxicol Sci 2004; 80:161-9.

[25] Hayes KR, Zastrow GM, Nukaya M, *et al.* Hepatic transcriptional networks induced by exposure to 2,3,7,8-tetrachlorodibenzo-p-dioxin. Chem Res Toxicol 2007; 20(11): 1573-81.

[26] McMillan BJ, McMillan SN, Glover E, Bradfield CA. 2,3,7,8-tetrachlorodibenzo-p-dioxin induces premature activation of the KLF2 regulon during thymocyte development. J Biol Chem 2006; 262(10): 12580-97.

[27] McMillan BJ, Bradfield CA. The aryl hydrocarbon receptor sans xenobiotics:endogenous function in genetic model systems. Mol Pharmacol 2007; 72(3): 487-98.

[28] Nebert DW, Dalton TP, Okey AB, Honzalez FJ. Role of aryl hycrocarbon receptor-mediated induction of the CYP1 enzymes in environmental toxicity and cancer. J Biol Chem 2004; 279: 23847-50.

[29] Schecter A, Birribaum L, Byan JJ, Constable JD Dioxins: an overview. Environ Res 2006; 101: 419-28.

[30] Belpomme D, Irigaray P, Hardell L, *et al.* The multitude and diversity of environmental carcinogens. Environ Res 2007; 105: 414-29.

[31] International Agency for Research on Cancer. Overall evaluations of carcinogenicity: an updating of IARC monographs volumes 1 to 42. IARC Monogr Eval Carcinog Risks Hum Suppl 1987; 7: 1-440.

[32] Lubbert M, Oster W, Ludwig WD, Ganser A, Mertelsmann R, Hermann F. A switch toward demethylation is associated with the expression of myeloperoxidase in acute myeloblastic and promyelocytic leukemias. Blood 1992; 80: 2066-73.

[33] Bollati V, Baccarelli A, Hou L, *et al.* Changes in DNA methylation patterns in subjects exposed to low-dose benzene. Cancer Res 2007; 67: 876-80.

[34] Yager JD, Davidson NE. Estrogen carcinogenesis in breast cancer. N Engl J Med 2006; 354: 270-82.

[35] Henderson BE, Feigelson HS. Hormonal carcinogenesis. Carcinogenesis 2000; 21: 427-33.

[36] Buterin T, Koch C, Naegeli H. Convergent transcriptional profiles induced by endogenous estrogen and distinct xenoestrogens in breast cancer cells. Carcinogenesis 2006; 27: 1567-78.

[37] Bolton JL, Thatcher RJ. Potential mechanisms of estrogen quinone carcinogenesis. Chem Res Toxicol 2008; 21: 93-101.

[38] Zahid M, Kohli E, Saeed M, Rogan E, Cavalieri E. The greater reactivity of estradiol-3,4quinone vs estradiol-2-3-quinone with DNA in the formation of depurinating adducts:Implications for tumor initiating activity. Chem Res Toxicol 2006; 19: 164-72.

[39] Kisselev P, Schunck WH, Roots L, Schwartz D. Association of CYP1A1 polymorphism with differential metabolic activation of 17beta estradiol and estrone. Cancer Res 2005; 65: 2972-8.

[40] IARC (International Agency for Research on Cancer), 1980. IARC Monographs on the evaluation of carcinogenic risk to humans. Some metals and metallic compounds, Vol. 23, IarcPress, Lyon.

[41] Chen CJ, Chen CW, Wu MM, Kuo TL. Cancer potential in liver, lung, bladder and kidney due to ingested inorganic arsenic in drinking water. Brit J Cancer 1992; 66: 888-92.

[42] Cantor KP, Ward MH, Moore L, Lubin J. Water contaminants. In: Schotenfield, D., Fraumeni Jr. F. (Eds). Cancer epidemiology and prevention, third ed. Kluwer Academic Publisher. Dondrecht, pp. 149-69.

[43] Witkiewicz-Kucharczyc A, Bal W. Damage of zinc fingers in DNA repair proteins, a novel molecular mechanism in carcinogenesis. Toxicol Lett 2006; 162: 29-42.

[44] Valko M, Izakovic M, Mazur M, Rhodes CJ, Telser J. Role of oxygen radicals in DNA damage and cancer incidence. Mol Cell Nicohem 2004; 266: 37-56.

[45] Valko M, Rhodes CJ, Moncol J, Izakovic M, Mazur M. Free radicals, metals and antioxidant in oxidative stress-induced cancer. Chem Biol Int 2006; 160: 1-40.

[46]   Liu KJ, Shi XL. *In vivo* reduction of chromium (V) and its related free radical generation. Moll Cell Biochem 2001; 222: 41-7.

[47]   Kilic E, Saraymen A, Demiroglu E. Chromium and manganese levels in the scalp hair of normals and patients with breast cancer. Biol Trace Elem Res 2004; 102: 19-25.

[48]   Kanat CD, Green DE, Curilla S, *et al.* Role of HIF signaling on tumorigenesis in response to chronic low-dose arsenic administration. Toxicol Sci 2005; 86: 248-57.

[49]   Eblin KE, Jensen TJ, Wnek SM, Buffington SE, Futscher BW, Gandolfi AJ. Reactive oxygen species regulate properties of transformation in UROtsa cells exposed to monomethylarsonous acid by modulating MAPK signaling. Toxicology 2009; 255(1-2): 107-14.

[50]   Waalkes MP, Liu J, Ward MJ, Diwan LA. Mechanisms underlying arsenic carcinogenesis:hypersensitivity of mice exposed to inorganic arsenic during gestation. Toxicology 2004; 198: 31-8.

[51]   Pope III CA, Burnett RT, Thun MJ, *et al.* Lung cancer, cardiopulmonary mortality, and long-term exposure to fine particulate air pollution. JAMA 2002; 287: 1132-41.

[52]   Vineis P, Forastiere F, Hoek G, Lipsett M. Outdoor air pollution and lung cancer: recent epidemiologic evidence. Int J Cancer 2004; 111: 647-52.

[53]   Alfaro-Moreno E, Martínez L, García-Cuellar C, *et al.* Biologic effects induced *in vitro* by PM10 from three different zones of Mexico City. Environ Health Perspect 2002; 110: 715-20.

[54]   de Kok TM, Hogervorst JG, Briedé JJ, *et al.* Genotoxicity and physicochemical characteristics of traffic-related ambient particulate matter. Environ Mol Mutagen 2005; 46: 71-80

[55]   De Vizcaya-Ruiz A, Gutierrez-Castillo ME, Uribe-Ramirez M, *et al.* Characterization and *in vitro* biological effects of concentrated particulate matter from Mexico City. Atmos Environ 2006; 40: S583-S92.

[56]   Gutiérrez-Castillo ME, Roubicek DA, Cebrián-García ME, De Vizcaya-Ruíz A, Sordo-Cedeño M, Ostrosky-Wegman P. Effect of chemical composition on the induction of DNA damage by urban airborne particulate matter. Environ Mol Mutagen 2006; 47: 199-211.

[57]   Valavanidis A, Fiotakis K, Vlachogianni T. Airborne particulate matter and human health: toxicological assessment and importance of size and composition of particles for oxidative damage and carcinogenic mechanisms. J Environ Sci Health C Environ Carcinog Ecotoxicol Rev 2008; 26: 339-62.

[58]   Risom L, Møller P, Loft S. Oxidative stress-induced DNA damage by particulate air pollution. Mutat Res 2005; 592: 119-37.

[59]   Klaunig JE, Kamendulis LM. The role of oxidative stress in carcinogenesis. Annu Rev Pharmacol Toxicol 2004; 44: 239-67.

[60]   Soberanes S, Urich D, Baker CM, *et al.* Mitochondrial complex III-generated oxidants activate ASK1 and JNK to induce alveolar epithelial cell death following exposure to particulate matter air pollution. J Biol Chem 2009; 284: 2176-86.

[61]   Møller P, Folkmann JK, Forchhammer L, *et al.* Air pollution, oxidative damage to DNA, and carcinogenesis. Cancer Lett 2008; 266: 84-97.

[62]   Vineis P and Husgafvel-Pursiainen K. Air pollution and cancer: biomarker studies in human populations. Carcinogenesis 2005; 26: 1846-55.

[63]   Sørensen M, Autrup H, Møller P, *et al.* Linking exposure to environmental pollutants with biological effects. Mutat Res 2003; 544: 255-71.

CHAPTER 2

Causes of Cancer

II. Obesity and Cancer

Ranier Gutiérrez[*]

Department of Pharmacology, Centro de Investigación y de Estudios Avanzados del I.P.N., Avenida Instituto Politécnico Nacional 2508, 07360 Mexico City, Mexico

Abstract: Obesity is the largest pandemic, the human being has undergone. Obesity has been linked to several health-related problems, but recent epidemiological studies have uncovered a link between excess body weight and certain types of cancers. We have begun to realize the complexity of the biological mechanisms that link obesity and being overweight to many forms of cancer. In this chapter, I briefly review these epidemiological findings and the three molecular pathways currently proposed to link body weight gain and cancer risk. Despite the fact that these molecular pathways, vary and depend on both sex and the type of cancer, I briefly discuss the possible roles of three hormonal systems, the adipose derived hormones, the Insulin-Like Growth Factor (IGF) axis and sex steroids, in linking obesity and cancer risk.

Keywords: Adiponectin, leptin, insulin, insulin-like growth factor, IGFBP, sex steroids, SHBG obesity, cancer.

OBESITY AND CANCER

The prevalence of obesity and being overweight has been increasing markedly over the past two decades. In US adults, 71% of men and 62% of women are overweight or obese [1]. It has long been recognized that excessive body weight is associated with various diseases, particularly cardiovascular diseases, diabetes mellitus type 2, sleep apnea, and osteoarthritis. However, the association between obesity and certain types of cancer has received much less attention.

Types of cancers related to obesity: Epidemiological data indicates that obesity is associated with increased risk of certain types of cancer. For example, *endometrial cancer* (cancer of the uterine lining) was the first cancer to be recognized as being related to obesity. In this regard, postmenopausal women show a linear increase in the risk of endometrial cancer with Body Mass Index (BMI). The BMI is the weight (in kg) divided by the square of the height (in meters) of an individual and adults with a BMI between 25 and 29.9 kg/m^2 are considered overweight, while those with a BMI equal to or greater than 30 kg/m^2 are obese. Using the BMI as a measure of adiposity, the International Agency for Research on Cancer (IARC) found that obesity and being overweight were consistently associated with *breast cancer* in postmenopausal women, with *colon cancer* in men, and with *adenocarcinoma of the esophagus* and *kidney cancer* (renal-cell cancer) in both men and women [2]. Further evidence, from a meta-analysis study [3], has also related obesity with *gallbladder cancer*, especially in women. A rigorous and comprehensive meta-analysis study recently uncovered that a 5 kg/m^2 increase in BMI (~15 kg weight gain in men and 13 kg in women) increases the risk of leukemia, malignant melanoma, multiple myeloma, non-Hodgkin lymphoma, and thyroid cancer [4].

Types of cancers not related to obesity: Recently the IARC concluded that there was not sufficient evidence for an association of obesity or being overweight with *prostate cancer* [5]. A cohort study of Swedish women found no association between obesity and *cervical cancer* [6]. In regards to *lung cancer*, an inverse correlation between BMI and lung cancer is reported in studies that do not exclude smokers from the analysis. The inverse relationship is explained by smoking itself, since BMI is also inversely related to smoking, probably because nicotine causes loss of appetite. No association between BMI and lung cancer has been found in non-smoking populations [7].

An epidemiological study estimated that 15-20% of all cancers deaths in the United States can be attributed to

---

*Address correspondence to Ranier Gutiérrez: Department of Pharmacology, Centro de Investigación y de Estudios Avanzados del I.P.N., Avenida Instituto Politécnico Nacional 2508, 07360 Mexico City, Mexico; E-mail: ranier@cinvestav.mx

obesity and being overweight [7]. Thus, excess body weight is a leading cause of cancer related deaths. Moreover, the epidemic of obesity has shown no signs of abating and in fact a ramping up in the frequency of obese children is currently observed worldwide [8]. Although it is clear that obesity is associated with certain types of cancers, there is currently no direct evidence that weight loss decreases the incidence of cancer. This is because current pharmacological treatments for obesity have a limited effectiveness and because dieting is generally ineffective in achieving significant weight loss over the long term [9].

MOLECULAR MECHANISMS THAT LINK OBESITY AND CANCER RISK

Although the molecular mechanisms that link excess weight and increased cancer risk are not well understood, at least, three hormonal systems may be implicated:

- Adipose derived hormones.

- The insulin and Insulin-like Growth Factor (IGF) axis.

- Sex steroids.

All three hormonal systems are related to insulin, but their particular roles in carcinogenesis vary and depend on the cancer type.

Adipose Derived Hormones

The main function of adipose tissue is to store lipids. However, increasingly, it is recognized that adipose tissue is a highly active endocrine organ and that the secretion of adipose derived hormones might be relevant for cancer development. Specifically, leptin and adiponectin have been studied most [10]. Leptin is an adipose derived hormone that regulates energy balance. Leptin circulates in the blood stream and acts on the brain to regulate food intake and energy expenditure. Specifically, when fat mass decreases, plasma leptin concentrations decrease, which stimulates appetite and suppresses energy expenditure until fat mass is restored. When fat mass increases, leptin concentrations increase, which suppresses appetite until weight is lost [11]. Although leptin can reduce appetite, in general, obese individuals have an unusually high circulating concentration of leptin. These people are said to be resistant to the anorectic effect of leptin. Thus, in humans, high BMI is directly associated with elevated circulating levels of the hormone leptin [11]. In addition to its endocrine functions, leptin can act as a mitogen and an angiogenic factor [10]. Leptin activates JAK2/STAT3 (Janus Kinase/ Signal Transducer and Activation of Transcription) signaling pathway, but it can also activate phosphatidylinositol 3-kinase/Akt (PI3K/Akt) and extracellular-signal-regulated kinase (ERK1/2) pathways, which are crucial for cell survival, proliferation and differentiation [10, 12]. To date, the best evidence that leptin may indeed be involved in neoplastic processes has been provided by studies on breast and colorectal cancer models, while the results for other cancer types are very limited and often inconsistent or inconclusive [10, 13, 14].

Adiponectin, the most abundant adipose derived hormone, is secreted mainly from visceral adipose tissue and is related inversely to BMI. Adiponectin circulates in plasma in high concentrations in healthy subjects, and in low levels in obese individuals. A reduction in adiponectin expression is associated with insulin resistance [15]. Administration of adiponectin has been accompanied by a reduction in plasma glucose and an increase in insulin sensitivity. On the other hand, this adipocyte protein seems to play a protective role in experimental models of vascular injury and anti-tumor activity [16]. Of importance to tumor development, adiponectin is a negative regulator of angiogenesis [17] and is associated with inhibition of transplanted fibrosarcoma tumor cells in mice [18].

Insulin-IGF Cancer Hypothesis

Insulin is a peptide secreted from pancreatic β-cells. Activation of the Insulin Receptor (IR) by insulin triggers intracellular activation of ERK and PI3K pathways. Both pathways are related to cell proliferation. Thus, hyperinsulinemia has the potential to be both mitogenic and anti-apoptotic. However, insulin is thought to be mitogenic at supraphysiologic levels. The IGF axis is a complex molecular network that includes two ligands (IGF-1 and IGF-2), two receptors (IGF-1R and IGF-2R), six high-affinity-binding proteins (IGFBP-1 to IGFBP6) and several proteases [19]. In a simplified form, the insulin-IGF cancer hypothesis postulates that prolonged hyperinsulinemia reduces the production of IGFBP-1 and IGFBP-2 (which normally bind to and inhibit the action of IGF-1); in turn, this increases the level of free, "bioactive" IGF-1, which might favor tumor development (Fig. **1A**) [13].

Sex Steroids

Adipocyte cells express the enzyme aromatase, whose function is to aromatize androgens producing estrogens. In men and postmenopausal women, adipose tissue is the main site of estrogen synthesis. Thus, adiposity influences the synthesis and bioavailability of endogenous sex steroids-estrogens and androgens. In particular, the levels of free estradiol increased with obesity in men and postmenopausal women, likewise the levels of androgens (free testosterone) increased with obesity in woman (See Fig. **1B**). Furthermore, it has been shown that leptin can also increase estrogen levels through the activation of aromatase [10].

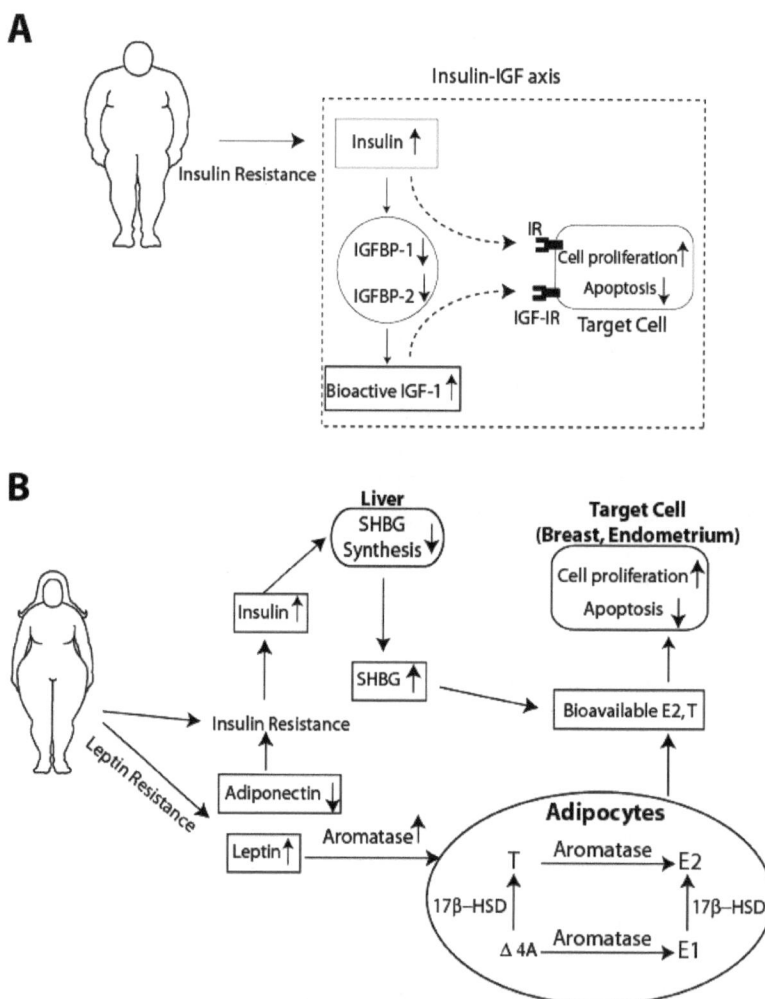

Figure 1: Molecular mechanisms relating obesity to cancer risk. **A.** In obesity, increased release of tumor-necrosis factor alpha (TNF-α) and reduced release of adiponectin lead to the development of insulin resistance and compensatory, chronic hyperinsulinemia. Increased insulin levels, in turn, lead to reduced blood levels of insulin-like growth factor binding protein 1 (IGFBP1) and IGFBP2. This results in increased levels of bioactive (unbound) IGF1. Insulin and IGF1 signal through the insulin receptors (IRs) and IGF1 receptor (IGF1R), respectively, to promote cellular proliferation and inhibit apoptosis in many tissue types. These effects might contribute to tumorigenesis. Modified from [13]. **B.** In men and women, the hallmark of obesity is the development of leptin resistance, which results in an increase in circulating leptin and a reduction of adiponectin. Low levels of adiponectin are associated with insulin resistance, whereas hyperleptinemia can upregulate the activity of the enzyme aromatase. Adipose tissue produces the enzymes aromotase and 17β-hydroxysteroid dehydrogenase (17β-HSD). Therefore, in obese individuals, there is typically an increased conversion of the androgens Δ4-androstenedione (Δ4A) and testosterone (T) into the

estrogens estrone (E1) and estradiol (E2), respectively, by aromatase. 17β-HSD converts the less biologically active hormones Δ4A and E1 into the more active hormones T and E2, respectively. In parallel, obesity leads to hyperinsulinemia, which in turn causes a reduction in the hepatic synthesis and circulating levels of sex-hormone-binding globulin (SHBG). The combined effect of increased formation of estrone and testosterone, along with reduced levels of SHBG, leads to an increase in the bioavailable fractions of estradiol (E2) and testosterone (T) that can diffuse to target cells, where they bind to estrogen and androgen receptors. The effects of sex steroids binding their receptors can vary, depending on the tissue types, but in some tissues (for example, breast epithelium and endometrium) they promote cellular proliferation and inhibit apoptosis. Modified from [7].

Alternatively and as mentioned above, adipose cells increase the circulating levels of insulin and increase IGF-1 bioactivity. This results in reduced hepatic synthesis and blood concentrations of sex-hormone binding globulin (SHBG), a plasmatic binding glycoprotein with high specific affinity for testosterone and estradiol. The SHBG inhibits the function of sex hormones estradiol and testosterone. Thus, the level of SHBG influences bioavailability of sex hormones. In both men and women, adiposity decreases SHBG levels, which increases the fraction of bioactive estradiol. In women, decreases in SHBG generally also lead to increased levels of bioactive testosterone. Furthermore, epidemiological studies suggests that these obesity-induced alterations in circulating levels of sex steroids explains large part of the association between excess weight and risk of the breast (post-menopausal women only) and endometrium cancer (both pre- and post-menopausal women).

Final Remarks

We are beginning to realize the complexity of the biological mechanisms that link obesity and being overweight to many forms of cancer. However, further research aimed to define the causal role of obesity in various types of cancers is desperately needed. A better understanding of these molecular mechanisms will be of great help in our battle to defeat obesity and cancer.

GRANTS

We thank Mike C. Wiest for general comments to the manuscript. This work was partially supported by CONACYT 78879, CONACYT 82175-M and SALUD-2010-02-151001

REFERENCES

[1]   Ogden CL, Carroll MD, Curtin LR, McDowell MA, Tabak CJ, Flegal KM. Prevalence of overweight and obesity in the United States, 1999-2004. JAMA 2006; 295(13): 1549-55.

[2]   IARC. Handbooks of Cancer Prevention. In: Weight Control and Physical Activity (International Agency for Research on Cancer). 2002. Lyon. France.

[3]   Larsson SC, Wolk A. Obesity and the risk of gallbladder cancer: a meta-analysis. Br J Cancer 2007; 96(9): 1457-61.

[4]   Renehan AG, Tyson M, Egger M, Heller RF, Zwahlen M. Body-mass index and incidence of cancer: a systematic review and meta-analysis of prospective observational studies. Lancet 2008; 371(9612): 569-78.

[5]   IARC, ed. World Cancer Report 2008. ed. P.a.L. Boyle, B. Vol. Section 2, Etiology of Cancer 2008; 154-158.

[6]   Tornberg SA, Carstensen JM. Relationship between Quetelet's index and cancer of breast and female genital tract in 47,000 women followed for 25 years. Br J Cancer 1994; 69(2): 358-61.

[7]   Calle EE, Kaaks R. Overweight, obesity and cancer: epidemiological evidence and proposed mechanisms. Nat Rev Cancer 2004; 4(8): 579-91.

[8]   Hedley AA, Ogden CL, Johnson CL, Carroll MD, Curtin LR, Flegal KM. Prevalence of overweight and obesity among US children, adolescents, and adults, 1999-2002. JAMA 2004; 291(23): 2847-50.

[9]   Friedman JM. A war on obesity, not the obese. Science 2003; 299(5608): 856-8.

[10]   Garofalo C. and Surmacz E. Leptin and cancer. J Cell Physiol 2006; 207(1): 12-22.

[11]   Friedman JM. Leptin at 14 y of age: an ongoing story. Am J Clin Nutr 2009; 89(3): 973S-9S.

[12]   Carnero A, Blanco-Aparicio C, Renner O, Link W, Leal JF. The PTEN/PI3K/AKT signalling pathway in cancer, therapeutic implications. Curr Cancer Drug Targets 2008; 8(3): 187-98.

[13]   Renehan AG, Frystyk J, Flyvbjerg A. Obesity and cancer risk: the role of the insulin-IGF axis. Trends Endocrinol Metab 2006; 17(8): 328-36.

[14]   Sauter ER, Garofalo C, Hewett J, Hewett JE, Morelli C, Surmacz E. Leptin expression in breast nipple aspirate fluid (NAF) and serum is influenced by body mass index (BMI) but not by the presence of breast cancer. Horm Metab Res 2004; 36(5): 336-40.

[15]   Kern PA, Di Gregorio GB, Lu T, Rassouli N, Ranganathan G. Adiponectin expression from human adipose tissue: relation to obesity, insulin resistance, and tumor necrosis factor-{alpha} expression. Diabetes 2003; 52(7): 1779-85.

[16]   Diez JJ, Iglesias P. The role of the novel adipocyte-derived hormone adiponectin in human disease. Eur J Endocrinol 2003; 148(3): 293-300.

[17]   Bråkenhielm E, Veitonmäki N, Cao R, *et al.* Adiponectin-induced antiangiogenesis and antitumor activity involve caspase-mediated endothelial cell apoptosis. Proc Natl Acad Sci USA 2004; 101(8): 2476-81.

[18]   Rose DP, Komninou D, Stephenson GD. Obesity, adipocytokines, and insulin resistance in breast cancer. Obes Rev 2004; 5(3): 153-65.

[19]   Rajaram S, Baylink DJ, Mohan S, Insulin-like growth factor-binding proteins in serum and other biological fluids: regulation and functions. Endocr Rev 1997; 18(6): 801-31.

Molecular Oncology: Principles and Recent Advances, 2012, 33-43

Causes of Cancer

III. Estrogens and Cancer

Jesús Adrián Rodríguez-Rasgado[1], Flavia Morales-Vásquez[2], Luz María Hinojosa[3] and Javier Camacho[1,*]

[1]*Department of Pharmacology, Centro de Investigación y de Estudios Avanzados del IPN, México,* [2]*Instituto Nacional de Cancerología, México,* [3]*Hospital General "Dr. Manuel Gea González", México*

Abstract. Estrogens are compounds that have a wide range of activities in the human body. These hormones regulate processes, such as the ovarian cycle, sexual development, preparation for implantation of fertilized embryos, and others. The most abundant estrogen in humans is estradiol. It exerts its effects through an estrogen receptor that functions as a transcriptional factor. The mechanism of action of estrogens involves the recruitment of co-regulator proteins that allow, or not, classical transcriptional activity and the transcriptional activation or repression of target genes. Non-genomic actions of estrogens have been reported, and these effects are mediated by a G-coupled protein receptor. Estrogens not only participate in physiological processes, they are also involved in pathology, such as cancer. Breast cancer is one of the main cancers that is affected by estrogens, as there is a higher expression of estrogen receptor α in breast cancer than in normal breast tissue. In this way, estrogens also participate in the development of other cancers including colon, ovarian and cervical cancer. Pharmacological strategies for estrogen related cancer treatments have been developed. Selective Estrogen Receptor Modulators (SERMs) and Aromatase Inhibitors (AIs) have been developed to antagonize the effects of estrogens, or estrogen synthesis, respectively. The use of tamoxifen and other compounds are effective in the treatment of some cancers, including breast cancer. Furthermore, change in lifestyle choices to help reduce xenoestrogen exposure is also a step that a woman can take to control total estrogen exposure.

Keywords: Estrogens, estrogen receptors, hormones, nuclear receptors, tamoxifen, breast cancer, aromatase.

INTRODUCTION

A wide range of physiological processes are regulated by estrogens. These hormones have an important role in the maintenance of normal reproductive function; and they also exert biological effects in the cardiovascular, immune and central nervous systems. The most important estrogen produced in the body is estradiol (E2), and it exerts its effects through nuclear receptors. In this way, estradiol can modulate target genes. Some genes that estrogens modulate are related to cellular proliferation and differentiation. Growing evidence has shown that estrogen receptor expression profile is altered when an estrogen target tissue becomes cancerous. Substantial evidence indicates that hormones play a major role in the etiology of several human cancers. The concept that hormones can increase the incidence of neoplasia was first proposed by Bittner (Bittner HL 1947) [1]. This theory has been refined into epidemiologic hypotheses related to cancers of the breast, endometrium, prostate, ovary, thyroid, bone and testis (Henderson CR 1988) [2] (Henderson CR 1982) [3]. The underlying mechanism proposed for all of these cancers is that neoplasia is the consequence of prolonged hormonal stimulation of the target organ, the normal growth and function of which are controlled by one or more steroid or polypeptide hormones. Evidence shows that the amount of hormone to which a tissue is effectively exposed is under strong genetic control (Feigelson JCBS 1996) [4]. Therefore, in addition to external factors, such as diet or exogenous hormone use which may modify hormone profiles, polymorphisms in genes encoding proteins involved in steroid-hormone biosynthesis, metabolism or extra- and intracellular transport, and DNA binding are important determinants of individual cancer risk (Feigelson JCBS 1996) [4] (Ross CR 1998) [5]. In the uterus, estrogen triggers the proliferation of endometrial cells during each month of the menstrual cycle, followed by death of these cells during menstruation. Similarly, during each menstrual

*Address correspondence to Javier Camacho:** Department of Pharmacology, Centro de Investigación y de Estudios Avanzados del I.P.N., Avenida Instituto Politécnico Nacional 2508, 07360 Mexico City, Mexico; Email: fcamacho@cinvestav.mx

cycle, estrogen normally triggers the proliferation of cells that form the inner lining of the ducts in the breast. Over a span of 40 years, from puberty to menopause, hundreds of cycles of cell division and cell death will occur. These repeated cycles of estrogen-induced cell division tend to increase the risk of developing cancer in two ways: estrogen can stimulate the division of uterine or breast cells that already have DNA mutations (oncogene or virus initiated), and it also increases the chances of developing new, spontaneous mutations (from carcinogens or radiation) (Feigelson JCBS 1996) [4] (Ross CR 1998) [5]. Whether the mutations are inherited or spontaneous, estrogen-driven proliferation increases the number of altered cells that can ultimately lead to the development of uterine or breast cancer. The historical perspective on the development of the estrogen-cancer association from early observations to recent conclusive reports began in 1896 with the Beatson report that ovary removal gives remission of breast cancer (Beatson Lancet 1896) [6]. However, the first time estrogen use was linked to endometrial cancer was in 1979 (Cramer OG 1979) [7]. In 1980, the effects of estriol on mammary carcinomas were debated (Lemon AES 1980) [8] (Bradlow JE 1996) [9]. In 1985, estrogen was reported to be a cause of endometrial cancer and likely a factor in breast cancer (Persson AOGSS 1985) [10]. It was also found that estrogens promoted mammary cancer in rodents and exert cell proliferative effects in humans (Lupulescu CI 1995) [11]. In the second half of the 1990's family history, sex hormones, diet, lifestyle, and environmental exposures were factors associated with breast cancer incidence (Hulka Lancet 1995) [12]. Differences in exposure to xenoestrogens, such as insecticides, weed killers, synthetic estrogens, and aromatic hydrocarbons may explain the five-fold higher rate of cancer in Canadian women compared to women in Asia (Robson CMAJ 1996) [13]. Multiple prospective studies strongly suggest that breast cancer risk in postmenopausal women is associated with relatively high concentrations of endogenous estradiol (Thomas CCC 1997) [14]. In 2000, it was noted that women with family history of breast cancer who used early oral contraceptive formulations have particularly high risk for the disease. (Grabrick JAMA 2000) [15]. In 2001, hormone replacement therapy was conclusively linked with breast cancer (Rodríguez JAMA 2001) [16]. Limiting exposure to environmental estrogens can reduce cancer risk. For example, estrogen activity has been found in nonylphenol and bisphenol. Nonylphenol is an antioxidant used in the manufacture of plastics, detergents, toiletries, lubricants, and spermicides. Bisphenol is leached from polycarbonate plastics when they are heated (Cotton JAMA 1994) [17]. Other xenoestrogens include DDT, aromatic hydrocarbons, and the common weed killer Atrazine which is widely used on corn crops. On the other hand, there is evidence that higher levels of estrogens can be found in breast and ovarian cancers compared to the normal tissues, thus aromatase levels also could be increased. Pharmacological strategies have been developed to inhibit the effects of estrogen and to offer more effective therapies for cancer patients. However, the estrogen dependent-tissue activity is a paradigm that continues under research.

BIOSYNTHESIS OF ESTROGENS

Cholesterol is the precursor of the five major classes of esteriod hormones: progestagens, glucocorticoids, mineralocorticoids, androgens, and estrogens. These hormones are signal molecules that regulate a host of organismal functions. Steroidal estrogens arise from androstenedione or testosterone by aromatization of the A ring. Testosterone is an androgen formed by the reduction of the 17-keto group of androstenedione. Estrogens are synthesized from androgens with the loss of the C-19 angular methyl group and the formation of an aromatic A ring. Estrone, an estrogen, is derived from androstenedione, whereas estradiol, another estrogen is formed from testosterone (Fig. 1). The final reaction is catalyzed by Cytochrome p450 enzyme complex named aromatase (CYP19), that uses NAPDH and molecular oxygen as co-substrates. Aromatase is localized in the endoplasmic reticulum of ovarian granulosa cells, Leydig and Sertolli cells, adipose stroma, various brain regions, and other tissues (Simpson ARP 2002) [18]. In premenopausal women, the ovaries are the principal source of estradiol, which functions as a circulating hormone to act on distal target tissues. Estradiol and other estrogens are required for the development of female secondary sex characteristics, and they also participate in the ovarian cycle. In postmenopausal women, the principal source of circulating estrogen is adipose tissue stroma. In men, estrogens are produced by Sertoli cells in the testes (Simpson JSBMB 2003) [19].

PHYSIOLOGICAL ACTIONS OF ESTROGENS

Estrogen plays a central role in the regulation of some aspects of female reproductive activity. Together with progesterone, estrogen acts at the level of the hypothalamus, pituitary, ovary and uterus to coordinate cyclic neuroendocrine gonadotropin production, ovulatory activity, and uterine development in preparation for implantation of fertilized embryos. The diverse physiological activities of estrogen are not restricted to the female reproductive system. Estrogen is essencial for male fertility; and this hormone has been implicated in the cardiovascular, immune, and central nervous systems and in bone function (Conneely Endocrinology 2001) [20]. Estrogens have also been shown to play an important role in protection against osteoporosis in postmenopausal women (Turner ER 1994) [21], in the prevention of coronary heart disease (Iafrati NM 1997) [22], and in the maintenance of cognitive function (Tang Lancet 1996) [23].

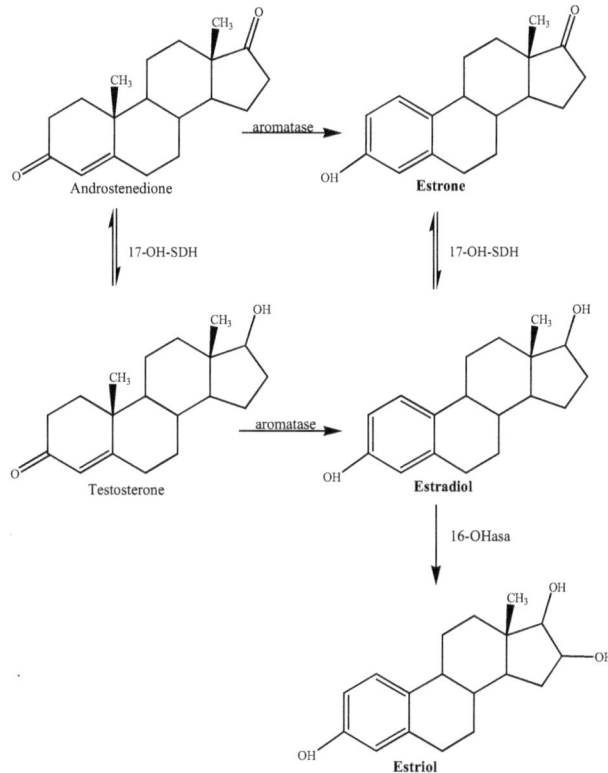

Figure 1: Estrogen biosynthetic route. 17-OH-SDH (17-hydroxysteroid dehydrogenase); 16-OHase (16α-hydroxylase).

ESTROGEN RECEPTORS

Estrogens are compounds that exert their effects by interaction with nuclear receptors. Estrogen Receptor α (ERα) and Estrogen Receptor β (ERβ) are transcription factors and promote a transcriptional response in target genes. Estrogen Receptors (ERs) contain conserved structurally and functionally distinct domains (Fig. **2**). The estrogen receptor is divided into six domains: NH_2 terminal A/B domain contains activation function 1 (AF-1), which can activate a transcriptional response independently of ligand. The DNA Binding Domain (DBD) that is present in C domain is involved in DNA recognition and binding; the D domain is a hinge region and contains the nuclear localization signal. Whereas ligand binding occurs in the Ligand-Binding Domain (LBD) that is present at E/F segment, other activation function (AF-2) resides in the COOH terminal LBD and is ligand-dependent. AF domains recruit a range of coregulatory protein complexes to the DNA bound receptor. The estrogen receptors have similar affinities for estradiol and bind the same DNA response elements (Heldring PR 2007) [24]. Both ERα and ERβ exist as multiple mRNA isoforms due to differential promoter use and alternative splicing (Lewandowski FEBSL 2002) [25] (Kos ME 2001) [26]. Ligand-dependent estrogen signaling begins with the binding of estrogen to estrogen receptor and the transcriptional response is cell specific and needs multiple factors. Some of these factors are: the composition of coregulatory proteins in a given cell and the characteristics of the promoters of estrogen responsive genes (Heldring PR 2007) [24]. At the promoters of some genes, particulary those involved in proliferation, ERα and ERβ can have opposite actions (Liu JBC 2002) [27], which suggests that the proliferative response to estradiol is the result of a balance between ERα and ERβ signalling. There is evidence that an ERβ isoform can induce proteosome-dependent degradation of ERα, presumably through the formation of ERβ/ERα heterodimers (Zhao CR 2007) [28].

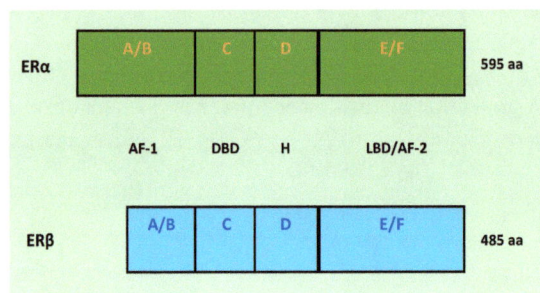

Figure 2: Estrogen receptor subtypes.

In addtion, estrogen may elicit effects through non-genomic mechanism where estrogen has been claimed to bind to ERs localized on the plasma membrane of target cells (Razandi ME 1999) [29] (Razandi ME 2004) [30]. In this respect, GPR30 is a G-coupled protein receptor, and the transcripts were reported in normal and malignant tissues, with high levels of expression found in heart, lung, liver, intestine, ovary, brain and breast (O´Dowed Genomics 1998) [31] (Prossnitz ARP 2008) [32]. Several primary breast cancers and lymphomas also express GPR30 transcripts (Carmeci Genomics 1998) [33] (Owman BBRC 1996) [34]. A number of reports demonstrated estrogen-mediated cell proliferation to be dependent on GPR30 (Vivacqua ME 2006) [35] (Albanito CR 2007) [36] (Vivacqua MP 2006) [37].

MOLECULAR MECHANISM OF ESTROGENS

Estrogens have functions in both female and male physiology (Hall JBC 2001) [38]. Estradiol has a central role in the proliferation and differentiation of responsive cells through changing the expression profile of target genes within responsive tissues (Métivier Cell 2003) [39]. As mentioned above both estrogen receptors are transcription factors that increase or decrease the transcription of target genes (Fig. **3**). The hormone enters into the cell by passive diffusion through the plasma membrane; in the nucleus ER is present as an inactive monomer bound to heat-shock proteins. Upon binding estrogen, a change in ER conformation dissociates the heat-shock proteins and promotes receptor dimerization. ER dimer binds to Estrogen Response Elements (ERE) GGTCAnnnTGACC localized in promoter regions of target genes; although there are other sequences that can act as ERE, which bind ER dimers in a promoter specific manner (Hall ME 2002) [40] (O´Lone ME 2004) [41]. Ligand-bound ER can interact with other transcription factor complexes like Fos/Jun or stimulating protein 1 (SP-1) and influence transcription of genes whose promoters do not harbor EREs (Kushner JSBMB 2000) [42] (Saville JBC 2000) [43] (Bjornstrom ME 2005) [44]. This ligand-dependent activation triggers recruitment of a variety of coregulators to the receptor. The first recruited proteins have the ability to modify nucleosome structure like SWI/Snf, or Histone Methyltransferase (HMT) activity provided by proteins as PRMT1 o CARM1. Other proteins that are recruited to this complex are steroid receptors co-activator (SRC-1) and cyclic AMP response Element Binding Protein (CBP). Co-activators have Histone Acetylase (HAT) activity and this complex alters chromatin estructure and facilitates recruitment of the RNA polymerase II transcriptional machinery, thus promoting transcription (Métivier Cell 2003) [39]. An antagonist can interact with ERs, and also promote dimerization and DNA binding. However, the ER conformation produced by an antagonist interaction is different from an agonist conformation. The antagonist-induced conformation facilitates binding of co-repressors such as nuclear hormone receptor co-repressor/silencing mediator of retinoid and thyroid receptors (NcoR/SMRT), and then the co-repressor/ER complex recruits proteins with deacetylase activity such as HDAC1 altering chromatin conformation and reducing the ability of the transcriptional machinery to form initiation complexes. On the other hand, the GPR30 signaling pathway has been studied in a variety of cell lines. GPR30 couples to a trimeric G protein, stimulating Src through Gβγ subunits. Subsequently, Src promotes the shedding of heparin-binding EGF-like growth factor and activation of the EGF receptor (Filardo JSBMB 2002) [45] (Filardo ME 2000) [46]. This in turn activates a whole series of intracellular signaling events, most notably the activation of Mitogen-Activated Protein Kinases (MAPK) (Prossnitz ARP 2008) [32]. Further cellular responses lie down-stream of these signals, including the activation of the gene fos, that accounts for all of the biological effects of GPR30 signaling that have been reported (Prakash EMBO 2009) [47].

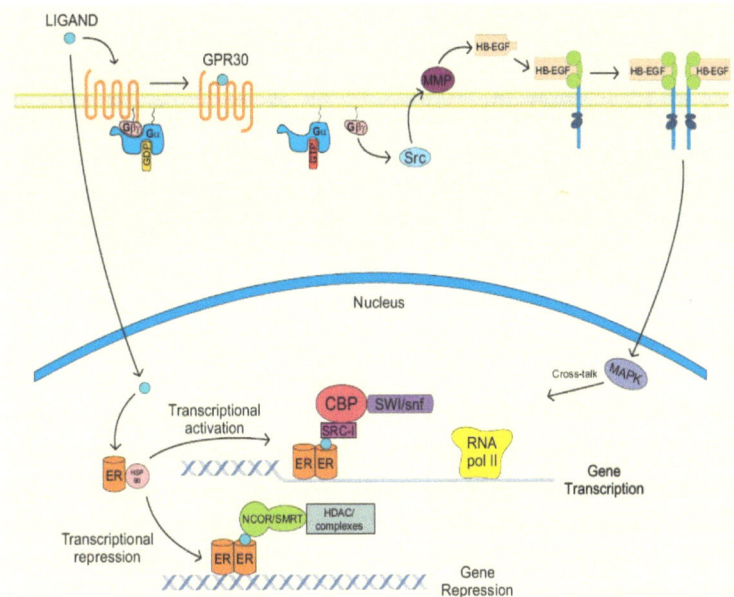

Figure 3: Estrogen-mediated transcriptional regulation.

CANCER-ESTROGEN IMPLICATIONS

Cancer is a disease that is produced by many factors. Estrogen is one of the etiological factors that can produce cancer that has been well studied. Estrogen is essential for growth and development of the mammary glands and has been associated with the promotion and growth of breast cancer (Zhao NRS 2008) [48]. ERα expression is found in only 6-10% of normal breast epithelial cells, whereas 60% of primary breast cancers are ERα positive (Hanstein EJE 2004) [49]. It has been largely reported that ERα mediates the mitogenic action of estrogens in breast cancer by inducing a variety of genes involved in cell proliferation (Zhao NRS 2008) [48]. A protective role of ERβ against breast cancer development has been proposed during the recent years. ERβ is lost in a majority of breast tumors (Bardin ERC 2004) [50] (Skiliris JP 2003) [51], apparently by ERβ promoter methylation in breast cancer cells (Rody ERC 2005) [52]. These data suggest that ERβ is a possible tumor supresor gene (Garinis HG 2002) [53]. Colon cancer incidence and mortality rates are lower in females compared with males, and numerous epidemiological studies suggest that estrogen replacement therapy reduces the incidence of colorectal cancer in postmenopausal women. ERβ is the predominant ER in the colonic epithelium (Campbell CR 2001) [54] (Konstantinopoulos EJC 2003) [55] suggesting that effects of estrogen in the colon are mediated by ERβ. Estrogens are major regulators of growth and differentiation in normal ovaries and also play an important role in the progression of ovarian cancer (O′Donell ERC 2005) [56]. In normal ovary, the levels of ERβ are high and predominate over ERα, whereas an opposite pattern characterizes the development of ovarian cancer, which often express ERα levels similar to those found in breast carcinoma (Bardin 2004 ERC) [50] (Jordan ER 1999) [57]. A marked proliferative response to estrogens was shown in ovarian surface epithelial cells representing the site of 90% of malignances (Bai IVCDBA 2000) [58], and an increased risk of ovarian tumor was observed in postmenopausal women receiving estrogen replacement therapy (Rodriguez JAMA 2001) [16] (Lacey JAMA 2002) [59]. Cervical cancer is the second leading cause of cancer morbidity and mortality for women around the world, especially in developing countries. It is well known that infection with high risk Human Papilloma Virus (HPV) is the predominant risk factor for cervical cancer. Since most infected females do not develop the disease, other factors must contribute to the initiation of the cancer (Au GO 2008) [60]. A contributing risk factor is chronic estrogen exposure since the risk of cervical cancer is increased 2-4 times for women with extended use of oral contraceptives and 4 times for women having 7 or more children (Elson CR 2000) [61] (Moodley IJGC 2003) [62]. In this way, estrogens have been shown to increase gene expression of HPV 16 and HPV 18, the two HPV subtypes most associated with cervical cancer (Kim IJGC 2000) [63]. All these data are related to an *in vivo* experiment, in which Brake & Lambert demonstrated that both K14E7 and K14E6/K14E7 transgenic mice treated for 6 and 9 months with exogenous estrogen developed cervical cancer, and those mice treated for 6 months followed by 3 months with no estradiol treatment showed a lower degree of dysplasia (Brake PNAS 2005) [64]. As above mentioned, aromatase is the enzyme responsible for the conversion of adrogens to estrogens. Although aromatase expression occurs mainly in the ovaries, other tissues have been shown to express this enzyme. Overexpression of aromatase is a potencial etiologic factor in hormone-sensitive cancers. Nair *et al.* reported that cervical carcinomas express aromatase, and both precancerous and normal cervical tissues do not express this enzyme (Nair CR 2005) [65]. On the other hand, a number of endometrial carcinomas also express aromatase as do endometriotic plaques, although healthy endometrium does not express aromatase (Bulun JCEM 1994) [66] (Noble JCEM 1996) [67]. Other carcinomas, as adrenocortical and non-small cell lung cancers also present a high expression of aromatase, which can be related with high levels of estrogen and the progression of the malignancy (Nicol MCE 2009) [68] (Oyama FB 2008) [69]. Interestingly, in all these pathological situations, the major promoter employed to drive aromatase expression is the gonodal-type promoter, promoter II, regardless of the tissue of origin of the tumor (Simpson ARP 2002) [18].

Estrogen Metabolite-Cancer Connections

In 1982, 16α-hydroxylated estrogens were associated with breast cancer and suggested to have an etiological role. Women with breast or endometrial cancer have increased estrogen-16α-hydroxylase activity. Daily excretion of urinary estrogen metabolites was quantified and total metabolite excretion was lowered by dietary fiber (Adlercreutz JSB 1986) [70]. The 16α-OHE1 has a unique capacity to bind covalently and irreversibly with the endoplasmic reticulum (Swaneck PNAS 1988) [71]. In 1992 the evidence that both genotoxic damage and aberrant proliferation caused by 16α-hydroxyestrone is found in mouse mammary cells (Telang JNCI 1992) [72]. The agents that increase 2-OHE1 inhibit carcinogenesis (Tuwari JNCI 1994) [73]. The ratio of 16-αOHE1 to 2-OHE1 was elevated in women and animals with high rates of mammary tumors. The Organochlorine pesticides activated CYP enzymes responsible for 16α-hydroxestrone formation (Bradlow EHP 1995) [74]. In 1996 CYP1A1 polymorphism caused lower 2-OHE1/16α-OHE1 ratios in African-American women compared to Caucasian women (Taioli JNCI 1996) [75]. The exposure of mammary epithelial cells to 16α-OHE1 resulted in genotoxic DNA damage and increased cell proliferation similar to that induced by the carcinogen 7,12-dimethyl-(α)benzanthracene (DMBA). A bifunctional pathway of genotoxic and estrogen receptor modulation was proposed for carcinogenesis of 16α-OHE1 (Davis EHP 1997) [76]. Data from women with breast cancer and age-matched controls showed a strong inverse association of the 2/16α ratios with cancer. Favorable clinical outcomes was predicted for women with high 2/16α ratios in a 9.5 year follow up prospective study of 5104 women (Guernsey III study) (Meilahn BJC 1998) [77].

METABOLIC FATE OF ESTROGENS

Normal premenopausal women produce several hundred micrograms of estradiol (E2) daily. A portion of the roughly 10^{17} newly synthesized molecules find their way to binding sites in the nucleus and other organelles of many tissues. Once bound to estrogen receptors, the estrogen hormones elicit an increased rate of DNA synthesis, resulting in gene transcription and cell division. Meanwhile, a similar number of estrone/estradiol molecules are removed from the body, maintaining a relatively constant stimulation of cell division in estrogen-sensitive tissues. Much of the estradiol is converted into estrone (E1) and estriol (E3), but these are only two of the best known metabolites. The half-life of E2 is about three hours. Its removal is accomplished by irreversible conversion into metabolites that may be passed into urine or bile. There are multiple pathways that convert E2 to products that have widely different biological activities. Some products are powerful carcinogens while others act as estrogen antagonists. The relative amounts of these metabolites control the overall cancer risk from estrogen exposure. Oxidation to form hydroxy derivatives is the principal route of endogenous steroid metabolism. Isoenzymes of the Cytochrome p450 (CYP) class can insert hydroxyl groups at the 2-, 4-, or 16- positions of E1. The iso-enzyme that catalyzes 2-hydroxylation of E2 (CYP1A1) is an inducible enzyme. It is formed in greater amounts in hepatic microsomes in response to dietary ingredients and cigarette smoke. A separate enzyme, CYP1B1, catalyzes 16α-hydroxylation. This enzyme is not inducible by diet, but xenobiotic carcinogens and pesticides may stimulate its activity (Fishman ANYAS 1995) [78]. As a result, a preferential increase in 2-hydroxylation can occur through dietary manipulation. After estrone hydroxylation, the various poly-hydroxy derivatives are conjugated with glucuronate or sulfate, or methylation occurs prior to excretion in urine. The catechol-O-methyl transferase (COMT) enzymes that catalyze the methylation reactions require S-adenosyl methionine. A portion of conjugated and unconjugated steroids also passes into bile, some of which may be reabsorbed *via* enterohepatic circulation. Lower intestinal re-uptake rates can explain why total estrogen loads are decreased by high fiber diets and especially by the lignans contained in flax seed. The principal hydroxylation products are 2-hydroxyestrone (2-OHE1), 2-hydroxyestradiol (2-OHE2), 4-hydroxyestrone (4-OHE1), 4-hydroxyestradiol (4-OHE2), and 16α-hydroxyestrone (16α-OHE1). The 2-hydroxy derivatives and 16α-OHE1 have opposite biological properties. Cell proliferative activity of the 2-hydroxy metabolites is nil, while 16α-OHE1 is a powerful estrogen agonist. The 4-hydroxy derivatives are also estrogen agonists, but their relative concentrations are smaller, so they may have less impact on cancer risk compared to the more abundant 2- and 16α-derivatives. The carcinogenic affects of 4-OHE1 may be due to the effects of toxic quinone metabolites rather than to estrogen agonist effects. Note that the 16α-derivative of estrone is the precursor to relatively inactive estriol. Apparently, it is the unique orientation of the 16α-OH group with the keto group of estrone that leads to the potent effects of this metabolite (Davis EHP 1997) [76]. 16-α-OHE1 can bind covalently to sites in the endoplasmic reticulum while becoming simultaneously bound to nuclear estrogen receptor sites. This binding stimulates heightened activity for days instead of hours. The 16α-OHE1 effects persist until the binding proteins are degraded. Such increased cell proliferative and genotoxic effects appear to be a mechanism of cancer induction by tumor viruses, carcinogens, and oncogenes associated with cancer, mainly in breast cancer. Early evidence suggested that 2-OHE1, at most, behaved as a weak estrogen and probably more as an anti-estrogen in several models. Cell culture studies in subsequent years also identified 2-OHE1 as a weak promotional estrogen that was less potent than 16α-OHE1 at initiating cell proliferation. Comparison of the relative potencies of 2-OHE1 and 16α-OHE1 at transforming cells showed that 16α-OHE1 exhibited increased unscheduled DNA synthesis, proliferation, and anchorage-independent growth relative to 2-OHE1, which showed less activity than estradiol in each of these parameters. In long-term proliferation studies, persistent proliferation was observed after treatment of human ER positive cancer cells with 16α-OHE1 but not with 2-OHE1 (Lustig ESP 1994) [79].

SELECTIVE ESTROGEN RECEPTOR MODULATORS AND AROMATASE INHIBITORS

Selective Estrogen Receptor Modulators (SERMs) are characterized by their diverse range of agonist/antagonist actions on estrogen receptor-mediated processes. They have the ability to act as either ER antagonists by blocking estrogen action through its receptor, or ER agonists by displaying estrogen-like actions, or as ER partial agonists/antagonists with mixed activity (Frasor CR 2004) [80]. However, these differences in SERM activity depend upon the target gene promoter, as well as the cell or tissue background (McKenna NM 2000) [81]. Many of the growth-stimulatory effects of estrogens in breast cancer have been linked to ERα (Beral Lancet 2003) [82]. Today, ERα expression is routinely checked in pathological diagnosis, and if ERα is expressed in the tumor, the patient receives the antiestrogen tamoxifen. The usefulness and importance of tamoxifen in breast cancer therapy is well established, and the disease-free survival rate has increased dramatically due to the widespread use of tamoxifen (Chia Lancet 2005) [83]. The benefical effects of SERMs on breast cancer were originally attributed to their ability to antagonize the actions of endogenous estrogens by competition for ER binding. X-ray structural work demonstrated that when different ER ligands such as estradiol, tamoxifen, raloxifen and the antiestrogen ICI 182,780 (ICI) interact with the ligand binding domain of the receptor, distinctly different conformations of the receptor are induced (Brzozowski Nature 1997) [84] (Shiau Cell 1998) [85] (Pike EMBO 1999) [86] (Kong BST 2003) [87]. When clinically used as antiprolifeative agents in the treatment of breast cancer, the agonist action of antiestrogens is desirable in certain tissues like bone and cardiovascular system, while highly non-desirable in tissues like uterus or breast (Heldring PR 2007) [24]. In this way, raloxifene and toremifene are therapeutically established antiestrogens, available for prevention of osteoporosis (Bilezikian IJFWM 2005) [88] and for the treatment of advanced hormone-sensitive breast cancer (Harvey Breast 2006) [89]. On the other hand, the recognition that locally produced, as well as circulating, estrogens may play a significant role in breast cancer has greatly stimulated interest in the use of Aromatase Inhibitors (AIs) to selectively block production of estrogens. Steroidal agents are substrate analogs that act as suicide inhibitors to irreversibly inactivate aromatase; examples of these drugs are formestane and exemestane. Nonsteroidal agents interact reversibly with the heme groups of CYPs (Haynes JSBMB 2003) [90]; examples of these drugs are anastrazole, letrozole and vorozole, which have been tested in several breast cancer clinical trials.

CONCLUSIONS

The role of estrogens in the origin and development of some kind of cancers is well established. In accordance some dietary means have been suggested to reduce cancer risk by improving estrogen metabolism (Lord RS Altern Med Rev 2002) [91]. The expression profile of estrogen receptors and the co-activators or co-repressors expression patterns present in the tissues are responsible for targeted gene expression and thus for the development of this malignancy. More studies are necessary in order to understand the changes in the ERs expression profile from normal tissue to cancer tissue, and the factors that could modulate estrogens activity. The evidence points to the xenobiotic contribution to excessive cell proliferation due to the total load of estrogen-receptor stimulators. In addition, some compounds like DDT can exert direct effects on procarcinogenic estrogen metabolites. Adjustment of lifestyle to reduce xenoestrogen exposure is a step a woman can take to control total estrogen exposure. SERMs, ER pure antagonists and aromatase inhibitors have served as a better and more effective treatment for many cancer patients. However, more studies are needed in order to offer alternative therapies for example for patients carrying either ER-negative or antiestrogen-resistant tumors.

ACKNOWLEDGEMENTS

The preparation of this book is part of a group research project supported by Conacyt (Grant 82175-M to JC). We thank Cynthia Chow for revising the English language.

REFERENCES

[1]   Bittner JJ. The causes and control of mammary cancer in mice. Harvey Lect 1947; 42: 221.

[2]   Henderson BE, Ross RK, Berstein L. Estrogens as a cause of human cancer:the Richard and Hinda Rosenthal Foundation Award Lecture. Cancer Res 198; 48: 246-53.

[3]   Henderson BE, Ross RK, Pike MC, *et al.* Endogenous hormones as a major factor in human cancer. Cancer Res 1982; 42: 3232-9.

[4]   Feigelson HS, Ross RK, Yu MC, *et al.* Genetic Susceptibility to cancer from exogenous and endogenous esposures. J Cell Biochem Suppl 1996; 25: 15-22.

[5]   Ross RK, Pike MC, Coetzee GA, *et al.* Androgen metabolism and prostate cancer:establishing a model of genetic susceptibility. Cancer Res 1998; 58: 4497-504.

[6]   Beaton G. On the treatment of inoperable cases of carcinoma of the mamma:suggestions for a new method of treatment, with illustrative cases. Lancet 1896; 2: 104-7.

[7]   Cramer DW, Knapp RC. Review of epidemiologic studies of endometrial cancer and exogenous estrogen. Obstet Gynecol 1979; 54: 521-6.

[8]   Lemon HM. Pathophysiologic considerations in the treatment of menopausal patients with oestrogens; the role of oestriol in the prevention of mammary carcinoma. Acta Endocrinol Suppl 1980; 233: 17-27.

[9]   Bradlow HL, Telang NT, Sepkovic DW, *et al.* 2-hydroxyestrone:the good estrogen. J Endocrinol 1996; 150: S259-S65.

[10]   Persson I. The risk of endometrial and breast cancer after estrogen treatment. A review of epidemiological studies. Acta Obstet Gynecol Scand Suppl 1985; 130: 59-66.

[11]   Lupulescu A. Estrogen use and cancer incidence:a review. Cancer Invest 1995; 13: 287-95.

[12]   Hulka BS, Stark At. Breast cancer: cause and prevention. Lancet 1995; 346: 883-7.

[13]   Robson B. Conferenses point to growing concern about possible links between breast cancer, enviroment. CMAJ 1996; 154: 1253-5.

[14]   Thomas HV, Reeves GK, Key TJ. Endogenous estrogen and postmenopausal breast cancer: a quantitative review. Cancer Causes Control 1997; 8: 922-8.

[15]   Grabrick DM, Hartmann LC, Cerhan JR, *et al.* Risk of breast cancer with oral contraceptive use in women with a family history of breast cancer. JAMA 2000; 284: 1791-8.

[16]   Rodriguez C, Patel AV, Calle EE, *et al.* Estrogen replacement therapy and ovarian cancer mortality in a large prospective study of US women. JAMA 2001; 285: 1460-5.

[17]   Cotton P. Enviromental estrogenic agents area of concern. JAMA 1994; 27: 414-6.

[18]   Simpson ER, Clyne C, Rubin G, *et al.* Aromatase-a brief overview. Annu Rev Physiol 2002; 64: 93-127.

[19]   Simpson ER. Sources of estrogen and their importance. J Steroid Biochem Mol Biol 2003; 86: 225-30.

[20]   Conneely OM. Perspective: Female steroid hormone action. Endocrinology 2001; 142: 2194-9.

[21]   Turner RT, Riggs BL, Spelsberg TC. Skeletal effects of estrogens.Endocr Rev 1994; 15: 275-300.

[22]   Iafrati MD, Karas RH, Aronovitz M, *et al.* Estrogen inhibits the vascular injury response in estrogen receptor α-deficient mice. Nature Med 1997; 3: 545-8.

[23]   Tang MX, Jacobs D, Stern Y, *et al.* Effect of oestrogen during menopause on kisk and age at onset of Alzheimer´s disease. Lancet 1996; 348: 429-32.

[24]   Heldring N, Pike A, Andersson S, *et al.* Estrogen receptors: How do they signal and what are their targets. Physiol Rev 2007; 87: 905-31.

[25]   Lewandowski S, Kalita K, Kaczmarek L. Estrogen receptor β Potencional functional significance of a variety of mRNA isoforms. FEBS Letters 2002; 524: 1-5.

[26]   Kos M, Reid G, Denger S, *et al.* Genomic organization of the human ERα gene promoter region. Mol Endocrinol 2001; 15(12): 2057-63.

[27]   Liu M, Albanese C, Anderson C, *et al.* Opposing action of estrogen receptors α and β on cyclin D1 gene expression. The J Biol Chem 2002; 277(27): 24353-60.

[28]   Zhao C, Matthews J, Tujague M, *et al.* Estrogen receptor beta2 negatively regulates the transactivation of estrogen receptor α in human breast cancer cells. Cancer Res 2007; 67: 3955-62.

[29]   Razandi M, Pedram A, Greene G, *et al.* Cell membrane and nuclear estrogen receptors (ERs) originate from a single transcript:Estudies of ERα and ERβ expressed in Chinese hamster ovary cells. Mol Endocrinol 1999; 13(2): 307-19.

[30]   Razandi M, Pedram A, Merchenthaler I, *et al.* Plasma membrane estrogen receptors exist and functions as dimers. Mol Endocrinol 2004; 18(12): 2854-65.

[31]   O´Dowed BF, Nguyen T, Marchese A, *et al.* Discovery of three novel G-protein-coupled receptor genes. Genomics 1998; 47: 310-3.

[32]   Prossnitz E, Arterburn J, Smith H, *et al.* Estrogen signaling through the transmembrane G protein-coupled receptor GPR30. Annu Rev Physiol 2008; 70: 165-90.

[33]   Carmeci C, Thompson D, Ring H, *et al.* Identification of a gene (GPR30) with homology to the G-protein-coupled receptor superfamily associated with estrogen receptor expression in breast cancer. Genomics 1997; 45: 607-17.

[34]   Owman C, Blay P, Nilsson C, *et al.* Cloning of the human cDNA encoding a novel heptahelix receptor expressed in Burkitt´s lymphoma and widely distributed in brain and peripheral tissues. Biochem Biophys Res Commun 1996; 228: 285-92.

[35]   Vivacqua A, Bonofiglio D, Recchia A, *et al.* The G-protein coupled receptor GPR30 mediates the proliferative effects induced by 17β-estradiol and hydroxytamoxifen in endometrial cancer cells. Mol Endocrinol 2006; 20: 631-46.

[36]   Albanito L, Madeo A, Lappano R, *et al.* G protein coupled receptor 30 (GPR30) mediates gene expresión changes and growth response to 17β-estradiol and selective GPR30 ligand G-1 in ovarian cancer cells. Cancer Res 2007; 67: 1859-66.

[37]   Vivacqua A, Bonofiglio D, Albanito L, *et al.* 17β-estradiol, genistein and 4-hydroxytamoxifen induce the proliferation of thyroid cáncer cells through the G protein-coupled receptor GPR30. Mol Pharmacol 2006; 70: 1414-23.

[38]   Hall J, Couse J, Korach K. The multifaceted mechanisms of estradiol and estrogen receptor signaling. The J Biol Chem 2001; 276(40): 36869-72.

[39]   Métivier R, Penot G, Hübner M, *et al.* Estrogen receptor-α directs, ordered, cyclical, and combinatorial recruitment of cofactors on a natural target promoter. Cell 2003; 15: 751-63.

[40]   Hall J, Mcdonnell D, Korach K. Allosteric regulation of estrogen receptor structure, function, and coactivator recruitment by different estrogen response elements. Mol Endocrinol 2002; 16(3): 469-86.

[41]   O´Lone R, Frith M, Karlsson E, *et al.* Genomic targets of nuclear estrogen receptors. Mol Endocrinol 2004; 18: 1859-75.

[42]   Kunsner P, Agard D, Greene G, *et al.* Estrogen receptor pathways to AP-1. J Steroid Biochem Mol Biol 2000; 74: 311-7.

[43]   Saville B, Wormke M, Wang F, *et al.* Ligand-, cell-, estrogen receptor subtype (alpha/beta)-dependent activation at GC-rich (Sp1) promoter elements. J Biol Chem 2000; 275: 5379-87.

[44]   Bjornstrom L, Sjoberg M. Mechanisms of estrogen receptor signaling: convergence of genomic and nongenomic actions on target genes. Mol Endocrinol 2005; 19: 833-42.

[45]   Filardo E. Epidermal growth factor receptor (EGFR) transactivation by estrogen *via* the G-protein-coupled receptor, GPR30: a novel signaling pathway with potencial significance for breast cancer. J Steroid Biochem Mol Biol 2002; 80: 231-8.

[46]   Filardo E, Quinn J, Bland K, *et al.* Estrogen-induced activation of Erk-1 and Erk-2 requires the G-protein-coupled receptor homolog, GPR30, and occurs *via* trans-activation of the epidermal growth factor receptor through release of HB-EGF. Mol Endocrinol 2000; 14: 1629-60.

[47]   Prakash D, Lappano R, Albanito L, *et al.* Estrogenic GPR30 signalling induces proliferation and migration of breast cancer cells through CTGF. The EMBO J 2009; 1-10.

[48]   Zhao C, Dahlman-Wright K, Gustafsson J. Estrogen receptor β: an overview and update. Nuc Rec Signaling 2008; 6,e003.

[49]   Hanstein B, Djahansouzi S, Dall P, *et al.* Insights into the molecular biology of the estrogen receptor define novel therapeutic targets for breast cancer. Eur J Endocrinol 2004; 150: 243-55.

[50]   Bardin A, Boulle N, Lazennec G, *et al.* Loss of ERbeta expression as a common step in estrogen-dependent tumor progression. Endocr Relat Cancer 2004; 11: 537-51.

[51] Skiliris G, Munot K, Bell S, *et al.* Reduced expression of oestrogen receptor β in invasive breast cancer and its re-expression using DNA methyl transferase inhibitors in a cell line model. J Pathol 2003; 201: 213-20.

[52] Rody A, Holtrich U, Solbach, *et al.* Methylation of estrogen receptor β promoter correlates with loss of ER-β expression in mammary carcinoma and is an early indication marker in premalignant lesions. Endocr Relat Cancer 2005; 12: 903-16.

[53] Garinis G, Patrinos G, Spanakis N, *et al.* DNA hypermethylation: when tumour supressor genes go silent. Hum Genet 2002; 111: 115-27.

[54] Campbell-Thompson M, Lynch I, Bhardwaj B. Expression of estrogen receptor (ER) subtypes and ERbeta isoforms in colon cancer. Cancer Res 2001; 61: 632-40.

[55] Konstantinopoulos P, Kominea A, Vandoros G, *et al.* Oestrogen receptor β (ERbeta) is abundantly expressed in normal colonic mucosa, but declines in colon adenocarcinoma paralleling the tumour's dedifferentiation. Eur J Cancer 2003; 39: 1251-8.

[56] O'Donell A, Macleod K, Burns D, *et al.* Estrogen receptor α mediates gene expression changes and growth response in ovarian cancer cells exposed to estrogen. Endocr Relat Cancer 2005; 12: 851-66.

[57] Jordan V, Morrow M. Tamoxifen, raloxifen, and the prevention of breast cancer. Endocr Rev 1999; 20: 253-78.

[58] Bai W, Oliveros-Saunders B, Wang Q, *et al.* Estrogen stimulation of ovarian surface epithelial cell proliferation. *In vitro* Cell Dev Biol Anim 2000; 36: 657-66.

[59] Lacey J, Mink P, Lubin J, *et al.* Menopausal hormone replacement therapy and risk of ovarian cancer. JAMA 2002; 288: 334-41.

[60] Au W, Abdou-Salama S, Al-Hendy A. Inhibition of growth of cervical cancer cells using a dominant negative estrogen receptor gene. Gynecol Oncol 2008; 104(2): 276-80.

[61] Elson D, Riley R, Lacey A, *et al.* Sensitivity of the cervical transformation zone to estrogen-induced squamous carcinogenesis. Cancer Res 2000; 60: 1267-75.

[62] Moodley M, Sewart S, Herrington C, *et al.* The interaction between steroid hormones, human papillomavirus type 16, E6 oncogene expression, and cervical cancer. Int J Gynecol Cancer 2003; 13: 834-42.

[63] Kim C, Um S, Kim T, *et al.* Regulation of cell growth and HPV genes by exogenous estrogen in cervical cancer cells. Int J Gynecol Cancer 2000; 10: 157-64.

[64] Brake T, Lambert P. Estrogen contributes to the onset, persistence, and malignant progression of cervical cancer in a human papillomavirus-transgenic mouse model. PNAS 2005; 102(7): 2490-5.

[65] Nair H, Luthra R, Kirma N, *et al.* Induction of aromatase espression in cervical carcinomas: Effects of endogenous estrogen on cervical cancer cell proliferation. Cancer Res 2005; 65(23): 11164-73.

[66] Bulun S, Economos K, Miller D, *et al.* CYP19 (aromatase) gene expression in human malignant endometrial tumors. J Clin Endocrinol Metab 1994; 79: 1831-4.

[67] Noble L, Simpson E, Johns A, *et al.* Aromatase expression in endometriosis. J. Clin. Endocrinol. Metab. 1996; 81:174-179.

[68] Nicol M, Papacleovoulou G, Evans D, *et al.* Estrogen biosynthesis in human H295 adrenocortical carcinoma cells. Mol Cel Endocrinology 2009; 300: 115-20.

[69] Oyama T, Sugio K, Isse T, *et al.* Expression of cytochrome P450 in non-small cell lung cancer. Front in Bioscience 2008; 13: 5787:93.

[70] Adlercreutz H, Fotsis T, Bannwart C, *et al.* Urinary estrogen profile determination in young Finnish vegetarian and omnivorous women. J Steroid Biochem 1986; 24: 289-96.

[71] Swaneck GE, Fishman J. Covalent binding of the endogenous estrogen 16-alphahydroxyestroneto estradiol receptor in human breast cancer cells: characterization and intracellular localization. Proc Natl Acad Sci USA 1988; 85: 7831-5.

[72] Telang NT, Suto A, Wong GY, *et al.* Induction by estrogen metabolite 16-alphahydroxyestrone of genotoxic damage and aberrant proliferation in mouse mammary epithelial cells. J Natl Cancer Inst 1992; 84: 634-8.

[73] Tiwari RK, Guo L, Bradlow HL, *et al.* Selective responsiveness of human breast cancer cells to indole-3-carbinol, a chemopreventive agent. J Natl Cancer Inst 1994; 86: 126-31.

[74] Bradlow HL, Davis DL, Lin G, *et al.* Effects of pesticides on the radio of 16 apha/2-hydroxyestrone: a biologic marker of breast cancer risk. Environ Health Perspect 1995; 103: 147-50.

[75] Taioli E, Garte SJ, Trachman J, *et al.* Ethnic differences in estrogen metabolism in healthy women. J Natl Cancer Inst 1996; 88: 617.

[76] Davis DL, Telang NT, Osborne MP, *et al.* Medical hypothesis: bifunctional genetic hormonal pathways to breast cancer. Environ Health Perspect 1997; 105: 571-6.

[77] Meilahn EN, De Stavola B, Allen DS, *et al.* Do urinary oestrogen metabolites predict breast cancer? Guernsey III cohort follow-up. Br J Cancer 1998; 78: 1250-5.

[78] Fishman J, Osborne MP, Telang NT. The role of estrogen in mammary carcinogenesis. Ann N Y Acad Sci 1995; 768: 91-100.

[79] Lustig R, Kendrick-Parker C, Jordan V. Effects of 16α-hydroxyestrone on MCF-7 cell proliferation and estrogen receptor regulation *in vitro*. Endocr Soc Proc 1994; 75: 317.

[80] Frasor J, Stossi F, Danes J, *et al.* Selective estrogen receptor modulators: Discrimination of agonistic *versus* antagonistic activities by gene expression profiling in breast cancer cells. Cancer Res 2004; 64: 1522-33.

[81] McKenna N, O´Malley B. An issue of tissues: divining the split personalities of selective estrogen receptor modulators. Nat Med 2000; 6: 960-2.

[82] Beral V. Breast cancer and hormone replacement therapy in the million women study. Lancet 2003; 362: 419-27.

[83] Chia S, Bryce C, Gelmon K. The 2000 EBCTCG overview: a widening gap. Lancet 2005; 365: 1665-6.

[84] Brzozowski A, Pike A, Dauter Z, *et al.* Molecular basis of agonism and antagonism in the oestrogen receptor. Nature 1997; 389: 753-8.

[85] Shiau A, Barstad D, Loria P, *et al.* The structural basis of estrogen receptor/coactivator recognition and the antagonism of this interaction by tamoxifen. Cell 1998; 95: 927-37.

[86] Pike A, Brzozowski A, Hubbard R, *et al.* Structure of the ligand-binding domain of oestrogen receptor beta in the presence of a partial agonist and a full antagonist. The EMBO J 1999; 18: 4608-18.

[87] Kong E, Pike A, Hubbard R. Structure and mechanism of the oestrogen receptor. Biochem Soc Trans 2003; 31: 56-59.

[88] Bilezikian J. Anabolic therapy for osteoporosis. Int J Fertil Womens Med 2005; 50: 53-60.

[89] Harvey H, Kimura M, Hajba A. Toremifene: an evaluation of its safety profile. Breast 2006; 15: 142-57.

[90] Haynes B, Dowsett M, Miller W, *et al.* The pharmacology of letrozole. J Steroid Biochem Mol Biol 2003; 87: 35-45.

[91] Lord RS, Bongiovanni B, Bralley JA. Lord RS. Estrogen metabolism and the diet-cancer connection: rationale for assessing the ratio of urinary hydroxylated estrogen metabolites. Altern Med Rev 2002; 7: 112-29.

CHAPTER 2

Causes of Cancer

IV. Example 1: Hepatocellular Carcinoma

Pablo Muriel[*]

Department of Pharmacology, Centro de Investigación y de Estudios Avanzados del I.P.N., Avenida Instituto Politécnico Nacional 2508, 07360 Mexico City, Mexico

Abstract. Primary liver cancer is the sixth most common cancer in the world and the third cause of death by cancer due to its bad prognosis. Most primary liver cancers are Hepatocellular Carcinomas (HCC). The major risk factors for HCC are chronic liver diseases (especially cirrhosis) including hepatitis B and C, alcoholic liver disease, non-alcoholic steatohepatitis, estrogens, and well documented environmental preventable risk factors, among others. Rho, hepatocyte growth factor, and metalloproteinases are associated with metastasis and death from HCC.

Kewwords: Cancer, fibrosis, necrosis, cirrhosis NF-κB, alcoholic liver disease, metalloproteinases, HBV, HCV, aflatoxins, hemochromatosis.

INTRODUCTION

Hepatocellular carcinoma (HCC) is the sixth most common tumor worldwide. However, because of its poor prognosis it ranks as the third most common cause of death from cancer [1, 2]. HCC constitutes more than 90% of primary liver malignancies followed by cholangiocarcinoma and haemangioendotelioma [3, 4]. The major risk factor for HCC is cirrhosis derived from alcohol consumption, hepatitis B and C, non-alcoholic steatohepatitis, hormones, and environmental factors [2] (Fig. **1**).

STEROID HORMONES AND HCC

The incidence of HCC is higher in males than in females (between 2:1 and 4:1, depending on the population studied) [1]. Predominance of this disease in men is associated to the clinical observation that cirrhosis is more frequently observed in males than in females and HCC development is largely considered to be the disease of men and postmenopausal woman [5]. Because this gender disparity, various *in vitro* and *in vivo* studies have been exploring the role of sex hormones in HCC. However the exact role of sex hormones and their receptors in HCC are still poorly understood. Androgens were suggested to induce and promote HCC [6], while androgen metabolism alteration has been associated with HCC [7]. In contrast, evidence on the role of estrogen in HCC has been controversial, suggesting both protective and carcinogenic effects in the liver [8].

Recently, Kalra *et al.* [8] have reviewed the role of sex steroids in HCC. They found that studies on animal models of hepatocarcinogenesis, hepatoma cell lines and HCC tissues highlight the importance of sex hormones and their receptors in HCC pathogenesis. New investigations are urgently required to elucidate the precise action mechanisms of androgens, estrogens and their receptors in regulating normal liver physiology and pathophysiology of the chronic hepatic injury leading in HCC. The reader interested in a deeper review of this topic may refer to the article by Kalra *et al.* [8].

HCC GEOGRAPHIC DISTRIBUTION AND ITS RELATION WITH ETIOLOGY

The geographic distribution of HCC is variable and overlaps the geographic distribution of Hepatic B Virus (HBV) and Hepatic C Virus (HCV) infections, alcoholism and poverty [9]. Eastern Europe and sub-Saharan Africa have the

*****Address correspondence to Pablo Muriel:** Department of Pharmacology, Centro de Investigación y de Estudios Avanzados del I.P.N., Avenida Instituto Politécnico Nacional 2508, 07360 Mexico City, Mexico; E-mail: pamuriel@cinvestav.mx

largest potential for the development of HCC followed by Europe and USA [3, 4, 10].

HCC geographic distribution is determined by specific etiologic factors in the exposure to hepatitis viruses. The average annual risk of HCC is 3.2% in patients with cirrhosis from HCV [3]. The annual risk is also high in patients with chronic HBV infection ranging from 0.1 to 1.0% among patients positive for HBV surface antigen who do not present cirrhosis. In cirrhotics presenting positive HBV surface antigen the risk is 2.2-3.2 [3]. In addition to hepatic viruses, hereditary hemochromatosis and alcohol intake also play a role as HCC risk factors [11]. Alcohol represents an important risk factor inducing inflammatory mediators like cytokines which contribute to cirrhosis, a predisposing factor for HCC [12].

Contamination of food with aflatoxins is associated with a high incidence of HCC. This micotoxin that frequently contaminates corn, soybeans, and peanuts has been related to HCC in Taiwan, where there is a high incidence of this type of cancer [13].

GENE EXPRESSION IN HCC

It is well known that development and progression of cancers are accompanied by complex changes in the patterns of gene expression [14]. Micro-arrays of cDNA have been utilized to compare the gene expression of normal tissue and HCC and it was found to vary significantly among the HCC and non-tumorous hepatic samples [15-18]. The "proliferation cluster" that is comprised of genes associated with cell proliferation and mitosis, was found to be increased in HCC samples. In contrast, genes expressed at lower levels in HCC as compared to normal liver belong to the "liver-specific cluster" consists of differentiated hepatocyte specific genes [15, 17]. These data indicate that increased cell proliferation is accompanied by the upregulation of mitosis associated genes frequently related to hepatocarcinogenesis. On the other hand, down regulation of liver specific genes is probably associated to dedifferentiation of hepatocytes to cancer cells.

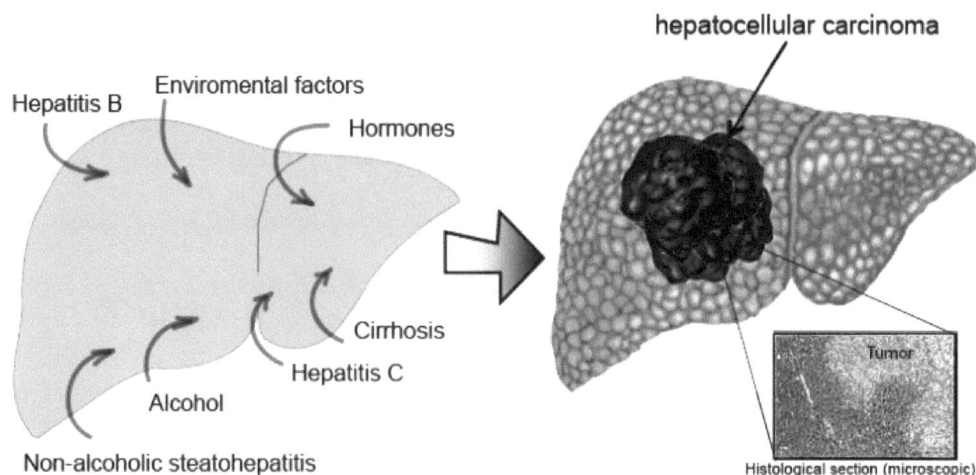

Figure 1: Risk factors for hepatocellular carcinoma.

cDNA micro-array, have been successfully used to compare the gene expression of different clinical and etiological characteristics of HCC. As mentioned earlier, HBV and HCV are the most important risk factors for HCC. In some investigations, researchers compared the gene expression profiles between HBV and HCV infected patients with HCC and showed significant differences between them [16, 17, 19]. These observations indicate that HBV and HCV associated HCC may result from distinct mechanisms. Angiogenesis is one of the most important factors promoting tumor metastasis and negatively affects the prognosis of the disease. Characterization of the genes involved in vascular invasion may contribute to find a treatment and patient management of HCC. The genes that regulate cell motility or extracellular matrix, like RhoC and Matrix Metalloproteinase (MMP) 14 increase their expression in HCC, carrying the vascular invasion phenotype [15, 17]. MMP, by degrading extracellular matrices, plays a relevant role in cancer cell invasion [20]. Cells derived from HCC that constitutively express MMP14 mRNA may induce cells to invade through matrix gel *in vitro* and this invasion, dependent on MMP14, is augmented in response to HGF (Hepatocyte Growth Factor) and as expected, blocked by MMP inhibitors [21]. In patients with HCC, on the other hand, the expression of MMP14 mRNA is associated to poorer differentiation of cancer cells and has a very significant statistical association to a bad prognosis [22]. Rho proteins, which are GTPase enzymes, are involved in cell morphology and motility by regulating the cytoskeletal organization; therefore Rho plays a crucial role in cancer metastasis [23, 24]. Accordingly, tumor metastasis and invasiveness is correlated to the expression of RhoC mRNA in human HCC [25, 26]. Furthermore, there is a significant inverse correlation between RhoC expression and survival of HCC patients [25]. Taken together, these observations indicate that cell motility and degradation of extracellular matrix play important roles in metastasis and mortality by HCC.

CONCLUSIONS

HCC is one of the most common and malignant cancers. To prevent it, it is necessary to fight against chronic liver diseases, especially viral hepatitis and alcoholism; surely vaccination against HBV and HCV and programs to reduce alcohol consumption will decrease HCC. Basic investigation on the factors that promote HCC cell invasion, like RhoC and HGF, along with the corresponding pharmacological developments will be accompanied by a better prognosis of this disease.

REFERENCES

[1]   El-Serag HB, Rudolph KL. Hepatocellular carcinoma: epidemiology and molecular carcinogenesis. Gastroenterology 2007; 132: 2557-76.

[2]   World Health Organization. Mortality database. WHO statistical information system. Available at http://www.who.int/whosis/. Accessed November, 2008.

[3]   Bosch FX, Ribes J, Diaz M, Cleries R. Primary liver cancer: worldwide incidence and trends. Gastroenterology 2004; 127: S5-S16.

[4]   Voiculescu M, Winkler RE, Moscovici M, Newman MG. Chemotherapies and targeted therapies in advanced hepatocellular carcinoma: from laboratory to clinic. J Gastrointest Liver Dis 2008; 17: 315-22.

[5]   Shimizu I. Impact of ostrogens on the progression of liver disease. Liver Int 2003; 23: 63-9.

[6]   Farinati F, De Maria N, Marafin C, Fagiuoli S, Della Libera G, Naccarato R. Hepatocellular carcinoma in alcoholic cirrhosis: is sex hormone imbalance a pathogenetic factor? Eur J Gastroenterol Hepatol 1995; 7: 145-50.

[7]   Shimizu I, Ito S. Protection of estrogens against the progression of chronic liver disease. Hepatol Res 2007; 37: 239-47.

[8]   Kalra M, Mayes J, Assefa S, Kaul AK, Kaul R. Role of steroid receptors in pathobiology of hepatocellular carcinoma. World J Gastroenterol 2008; 14: 5945-61.

[9]   LLovet JM, Burroughs A, Bruix J. Hepatocellular carcinoma. Lancet 2003; 262: 1907-17.

[10]   Kim WR, Brown RS Jr, Terrault NA, El-Serag H. Burden of liver disease in the United States: summary of a workshop. Hepatology 2002; 36: 227-42.

[11]   Bralet MP, Regimbeau JM, Pineau P, *et al.* Hepatocellular carcinoma occurring in nonfibrotic liver: epidemiologic and histopathologic analysis of 80 French cases. Hepatology 2000; 32: 200-4.

[12]   Muriel P. Cytokines in liver diseases. In: Sahu S. Ed. Hepatotoxicity: from genomics to *in vitro* and *in vivo* models. West Sussex, UK, John Wiley & Sons LTD. 2007; pp. 371-89.

[13]   Chen CJ, Wang LY, Lu SN, *et al.* Elevated aflatoxins exposure and increased risk of hepatocellular carcinoma. Hepatology 1996; 24: 38-42.

[14]   Wong CM, Ng OL. Molecular pathogenesis of hepatocellular carcinoma. Liver Int 2007; 160-74.

[15]   Chen X, Cheung ST, So S, *et al.* Gene expression patterns in human liver cancers. Mol Biol Cell 2002; 13: 1929-39.

[16]   Delpuech O, Trabut JB, Carnot F, Feuillard J, Brechot C, Kremsdorf D. Identification, using cDNA macroarray analysis, of distinct gene expression profiles associated with pathological and virological features of hepatocellular carcinoma. Oncogene 2002; 21: 2926-37.

[17]   Xu L, Hui L, Wang S, Gong J, *et al.* Expression profiling suggested a regulatory role of liver-enriched transcription factors in human hepatocellular carcinoma. Cancer Res 2001; 61: 3176-81.

[18]   Xu XR, Huang J, Xu ZG, *et al.* Insight into hepatocellular carcinogenesis at transcriptome level by comparing gene expression profiles of hepatocellular carcinoma with those of corresponding noncancerous liver. Proc Natl Acad Sci USA 2001; 98: 15089-94.

[19]   Iizuka N, Oka M, yamada-Okabe H, *et al.* Comparison of gene expression profiles between hepatitis B virus- and hepatitis C virus-infected hepatocellular carcinoma by oligonucleotide microarray data on the basis of a supervised learning method. Cancer Res 2002; 62: 3939-44.

[20]   Westermarck J, Kahari VM. Regulation of matrix metalloproteinase expression in tumor invasion. FASEB J 1999; 13: 781-92.

[21]   Murakami K, Sakukawa R, Ikeda T, Matsuura T, Hasumura S, Nagomori S. Invasiveness of hepatocellular carcinoma cell lines: contribution of membrane-type 1 matrix metalloproteinase. Neoplasia 1999; 1: 424-30.

[22]   Maatta M, Soini Y, Liakka A, Autio-Harmainen H. Differential expression of matrix metalloproteinase (MMP)-2, MMP-9, and membrane type 1-MMP in hepatocellular and pancreatic adenocarcinoma: implications for tumor progression and clinical prognosis. Clin Cancer Res 2000; 6: 2726-34.

[23]   Clark EA, Golub TR, Lander ES, Hynes RO. Genomic analysis of metastasis reveals an essential role for RhoC. Nature 2000; 406: 532-5.

[24]   Hakem A, Sanchez-Sweatman O, You-Ten A, *et al.* RhoC is dispensable for embryogenesis and tumor initiation but essential for metastasis. Genes Dev 2005; 19: 1974-9.

[25]   Wang W, Yang LY, Huang GW, *et al.* Genomic analysis reveals RhoC as a potential marker in hepatocellular carcinoma with poor prognosis. Br J Cancer 2004; 90: 2349-55.

[26]   Wang W, Yang LY, Yang ZL, Huang GW, Lu WQ. Expression and significance of RhoC gene in hepatocellular carcinoma. World J Gastroenterol 2003; 9: 1950-3.

Causes of Cancer

V. Example 2: Estrogens, Retinoids and Cervical Cancer Development *

Jorge Gutiérrez, Enoc Mariano Cortés, José Juan Vázquez, Patricio Gariglio*

Department of Genetics and Molecular Biology, Centro de Investigación y de Estudios Avanzados del Instituto Politécnico Nacional, México

Abstract: Cervical Cancer (CC) is a major cause of cancer mortality and is caused by persistent infection with High-Risk Human Papillomavirus (HR-HPVs). Infection occurs primarily at the transformation zone (the most estrogen and retinoid sensitive region of the cervix). Development of CC affects a small percentage of HR-HPV-infected women and often takes decades after infection suggesting that HR-HPV is a necessary but not sufficient cause of CC. Thus, other cofactors are necessary for progression from cervical HR-HPV infection to cancer such as long-term use of hormonal contraceptives, multiparity, smoking and retinoid deficiency which alter epithelial differentiation, cellular growth and apoptosis of malignant cells. Thereby, the early detection of HR-HPV and management of precancerous lesions together with a profound understanding of other risk factors could be a strategy to avoid this disease. In this review, we focus on the synergic effect of estrogens, retinoid deficiency and HR-HPVs in the development of CC. These risk factors may act in concert to induce neoplastic transformation in squamous epithelium of the cervix, setting the stage for secondary genetic or epigenetic events leading to carcinogenesis.

Keywords: Cancer, cervical, HR-HPV, estrogens, 17β-estradiol, hormones, nuclear receptors, retinoids, vitamin A, retinoic acid, gene expression, transcription, cofactors, apoptosis, cell proliferation, oncoproteins, epigenetic, tumor suppressor proteins.

INTRODUCTION

Cervical Cancer (CC) and precancerous cervical lesions constitute a major women health problem. Approximately 500,000 CC cases are diagnosed each year worldwide resulting in nearly 240,000 deaths (Parkin IJC 2001) [1]. Clinical, epidemiological and molecular investigations have identified oncogenic or High Risk Human Papillomavirus (HR-HPV) as the major cause of CC and cervical dysplasia (zur Hausen CTMI 1977) [2] (Walboomers JP 1999) [3] (zur Hausen Biochemistry 2008) [4]. Of the 120 subtypes of HPV, about 40 are known to infect the genital tract and epidemiological studies to date suggest that 14 of these are HR-HPV types and are significantly associated with progression to CC (Bosch JNCI 1995) [5] (Brown JCM 1999) [6]. Virtually all CCs (99%) contain HR-HPVs, mostly HPV16 and 18, which are also found in 50-80% of squamous intraepithelial lesions (SILs). The HPVs belong to a family of small (8-kb pairs) double stranded circular DNA viruses, whose genome has the coding capacity for at least six early proteins that are necessary for the replication of the viral DNA and cellular immortalization; two of these early proteins (E6 and E7) are oncogenic. The Long Control Region (LCR) is a noncoding region that regulates expression and viral gene function (Munoz Vaccine 2006) [7]. The HPV's life cycle is intimately coupled to the differentiation state of the infected epithelium. Since HPV lack most of the rate-limiting enzymes required for genome synthesis, they need to uncouple keratinocyte differentiation from cell cycle arrest and maintain or re-establish a replication competent state within terminally differentiated keratinocytes (McLaughlin-Drubin JV 2008) [8]. Oncoproteins E7 and E6 of HR-HPV inactivate the function of the retinoblastoma (Rb) and p53 tumor suppressor proteins, respectively (Boyer CR 1996) [9] (Scheffner Cell 1990) [10] and immortalize cells in culture (Band JV 1991) [11] (Halbert JV 1991) [12]. HPV16 E7 alone induces immortalization of human keratinocytes at a low frequency, but transfection with E6 and E7 together is more effective. Cells immortalized by E6 alone or E6 and E7 have normal levels of Rb protein, but have markedly less immunoprecipitable p53 protein than do parent cells

---

*Address correspondence to Patricio Gariglio: Department of Genetics and Molecular Biology, Centro de Investigación y de Estudios Avanzados del Instituto Politécnico Nacional, México; E-mail: vidal@cinvestav.mx

Javier Camacho (Ed)

(Halbert JV 1991) [12]. The most manifest function of the E6 protein is to promote the degradation of tumor suppressor protein p53 through its interaction with a cellular protein, the E6 associated protein (E6AP), an E3 ubiquitin ligase. The degradation of p53 leads to activation of proliferation and apoptosis inhibition. Besides p53, E6 interferes with other pro-apoptotic proteins, such as Bak, Bax, FADD, procaspase 8, GADD34/PP1 and c-Myc, to prevent apoptosis (Narisawa-Saito CS 2007) [13] (Boulet IJBCB 2007) [14]. Also, E6 induces expression of the E2F responsive genes, Mcm7 and cyclin E, in the absence of the E7 oncogene (Shai CR 2007) [15]. Some of the cellular proteins that interact with E6 can be grouped based on common amino-acid motifs in their E6-binding domains. One such group, the PDZ partners, binds to the carboxy-terminal four aminoacids of E6 through their PDZ domains and are degraded by E6 through E6AP (Nakagawa MCB 2000) [16]. The PDZ ligand domain of E6 is necessary for the induction of epithelial hyperplasia and differentiation inhibition (Nguyen JV 2003) [17], two important steps in carcinogenesis.

The E7 protein appears to be a major determinant for cell immortalization; this viral oncoprotein induces an aberrant S-phase entry through the inactivation of Rb and related pocket proteins (p107 and p130), the inhibition of the cyclin dependent kinase inhibitors p21 and p27, and the activation of cyclin A/cdk2, cyclin E and E2F1 (Munger Oncogene 2001) [18] (Hwang JBC 2002) [19] (He JV 2003) [20]. HR-HPV E7 proteins can associate with and repress activity of E2F6 (a component of polycomb group complexes, involved in chromatin silencing), thereby subverting another critical cellular defense mechanism. This may result in extended S-phase competence of HPV infected cells (McLaughlin-Drubin JV 2008) [8]. There are several E7 target proteins, such as AP1, TBP, c-Myc (Boulet IJBCB 2007) [14], pCAF, Smad 1 to 4, SRC-1 and Siva-1 (Avvakumov Oncogene 2003) [21] (Habig AV 2006) [22] (Baldwin JV 2006) [23] (Severino JCP 2007) [24] that may facilitate cellular transformation. Thus, E6 and E7 interact with many important cellular proteins, altering critical pathways like proliferation, apoptosis, and immune system (Mammas POR 2008) [25]. However, HR-HPV is a necessary but not sufficient cause of CC and other co factors must be considered in cervical carcinogenesis (Munoz Vaccine 2006) [7].

COFACTORS FOR CERVICAL CANCER

Development of CC often takes decades after initial infection (Walboomers JP 1999) [3] (Rangel AMR 1994) [26] and only a small percentage of women infected with HR-HPV develop CC, indicating that other factors are involved along with HR-HPV to induce cervical carcinogenesis (Munoz Vaccine 2006) [7] (Nair CR 2005) [27]. For example, dietary factors significantly influence the risk of gynecological cancer; fruits, vegetables and antioxidants reduce risk whereas high animal fat and energy intakes increase risk (Rieck BPRCOG 2006) [28]. Ghosh *et al.* investigated the relationship between intake of selected dietary nutrients belonging to several food groups and risk of CC. Odds ratios (OR) and 95% Confidence Intervals (CI) were estimated by unconditional logistic regression adjusting for age, education, smoking status, use of Oral Contraceptives (OCs), barrier contraceptives and spermicides, family history of CC, and energy intake. Significant reductions in risk of approximately 40-60% were observed for women in the highest vs lowest tertiles of dietary fiber, vitamin C, vitamin E, vitamin A, alpha-carotene, beta-carotene, lutein, folate, and total fruit and vegetable intake. These findings suggest that a diet rich in plant-based nutrients may be important in reducing the risk of CC (Ghosh NC 2008) [29]. Smoking is also associated with an increased risk of developing High Grade Squamous Intraepithelial Lesion (HSIL) in women infected with HR-HPV (Tolstrup AOGS 2006) [30]. Relative death risks due to CC among current smokers were two times higher compared with non-smokers (Odongua YMJ 2007) [31]. The mechanistic explanation of this increased risk of HR-HPV infections among smokers is most likely immunologic because cigarette smoke constituents impair the host cellular immunity; for example, Langerhans Cells (LCs) that are important in presenting HPV antigens to effector T-cells are abrogated by smoking (Syrjanen EJE 2007) [32].

Long-term use of hormonal contraceptives may increase the risk of progression from infection or LSILs to HSIL and CC (Munoz Vaccine 2006) [7]. High parity likely increase the risk of CC because it maintains the most estrogen sensitive region of the cervix, known as the Transformation Zone (TZ), on the exocervix for many years, facilitating the direct exposure to HR-HPV and, possibly, to other cofactors (Auborn IJC 1991) [33] (Autier BJC 1996) [34] (Jordan The Cervix 1976) [35].

A) ESTROGENS AND CERVICAL CANCER

Estrogens (alternate spellings: oestrogens) are a group of steroid compounds, named for their importance in the estrous cycle, and functioning as the primary female sex hormones (Dallenbach-Hellweg CTP 1981) [36]. The three major naturally occurring estrogens in women are estradiol, estriol and estrone (Fig. **1**); each contains a phenolic ring with a hydroxyl group at carbon 3 and a β-OH or ketone in position 17 of ring D (Auborn IJC 1991) [33] (Goodman MH 2006) [37]. From menarche to menopause the primary estrogen is 17β-estradiol, which arises from androstenedione or testosterone by aromatization of the ring. The reaction is catalyzed by cytochrome P450 monooxygenase enzyme complex (aromatase or CYP19); this enzyme, mainly expressed in ovaries and placenta, is essential for the conversion of androgens to estrogens, the rate-limiting and final step in estrogen biosynthesis (Santner JCEM 1997) [38].

Several studies have shown a link between hormonal exposure and risk of CC. An important study (Brisson AJE 1994) [39] has indicated that women consuming estrogen-containing OC for 6 years or more had increased risk of developing CC or HSIL. Serum 17β-estradiol levels were significantly higher in OC user women with an increased risk of cervical neoplasia compared with controls (Salazar GE 2001) [40]. In addition, the estrogen increases the rate of cells in S-phase (Bhattacharya BJC 1997) [41]. Interestingly, DNA damage induced by estrogen metabolites may lead to cervical carcinogenesis (Auborn IJC 1991) [33] (Newfield PSEBM 1998) [42]. Estrogen metabolites like the 16α-hydroxy-estrone is highly estrogenic and shown to be tumorigenic in mice (Swaneck PNAS USA 1988) [43] (Telang JNCI 1992) [44], whereas 2-hydroxy-estrone has been associated with a decreased risk of cancer as well as an antiproliferative effect (de Villiers IJC 2003) [45]. The 16α-hydroxy-estrone covalently binds to the Estrogen Receptors (ERs), thereby prolonging the effect of estrogen (de Villiers IJC 2003) [45]. Primary cells, particularly those explants from TZ are able to 16α-hydroxylate estrone. Both cervical and foreskin cells immortalized with HPV16 are greatly enhanced (about 8 fold) in 16α-hydroxylation of estrone in comparison to normal cells (Auborn IJC 1991) [33]. HR-HPV infection increases 16α-hydroxylation of estrone, providing a possible link between viral and hormonal elements, with regard to the etiology of CC (Salazar GE 2001) [40].

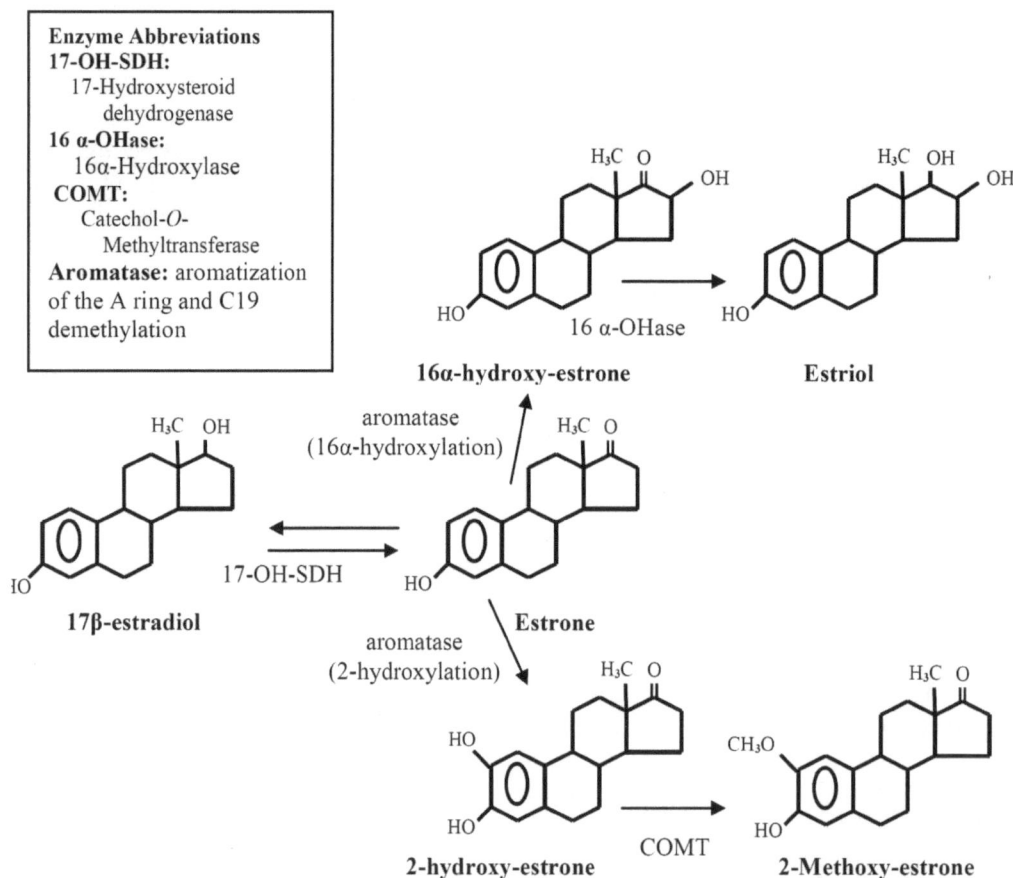

Overexpression of aromatase, a potential etiologic factor in hormone-sensitive cancers, is known to increase estrogenic activity in breast tissue (Santner JCEM 1997) [38]. Nair *et al.* reported that approximately 35% of human cervical carcinomas tested (n = 19) express aromatase, but no aromatase expression was detected in precancerous (n = 42) or normal cervical (n = 17) tissue samples. Aromatase overexpression induced the expression of cyclin D1, proliferating cell nuclear antigen and HPV oncogenes (Nair CR 2005) [27]. Stable transfectants overexpressing aromatase (C33A-Aro cells) showed less Estrogen Response Element (ERE) activity than CaSki cells in response to exogenous estrogen treatment or to endogenous estrogen synthesis by aromatase. This indicates that estrogenic response is higher in CaSki than in HPV negative C33A-Aro cells, and that in addition to the aromatase activity, other cell factors as well as HPV status are important for the estrogen response (Nair CR 2005) [27]. Thus, it is possible that estrogens (17β-estradiol or 16α-hydroxy-estrone) as well as elevated aromatase levels may be early events in the development of cervicovaginal neoplasia in humans, assuming that sufficient ER levels are present in TZ stem cells.

CERVICAL CANCER AND ESTROGEN RECEPTORS

The ERs are members of the nuclear receptor superfamily of transcription factors; two estrogen receptors have been identified: the originally described estrogen receptor alpha (ERα) and the more recently discovered Estrogen Receptor Beta (ERβ) (Gruber NEJM 2002) [46]. Normally, ERα is the predominant in rat uterus, oviduct and cervix. The ERβ is abundantly expressed in ovary, weakly expressed in uterus and vagina/cervix, and sparsely expressed in oviduct during the estrous cycle (Wang BR 2000) [47].

Immunohistochemical assays indicated that ERs are significantly higher in the human TZ compared with the ectocervix and hormone receptor-positive cells are mainly observed in suprabasal and intermediate cell layers in both the TZ and ectocervical epithelium (Remoue AJOG 2003) [48].

The presence of ERs in the normal uterine cervix and in CC, has been studied. Thus, Nair *et al.* observed an increase in ERα and ERβ in the tumors as compared with normal cervix, which may be a consequence of increased *in situ* estrogen synthesis due to aromatase expression (Nair CR 2005) [27]. They have also shown that aromatase overexpression induces ER levels and activity in HPV positive CC cells and that this increase is associated with expression of the viral oncogenes (Nair CR 2005) [27]. Related to HPV infection status it was observed that women who expressed higher levels of ERs transcripts are significantly more likely to have cervical HPV infection; it may be that the presence of the receptor allows cellular acquisition of HPV and increased viral transcription (Shew STI 2002) [49].

In order to investigate the effect of ERs on HPV oncogene expression, cell proliferation and apoptosis, an adenovirus system to deliver a dominant negative estrogen receptor mutant gene (Ad-ER-DN) into CC cells was used. In this study, disturbance of cell colony morphology, reduction of HPV E6 and E7 mRNA, interruption of cell proliferation, reduction of cyclin D1 protein and increased apoptosis was evident. These changes are consistent with the possible reactivation of p53 and Rb function (Au GO 2007) [50]. Besides, the cell death using Ad-ER-DN in combination with cisplatin and paclitaxel was investigated; the increase in cytotoxicity and apoptosis in CaSki cell line suggested a possible gene therapy approach (Heo AR 2008) [51].

Some studies have associated the importance of ERα in human colon, prostate and breast cancer (Chen MRR 2008) [52] (Cho CR 2007) [53] (Ricke Differentiation 2007) [54]. The ERα role in CC has been also investigated employing a transgenic mouse model (Chung CR 2008) [55]; these studies suggested that ERα is absolutely necessary for cervical carcinogenesis (see later).

ESTROGENS UPREGULATE E6/E7 IN CERVICAL CANCER CELLS

The growth stimulation of HR-HPV-positive CC cells by estrogen appeared to be related to the increased expression of HPV E6/E7 genes; for example, in SiHa cells 17β-estradiol stimulates both growth and the transcription of E6/E7 viral oncogenes (Mitrani-Rosenbaum JGV 1989) [56] (Kim IJGC 2000) [57]. Viral oncogene expression *via* HPV16-LCR was upregulated 2-3 fold under treatment with 10^{-7} M estriol, 17β-estradiol, and several progestins including pregnenolone, 17α-hydroxy-progesterone, norethynodrel and cyproterone acetate (Chen BBRC 1996) [58]; the transcription *via* HPV18-LCR was not or weakly stimulated by these analogs (Chen BBRC 1996) [58]. However, transient transfection experiments using the HPV18-LCR-CAT reporter plasmid in C33A cells indicated that expression was increased by 17β-estradiol and tamoxifen treatment (Kim IJGC 2000) [57]; co-transfection of ER and HPV18-LCR-CAT in C33A cells leads to a fourfold increase in CAT activity by 17β-estradiol or tamoxifen at physiologic concentrations, suggesting that estrogens are important for E6/E7 expression under the HPV18 promoter (Kim IJGC 2000) [57]. A progesterone-glucocorticoid responsive element in the HPV18-LCR has been suggested to account for the direct effects of estrogen and progesterone on HPV18 transcription enhancing transformation of cervical cells (Chen BBRC 1996) [58]. Other binding sites in the LCR of HPV18 and HPV16 have been identified such as NFI/CTF, OCT1, AP1, and SP1. AP1 is a heterodimer of the products of two protooncogenes, jun (c-jun, jun B, junD) and fos (c-fos, fosB, fra1, fra2) (Vogt ACR 1990) [59]; the transcription of c-fos and c-jun protooncogenes is stimulated by 17β-estradiol (Weisz NAR 1990) [60] (Weisz ME 1990) [61]. An element responsible for estrogen induction was mapped upstream of the transcription start site of the c-fos gene and sequence analysis revealed an imperfectly palindromic Estrogen Response Element (ERE) and two AP1 consensus sequences in this DNA region (Weisz NAR 1990) [60] (Weisz ME 1990) [61]. The estrogenic induction of *c-fos* and *c-jun* suggests that AP1 components play an early role in estrogen-induced proliferation in HR-HPV infected cells (Weisz NAR 1990) [60] (Weisz ME 1990) [61].

It has been shown that two Jun B specific AP1 sites are essential for HPV18 transcription in keratinocytes (Thierry JV 1992) [62]. HPV16 contains up to three binding sites for AP1 in the LCR (Nurnberg BJC 1995) [63]. In a study, using a CAT-reporter construct containing the HPV16 enhancer/promoter element was determined the trans-activating properties of nuclear proto-oncogene proteins c-Fos and c-Jun. The c-Fos and c-Jun overexpression resulted in a 3.3 and 3.1 fold up-regulation of CAT activity in HT3-cells. Based on these findings, it was investigated the expression of HPV DNA (16 and 18) as well as nuclear proto-oncogenes (c-fos and c-jun) in nine cervical cancers by *in situ* hybridization. In six out of nine carcinomas, HPV16 and/or HPV18 DNA expression was detectable and all tumours showed an intense and homogeneous expression of c-fos and c-jun mRNA. It is possible that deregulation of nuclear proto-oncogene expression may contribute to an overexpression of HPV-derived oncogenic proteins (E6 and E7), which is an important step in the malignant transformation of HPV-associated tumors (Nurnberg BJC 1995) [63].

The relationship between AP1 and ERs was investigated to know the transactivation properties of ERα and ERβ in AP1 sites using five ligands: estrogen (17β-estradiol), DES, as well as the antiestrogens ICI 164384, tamoxifen and raloxifen. This relation was examined by transfecting HeLa cells with either an ERα or ERβ expression plasmid and with AP1-driven luciferase reporter plasmid. With ERα, all five ligands stimulated luciferase transcription, including the antiestrogens ICI 164384, tamoxifen and raloxifen. This stimulation was dependent on transfected ERα. If 17β-estradiol is classified as a full activator of ERα at an AP1 element (ERα-AP1), then raloxifen functioned as a partial activator and tamoxifen functioned also as a full activator. In contrast to the results seen with ERα-AP1, a difference in the ligand activation profile of ERβ at an AP1 element (ERβ-AP1) was observed; in cells transfected with ERβ, treatments with 17β-estradiol and DES did not increase luciferase transcription over the control (no ligand added), whereas treatment with the antiestrogens ICI 164384, raloxifen and tamoxifen increased luciferase transcription. This suggests that ERα and ERβ respond differently to estrogens through an AP1 element (Paech Science 1997) [64].

On the other hand, it was reported that HPV18 E6 and E7 proteins directly interacted with Nuclear Receptors (NRs) such as Thyroid Receptor (TR), Androgen Receptor (AR) and ER through a hormone-independent mechanism (Wang BBRC 2003) [65]. Transient transfection of HEK 293 cells was used to test the ability of HPV18 E6 or E7 proteins to act as coregulator for AR, ER, and TR with reporter genes containing luciferase coding region. HPV18 E6 protein generally enhanced these three NRs reporter activities. In contrast, HPV18 E7 protein repressed these three NRs reporter activities either in the absence or presence of cognate ligands. However, in HeLa cells (compared with HEK 293 cells), in the absence of appropriate ligand, no coregulatory effect on AR, ER, and TR was detected, whereas these NR activities increased up to 7-fold in the presence of hormone (Wang BBRC 2003) [65]. With regard to apoptosis, it has been suggested that the stimulatory effects of 17β-estradiol on E2 and E7 induced cell death are mediated by 16α-hydroxy-estrone in HeLa cells (Webster JGV 2001) [66]. A significant increase in the levels of E2- and E7- induced apoptosis was observed in the presence of 2 μM progesterone and 100 nM 17β-estradiol (Webster JGV 2001) [66]. It is important to point out that both E2- and E7- induced apoptosis can be blocked by the HPV16 E6 protein *via* inactivation of p53 (Webster JBC 2000) [67]. In HPV-induced CC, viral DNA is often integrated into the host genome and this frequently results in the loss of the E2 protein; the loss of E2 repressor might be expected to induce E6 and E7 expression resulting in increased cell proliferation (Sanchez-Perez JGV 1997) [68]. One possibility is that in the presence of E2, estrogen and progesterone might be protective against CC *via* their upregulation of cell death. In contrast, in the absence of E2 these hormones might be a risk factor in cervical carcinogenesis either *via* their effects on HR-HPV or cellular gene expression. It was reported that 17β-estradiol reduced the percentage of CC cells undergoing apoptosis after exposure to the DNA-damaging agents UVB, mitomycin C and cisplatin. Protection was independent of HPV gene expression, and not specific to apoptosis induced by DNA damage, since 17β-estradiol also reduced the number of apoptotic cells produced after exposure to indole-3-carbinol (I3C), a non-genotoxic phytochemical effective in preventing HPV-induced tumors (Chen AR 2004) [69]. It has been reported a more efficient antiapoptotic effect of estrogen in normal cells, compared with CC cells (Wang Endocrinology 2004) [70]. On the other hand, progesterone increased cell proliferation in both CaSki and SiHa cells, while estrogen increased proliferation of SiHa cells only. Estrogen seemed to protect CaSki cells from apoptosis upregulating Bcl-2, and tamoxifen did not abrogate this effect. Progesterone slightly increased apoptosis of CaSki cells, and this effect was neutralized with the anti-progesterone compound RU486 which binds with high affinity to the progesterone receptor and acts as a partial antagonist (Ruutu IJGC 2006) [71]. In summary, the stimulation of proliferation in HPV-positive CC cells by 17β-estradiol may be related to the upregulation of HPV LCR-activity and in certain cell lines to the inhibition of apoptosis (Kim IJGC 2000) [57]. The above observations may be useful in understanding the crucial molecular pathways that can be exploited for the development of gene therapy for CC and other estrogen-dependent cancers.

THE EFFECT OF ESTROGENS IN HPV TRANSGENIC MICE

1) HPV18 Transgenic Mice

It is known that E6 and E7 expression from the HPV18 LCR is necessary for the development of genital hyperplasia and neoplasia in transgenic mice; approximately 41% of HPV18 LCR E6/E7 transgenic females developed cervical neoplasms between 1-2 years of age. Histologically, tumors were mesenchymal rather than epithelial in origin. The HPV18 LCR restricted E6 and E7 transcripts to cervix and kidney (Comerford Oncogene 1995) [72]. Transgenic mice carrying the bacterial lacZ gene under the control of the HPV18 LCR were constructed; β-galactosidase activity, analyzed employing immunohistochemical staining of tissue sections of four independent transgenic mice, showed that this viral promoter was specifically active in epithelial cells within a variety of organs (tongue, ovary, uterus, testis, and small intestine) (Cid JV 1993) [73]. In these mice, progesterone was found to activate the HPV18 LCR acutely, whereas RU 486 does not block progesterone activation. 17β-estradiol also activates the HPV18 LCR acutely compared to placebo (Michelin GO 1997) [74]. Dysplastic lesions of lower genital tract were more frequently seen in estrogen-treated HPV18 LCR E6/E7 transgenic mice compared to those of control groups (Park GO 2003) [75]; it is important to mention that the level of E6/E7 transcripts in these transgenic mice was increased in the presence of estrogen (Park GO 2003) [75], suggesting again that this hormone is involved in CC development.

2) HPV16 Transgenic Mice

Models for specifically studying CC were improved with the generation of the K14HPV16 transgenic mouse (Arbeit JV 1994) [76]. In this model, the human K14 promoter targets HPV entire early region gene expression to the basal layer of the squamous epithelium of uterine cervix. K14HPV16 transgenic mice developed various degrees of persistent epidermal and squamous mucosal hyperplasia (Arbeit JV 1994) [76]. When these virgin female mice were treated chronically with 17β-estradiol (0.25 mg) in the form of a 60 day continual release pellet starting at 4 weeks of age for a period of up to 6 months, they developed cervical and vaginal squamous carcinoma accompanied by an increase in the incidence and distribution of proliferating cells solely within the cervical and vaginal squamous epithelium (Arbeit PNAS USA 1996) [77]. Expression of the HPV transgenes in untreated transgenic mice was detectable only during estrus phase and estrogen treatment resulted in transgene expression that was persistent during the estrous cycle but not further upregulated, remaining at low levels during all stages of carcinogenesis. The data demonstrate a novel mechanism of synergistic cooperation between chronic estrogen exposure and viral oncogenes that coordinates squamous carcinogenesis in the female reproductive tract of K14HPV16 transgenic mice (Arbeit PNAS USA 1996) [77]. It is important to point out that this cooperation is independent of estrogen-responding viral LCR, suggesting that other properties of estrogens are involved in epithelial cancer induction. Transgenic mice treated with 0.05 mg/60-day 17β-estradiol induced squamous cancers that were almost exclusively localized in the TZ. The TZ cancers were first detected after 4 months of treatment in 30% of transgenic mice, and increased to 60% after 5 months and 91% after 6 months of hormone treatment. With longer hormone treatment (6 months), there was an increase in the number and stromal extension of TZ glands in nontransgenic mice and a more extensive glandular squamous metaplasia and stromal invasion by multifocal squamous carcinomas in transgenic mice (Elson CR 2000) [78]. Although the location of the TZ in mice is at the junction of the upper cervix and lower uterus, in contrast to the portio of the cervix in humans, squamous metaplasia appears to be the first stage of TZ carcinogenesis both in this model and in human disease (Elson CR 2000) [78].

Cervical tumors arising in HPV16 transgenic mice (K14E7 transgenic and K14E6/K14E7 doubly transgenic female mice) chronically treated for 9 months with 17β-estradiol (0.05 mg/60-day) were greatly increased in their size compared with tumors developing after 6 months of estrogen treatment. Transgenic mice treated 6 months with estrogen followed by 3 months without exogenous estrogen had significantly fewer tumors and the tumors were smaller and less aggressive than those arising in mice treated the full 9 months, suggesting reversibility. When treated chronically for 6 months with 17β-estradiol, the K14E7, but not the K14E6 or nontransgenic mice, developed CC; the E6 oncoprotein contributed only to increased tumor size in estrogen treated K14E6/K14E7 doubly transgenic mice (Brake PNAS USA 2005) [79]. It was recently found that the E6 oncogene synergizes with estrogen to induce CC in mice treated for 9 months and it is possible that the interactions of E6 with cellular α helix and PDZ partners correlate with its ability to induce cervical carcinogenesis (Shai CR 2007) [15]. In the presence of 17β-estradiol, E7 induced CC formation even when the E7-Rb interaction was disrupted by the use of a knock-in mouse carrying an E7-resistant mutant Rb allele (Balsitis CR 2006) [80]. Rb inactivation was necessary but not sufficient for E7 to overcome differentiation-induced or DNA damage-induced cell cycle arrest, and expression patterns of the E2F-responsive genes Mcm7 and cyclin E indicate that other E2F regulators besides Rb are important targets of E7. Together, these data indicate that non-Rb targets of E7 play critical roles in cervical carcinogenesis (Balsitis CR 2006) [80].

To evaluate the ERs role in CC, female reproductive tracts of K14E6, K14E7 or K14E6/K14E7 double transgenic mice were treated with exogenous estrogen during 6 or 9 months. Results showed that 94% of cancer cells and 57% of stromal cells surrounding the cancers were positive for ERα in all transgenic mice. In apparently normal cervix of transgenic mice the expression of ERα was evident in the basal and suprabasal epithelial cells (Chung CR 2008) [55]. In contrast, ERβ was not detected neither in normal cervical epithelial nor in cancer as well as the surrounding stroma (Chung CR 2008) [55]. Other work investigated whether ERα is required for the development of CC in a mouse model that express the E7 oncoprotein of HPV16 and additionally express ERα (K14E7/ERα$^{+/+}$) or fail to express ERα (K14E7/ERα$^{-/-}$). When K14E7/ERα$^{+/+}$ mice were treated chronically with estrogen they developed CC and HSIL. However, K14E7/ERα$^{-/-}$ mice treated with estrogen do not develop CC or any grade of dysplasia (Chung CR 2008) [55]. Thus, it is possible that the constant administration of estrogen in K14E7/ERα$^{+/+}$ female creates a favorable environment for tumor growth, whereas the cycling estrogen levels that arise normally in female mice are not as favorable. The higher range of estrogen concentration in women might be sufficient to contribute to CC development in concert with HR-HPV infection, although not as efficiently as seen when these levels are elevated through OC use or pregnancy. The elevated frequency of spontaneous high-grade cervical dysplasia regression in women is consistent with the likelihood that the natural range in estrogen concentrations in women is suboptimal for carcinogenesis. In summary, several studies in transgenic mice suggest that estrogens play a critical role not only in the genesis of CC but also in its persistence and continued development (Brake PNAS USA 2005) [79].

ESTROGENS ALTER THE IMMUNE MICROENVIRONMENT OF THE UTERINE CERVIX

It was previously reported that HPV early proteins inhibit specific components of the innate immune system (Woodworth FB 2002) [81] (Mendoza BMCC 2008) [82]. Indeed, several studies have described a localized immune dysfunction accompanying cervical HPV infections (Hughes JCP 1988) [83] (Frazer Virology 2009) [84]. Hormones could also sensitise the TZ to cervical cancer formation by altering the local immune microenvironment (Hughes JCP 1988) [83]. Sex hormones have been shown to influence the distribution of Dendritic Cells (DC) and a variety of immune cells in the epithelium of rat reproductive tract; the number and distribution of DCs vary in a tissue-specific manner with the stage of the estrous cycle (Kaushic AJRI 1998) [85]. 17β-estradiol inhibits antigen presentation and decreases the number of vaginal LCs in ovariectomized rodents without affecting the number of major histocompatibility complex class II positive cells (Wira Immunology 1995) [86]. In contrast, progesterone given together with 17β-estradiol reverses the inhibitory effect of 17β-estradiol on antigen presentation and increases the number of LC in ovariectomized rodents (Wira Immunology 1995) [86]. In other study, ovariectomized rats treated with estradiol showed a significant fourfold increase in antigen presentation by epithelial cells relative to that in saline-treated controls. (Prabhala JI 1995) [87]. This study demonstrates that the female reproductive tract is an inductive site for immune responses and that mucosal immune protection may be either enhanced or suppressed depending on the endocrine balance when the female reproductive tract is exposed to pathogens.

B) RETINOIDS AND CERVICAL CANCER

Retinoids is a generic term that includes both naturally dietary vitamin A (retinol) metabolites and active synthetic analogs (Sporn FP 1976) [88] (Chambon ME 2005) [89]. Natural retinoids are produced *in vivo* from the oxidation of vitamin A. Synthesis of retinoic acid (RA), also named all-trans retinoic acid (ATRA), from retinol is a two-step process. In this process, alcohol dehydrogenases perform the oxidation of vitamin A to all-*trans*-retinaldehyde, followed by oxidation of the latter to ATRA by retinaldehyde dehydrogenases, which is a rate-limiting step in its production. ATRA, the most potent biologically active metabolite of vitamin A, can both prevent and rescue the main defects caused by vitamin A deficiency in adult animals (Kastner Cell 1995) [90]. ATRA is in turn metabolized by CYP26 to hydroxylated metabolites; the main function of CYP26 is to degrade endogenous ATRA protecting cells from ATRA excess (Niederreither NG 2002) [91].

The physiological actions of the retinoids are mediated primarily by the Retinoic Acid Receptors (RARs) and Retinoic X Receptors (RXRs). The RARs and RXRs are members of the ligand-dependent transcription factor super-family of nuclear receptors (Robinson-Rechavi JCS 2003) [92]. Multiple isotypes (α, β and γ) of both RARs and RXRs have been identified. RARα (Giguere Nature 1987) [93], RARβ (Benbrook Nature 1988) [94], and RARγ (Krust PNAS USA 1989) [95] are activated by both ATRA and 9-cis-RA, whereas RXRα, RXRβ, and RXRγ (Mangelsdorf GD 1992) [96] have thus far been shown to be activated only by 9-cis-RA (Heyman Cell 1992) [97] (Allenby PNAS USA 1993) [98]. In the presence of the ligand, RARs function as homodimers or heterodimers (Mangelsdorf Cell 1995) [99] (Kastner Development 1997) [100] (Mark PNS 1999) [101], which in turn interact with RA Response Elements (RAREs) or Retinoid X Response Elements (RXREs) localized in ATRA or 9-cis-RA sensitive genes (Zhang Nature 1992) [102]. RAREs correspond to repeats of polymorphic arrangements of the canonical motif 5'-PuG(G/T)TCA (Mangelsdorf Cell 1995) [99] (Leid TBS 1992) [103].

In the absence of ligand, the RXR/RAR heterodimers recruit the corepressor proteins NCoR or SMRT and associated factors such as Histone Deacetylases (HDACs) or DNA-methyl transferases that may lead to an inactive condensed chromatin; this prevents transcription and therefore provides a direct functional link with the core transcriptional machinery and the modulation of the nucleosomal structure. Upon RAR agonist binding, corepressors are released, and coactivator complexes containing Histone Acetyltransferases (HATs, for example p300 or CREB-binding protein) or histone arginine methyltransferases are recruited to activate transcription (Hu TEM 2000) [104] (Aranda PR 2001) [105] (Privalsky CTMI 2001) [106] (McKenna Cell 2002) [107].

The concentration of multiple isotypes of RARs and RXRs varies among different tissues; the mouse simple cervical columnar epithelium, which is highly responsive to vitamin A status, expressed high levels of RARα, RARβ, and RXR (α and β) transcripts (Darwiche Endocrinology 1994) [108]. Only RARβ and RXR (α and β) transcripts were downmodulated by the condition of vitamin A deficiency and were expressed less in squamous metaplastic foci than in the simple columnar epithelium (Darwiche Endocrinology 1994) [108].

The role of RXRα or RARβ2 in epithelial homeostasis was studied using the Cre/loxP technology (Li Nature 2000) [109] (Metzger ME 2003) [110] (Chapellier Genesis 2002) [111]. Several histological alterations, such as ectocervical atrophy with moderate epidermoid metaplasia were found after RXRα gene ablation (Ocadiz Genesis 2008) [112]; a simultaneous increase of cell proliferation and apoptosis levels, as well as the alteration in the expression of important cancer related genes were also observed in these animals. Interestingly, mice in which RARβ2 gene was ablated show similar histological alterations (Albino unpublished observations). These results suggest that RARs or RXRs alterations may predispose mice to development of cevical neoplasia in combination with HR-HPV oncogenic activity (Ocadiz Genesis 2008) [112]. In fact, we have observed that some RXRα null conditional mice expressing E6/E7 oncogenes develop severe dysplasia, carcinoma *in situ* and invasive carcinoma (Ocadiz manuscript in preparation).

RETINOIDS INHIBIT CELLULAR PROLIFERATION AND INDUCE APOPTOSIS.

One of the major biological effects of RA is to inhibit cell proliferation in almost all cells tissues. This regulation occurs in the G1 phase of the cell cycle where it was shown that cyclin D1 was inhibited and p27 expression was increased blocking cell cycle progression (Zhou Oncogene 1997) [113] (Seewaldt ECR 1999) [114]. Retinoids have also been shown to inhibit the activity of the MAPKinase pathway; for example, the suppression of Erk1/2 activity by RA was observed in HPV-immortalized human ectocervical cells treated with EGF. In this case, RA inhibited Erk1/2 activation, which in turn eliminated the induction of cyclin D1 and the EGF-stimulated proliferation (Sah JBC 2002) [115].

Retinoids cause apoptosis in cervical carcinoma cells (Arany AR 2003) [116] employing a mechanism that involves STAT1, caspase-1 and IRF1 which in turn acts as a transcription factor for TRAIL (Altucci NRC 2001) [117] (Clarke EMBOJ 2004) [118]. Interestingly, it has been demonstrated that the combination of retinoids and Interferons (IFNs) resulted in a synergistic effect that induces apoptosis (Mascrez Development 1998) [119] and this is modulated by IFN-inducible gene expression after increasing the levels of STAT1 (Sucov GD 1994) [120]. Thus, increased level of STAT1 may be an early step in the cooperative antitumor effect of IFN and RA. However, the ability of RA to induce apoptosis is variable and is highly dependent on the type of cell (Nagy CDD 1998) [121].

RARβ2 ISOFORM IS A TUMOR SUPPRESSOR

In mice, the RARβ gene generates four distinct transcripts: splice variants RARβ1 or RARβ3 derived from transcription at promoter P1, and RARβ2 or RARβ4 from the RARE-containing P2 promoter (Chambon FASEB J 1996) [122] (Nagpal PNAS USA 1992) [123]. In humans, only RARβ2 and RARβ4 transcripts have been identified in normal adult cells (Sommer PNAS USA 1999) [124]. The RARβ2 and RARβ4 transcripts differ only in the 5' untranslated region. The 5' region of RARβ4 transcript is spliced out including the ATG start codon. Therefore, RARβ4 translation is initiated from an internal CUG codon and RARβ2 translation is initiated from the normal ATG codon (Nagpal PNAS USA 1992) [123].

Alterations in RARβ gene expression result in both abnormally low mRNA levels and loss of ligand inducibility; these alterations are a striking feature of human cancers and tumor-derived cell lines. The cancer types prone to RARβ abnormalities include lung (Gebert Oncogene1991) [125], head and neck (Xu CR 1994) [126], breast (Swisshelm CGD 1994) [127], oral (Crowe Differentiation 1991) [128] and uterine cervix carcinomas (Geisen CR 1997) [129].

Primary human cervical epithelial cells regularly express high basal levels of the RARβ gene, whereas this expression is either absent or strongly diminished in a high percentage of CC (Geisen CR 1997) [129]. It was found that RARs were expressed in all adjacent normal cervical epithelia, whereas all CIN lesions including CIN1, CIN2, and CIN3 exhibited decreased expression of RARα (56%), RARβ (65%) and RARγ (55%) (Xu CCR 1999) [130].

There is mounting evidence in epithelial cancer cell lines and animal models of the potent tumor suppressor role for RARβ2 (Houle PNAS USA 1993) [131] (Liu MCB 1996) [132] (Si ECR 1996) [133] (Bérard FASEB J 1996) [134] (Kaiser Gastroenterology 1997) [135] (Faria JBC 1999) [136] (Lin CR 2000) [137] (Toulouse LC 2000) [138]. Exogenous expression of RARβ2 in cancer cells presenting low or absent RARβ2 expression restored RA induced G1 phase inhibition and caused decreased tumorigenicity (Si ECR 1996) [133]. This expression of RARβ2 results both in RA-dependent and RA-independent apoptosis as well as growth arrest even in breast cancer cell lines with scanty amounts of RARα, the first effector of RARβ P2 promoter (Liu MCB 1996) [132] (Lin CR 2000) [137] (Swisshelm CGD 1994) [127]. Moreover, F9 teratocarcinoma cells RARβ2 null could not undergo growth arrest in the presence of RA, indicating that RARβ2 is required for the growth inhibitory action of RA (Faria JBC 1999) [136]. RARβ2 gene transfection in HeLa cells results in the reduction of clonal cell growth in a ligand-dependent manner (Geisen IJC 2000) [139]. Similarly, a pancreatic carcinoma cell line also showed reduced tumor growth *in vivo* after RARβ2 transfection (Kaiser Gastroenterology 1997) [135]. In addition, lung tumors were induced in mice expressing an antisense RARβ2 transgene (Bérard FASEB J 1996) [134].

In cervical epithelial cells, RARα is the major regulator of ligand inducibility of RARβ transcription. The RARα gene does not show any abnormalities in structure or expression in CC cells, indicating that loss or inactivation of the RARα gene is not the primary cause for loss of RA-inducibility of RARβ (Geisen CR 1997) [129]. Confirming this result, it has been observed that RARβ2 is not expressed due to epigenetic modifications such as promoter hypermethylation as demonstrated in several epithelial carcinomas (affecting the RARβ P2 promoter of one or more RARβ alleles) (Ivanova BMCC 2002) [140] (Virmani JNCI 2000) [141] (Youssef CCR 2004) [142]. In addition, one investigation about lung cancer cell lines reported that the lack of RARβ2 expression is linked to aberrant histone H3 acetylation (Suh CR 2002) [143].

RARβ2 BLOCKS AP1 ACTIVITY

Transcription factor AP1 regulates the expression of several cancer related genes and has been shown to play an important role in the preneoplastic to neoplastic progression in cell culture and CC biopsies (Wilson PNAS USA 1997) [144]. Accordingly, it was demonstrated *in vivo* that blocking AP1 activity is required for the antitumor effect of retinoids (Huang PNAS USA 1997) [145]. A mechanism by which RARβ2 can exert growth inhibitory function is based on its ability to repress the AP1 transcription factor; supporting this possibility, cDNA of RARβ2 was stably introduced into cervical carcinoma cells (HeLa) in order to induce a constitutive expression of this tumor suppressor (De Castro JBC 2004) [146]. Non-liganded RARβ2 abrogated both AP1 binding affinity and activity due to a selective degradation of the c-Jun protein, a major dimerization partner of AP1, without substitution by other members of the Jun family (De Castro JBC 2004) [146]. In this same model system, after ectopic expression of RARβ2, they were able to down-regulate HPV18 E6/E7 oncogenes transcription by selectively abrogating the binding of AP1 to the viral regulatory region in a ligand-independent manner. Aditionally, under these conditions they observed reinduction of cell cycle inhibitory proteins such as p53, p21 (CIP1), and p27 (KIP), as well as cessation of cellular growth, and decreased cyclin D1 expression (De Castro JBC 2004) [146] (De Castro JBC 2007) [147]. It is important to mention that the cyclin D1 promoter contains two AP1 binding sites and c-Jun has been found to induce its transcription (Shaulian Oncogene 2001) [148]. Thus, the cyclin D1 down regulation is consistent with the finding that c-Jun is selectively degraded upon RARβ2 restoration (De Castro JBC 2004) [146]. Depending on the cell system, different negative regulatory mechanisms for RARβ2/RXR on AP1 have been proposed: (a) direct interaction with Jun/Fos family members (Suzukawa Oncogene 2002) [149], (b) disruption of Jun-Fos dimerization (Zhou ME 1999) [150], (c) competition with AP1 to avoid recruitment of transcriptional co-activators such as p300 or CPB (Kamei Cell 1996) [151], or (d) inhibition of the c-Jun N-terminal Kinase (JNK), which prevents phosphorylation-dependent activation of c-Jun (De-Castro JBC 2004) [146] (Lee JBC 1998) [152].

CONCLUSION

In conclusion, there are many additional factors associated to HR-HPV-related cervical cancer. Chronical estrogen exposure is a key factor for the development of this disease. Estrogens upregulate HPV E6/E7 oncogenes expression, stimulate cell proliferation, inhibit apoptosis and their metabolites cause DNA damage. On the other hand, retinoids deficiency is implicated in cervical squamous metaplasia and the suppression of RARβ2 promotes AP1-dependent cellular proliferation. Synergistic activation of cell proliferation by viral oncoproteins, cell cycle dysregulation and estrogen receptor signaling, together with altered RARβ2 expression and other factors may conspire to support and promote neoplastic progression and cervical cancer.

ACKNOWLEDGEMENTS

We thank Enrique Garcia Villa, Rodolfo Ocadiz Delgado and Elizabeth Álvarez Ríos CINVESTAV-IPN, D. F., Mexico, city for their invaluable advices in this review, and CONACYT (Grant numbers: 83597, 45953-N and 53603) as well as ICyT-PGV for financial support.

DISCLOSURE

Part of information included in this chapter has been previously published in Arch Med Res. 2009 Aug; 40(6):449-65. http://www.ncbi.nlm.nih.gov/pubmed/19853185).

REFERENCES

[1]   Parkin DM, Bray F, Ferlay J, Pisani P. Estimating the world cancer burden: Globocan 2000. Int J Cancer 2001; 94: 153-6.

[2]   zur Hausen H. Human papillomaviruses and their possible role in squamous cell carcinomas. Curr Top Microbiol Immunol 1977; 78: 1-30.

[3]   Walboomers JM, Jacobs MV, Manos MM, *et al.* Human papillomavirus is a necessary cause of invasive cervical cancer worldwide. J Pathol 1999; 189: 12-9.

[4]   zur Hausen H. Papillomaviruses--to vaccination and beyond. Biochemistry 2008; 73: 498-503.

[5]   Bosch FX, Manos MM, Munoz N, *et al.* Prevalence of human papillomavirus in cervical cancer: a worldwide perspective. International biological study on cervical cancer (IBSCC) Study Group. J Natl Cancer Inst 1995; 87: 796-802.

[6]   Brown DR, Schroeder JM, Bryan JT, Stoler MH, Fife KH. Detection of multiple human papillomavirus types in Condylomata acuminata lesions from otherwise healthy and immunosuppressed patients. J Clin Microbiol 1999; 37: 3316-22.

[7]   Munoz N, Castellsague X, de Gonzalez AB, Gissmann L. Chapter 1: HPV in the etiology of human cancer. Vaccine 2006; 24 Suppl 3: S3/1-10.

[8]   McLaughlin-Drubin ME, Huh KW, Munger K. Human papillomavirus type 16 E7 oncoprotein associates with E2F6. J Virol 2008; 82: 8695-705.

[9]   Boyer SN, Wazer DE, Band V. E7 protein of human papilloma virus-16 induces degradation of retinoblastoma protein through the ubiquitin-proteasome pathway. Cancer Res 1996; 56: 4620-4.

[10] Scheffner M, Werness BA, Huibregtse JM, Levine AJ, Howley PM. The E6 oncoprotein encoded by human papillomavirus types 16 and 18 promotes the degradation of p53. Cell 1990; 63: 1129-36.

[11] Band V, De Caprio JA, Delmolino L, Kulesa V, Sager R. Loss of p53 protein in human papillomavirus type 16 E6-immortalized human mammary epithelial cells. J Virol 1991; 65: 6671-6.

[12] Halbert CL, Demers GW, Galloway DA. The E7 gene of human papillomavirus type 16 is sufficient for immortalization of human epithelial cells. J Virol 1991; 65: 473-8.

[13] Narisawa-Saito M, Kiyono T. Basic mechanisms of high-risk human papillomavirus-induced carcinogenesis: roles of E6 and E7 proteins. Cancer Sci 2007; 98: 1505-11

[14] Boulet G, Horvath C, Vanden Broeck D, Sahebali S, Bogers J. Human papillomavirus: E6 and E7 oncogenes. Int J Biochem Cell Biol 2007; 39: 2006-11.

[15] Shai A, Brake T, Somoza C, Lambert PF. The human papillomavirus E6 oncogene dysregulates the cell cycle and contributes to cervical carcinogenesis through two independent activities. Cancer Res 2007; 67: 1626-35.

[16] Nakagawa S, Huibregtse JM. Human scribble (Vartul) is targeted for ubiquitin-mediated degradation by the high-risk papillomavirus E6 proteins and the E6AP ubiquitin-protein ligase. Mol Cell Biol 2000; 20: 8244-53.

[17] Nguyen ML, Nguyen MM, Lee D, Griep AE, Lambert PF. The PDZ ligand domain of the human papillomavirus type 16 E6 protein is required for E6's induction of epithelial hyperplasia *in vivo.* J Virol 2003; 77: 6957-64.

[18] Munger K, Basile JR, Duensing S, *et al.* Biological activities and molecular targets of the human papillomavirus E7 oncoprotein. Oncogene 2001; 20: 7888-98.

[19] Hwang SG, Lee D, Kim J, Seo T, Choe J. Human papillomavirus type 16 E7 binds to E2F1 and activates E2F1-driven transcription in a retinoblastoma protein-independent manner. J Biol Chem 2002; 277: 2923-30.

[20] He W, Staples D, Smith C, Fisher C. Direct activation of cyclin-dependent kinase 2 by human papillomavirus E7. J Virol 2003; 77: 10566-74.

[21] Avvakumov N, Torchia J, Mymryk JS. Interaction of the HPV E7 proteins with the pCAF acetyltransferase. Oncogene 2003; 22: 3833-41.

[22] Habig M, Smola H, Dole VS, Derynck R, Pfister H, Smola-Hess S. E7 proteins from high- and low-risk human papillomaviruses bind to TGF-beta-regulated Smad proteins and inhibit their transcriptional activity. Arch Virol 2006; 151: 1961-72.

[23] Baldwin A, Huh KW, Munger K. Human papillomavirus E7 oncoprotein dysregulates steroid receptor coactivator 1 localization and function. J Virol 2006; 80: 6669-77.

[24] Severino A, Abbruzzese C, Manente L, *et al.* Human papillomavirus-16 E7 interacts with Siva-1 and modulates apoptosis in HaCaT human immortalized keratinocytes. J Cell Physiol 2007; 212: 118-25.

[25] Mammas IN, Sourvinos G, Giannoudis A, Spandidos DA. Human Papilloma Virus (HPV) and Host Cellular Interactions. Pathol Oncol Res 2008; 14: 345-54.

[26] Rangel LM, Ramirez M, Torroella M, Pedroza A, Ibarra V, Gariglio P. Multistep carcinogenesis and genital papillomavirus infection. Implications for diagnosis and vaccines. Arch Med Res 1994; 25: 265-72.

[27]   Nair HB, Luthra R, Kirma N, *et al.* Induction of aromatase expression in cervical carcinomas: effects of endogenous estrogen on cervical cancer cell proliferation. Cancer Res 2005; 65: 11164-73.

[28]   Rieck G, Fiander A. The effect of lifestyle factors on gynaecological cancer. Best Pract Res Clin Obstet Gynaecol 2006; 20: 227-51.

[29]   Ghosh C, Baker JA, Moysich KB, Rivera R, Brasure JR, McCann SE. Dietary intakes of selected nutrients and food groups and risk of cervical cancer. Nutr Cancer 2008; 60: 331-41.

[30]   Tolstrup J, Munk C, Thomsen BL, *et al.* The role of smoking and alcohol intake in the development of high-grade squamous intraepithelial lesions among high-risk HPV-positive women. Acta Obstet Gynecol Scand 2006; 85: 1114-9.

[31]   Odongua N, Chae YM, Kim MR, Yun JE, Jee SH. Associations between smoking, screening, and death caused by cervical cancer in Korean women. Yonsei Med J 2007; 48: 192-200.

[32]   Syrjanen K, Shabalova I, Petrovichev N, *et al.* Smoking is an independent risk factor for oncogenic human papillomavirus (HPV) infections but not for high-grade CIN. Eur J Epidemiol 2007; 22: 723-35.

[33]   Auborn KJ, Woodworth C, DiPaolo JA, Bradlow HL. The interaction between HPV infection and estrogen metabolism in cervical carcinogenesis. Int J Cancer 1991; 49: 867-9.

[34]   Autier P, Coibion M, Huet F, Grivegnee AR. Transformation zone location and intraepithelial neoplasia of the cervix uteri. Br J Cancer 1996; 74: 488-90.

[35]   Jordan JA, Singer A. The Cervix. London. Saunders 1976

[36]   Dallenbach-Hellweg G. Structural variations of cervical cancer and its precursors under the influence of exogenous hormones. Curr Top Pathol 1981; 70: 143-70.

[37]   Goodman LS, Gilman A, *et al.* Eds. Goodman & Gilman's the pharmacological basis of therapeutics. New York: McGraw-Hill 2006

[38]   Santner SJ, Pauley RJ, Tait L, Kaseta J. Santen RJ. Aromatase activity and expression in breast cancer and benign breast tissue stromal cells. J Clin Endocrinol Metab 1997; 82: 200-8.

[39]   Brisson J, Morin C, Fortier M, *et al.* Risk factors for cervical intraepithelial neoplasia: differences between low- and high-grade lesions. Am J Epidemiol 1994; 140: 700-10.

[40]   Salazar EL, Sojo-Aranda I, Lopez R, Salcedo M. The evidence for an etiological relationship between oral contraceptive use and dysplastic change in cervical tissue. Gynecol Endocrinol 2001; 15: 23-8.

[41]   Bhattacharya D, Redkar A, Mittra I, Sutaria U, MacRae KD. Oestrogen increases S-phase fraction and oestrogen and progesterone receptors in human cervical cancer *in vivo*. Br J Cancer 1997; 75: 554-8.

[42]   Newfield L, Bradlow HL, Sepkovic DW, Auborn K. Estrogen metabolism and the malignant potential of human papillomavirus immortalized keratinocytes. Proc Soc Exp Biol Med 1998; 217: 322-6.

[43]   Swaneck GE, Fishman J. Covalent binding of the endogenous estrogen 16 alpha-hydroxyestrone to estradiol receptor in human breast cancer cells: characterization and intranuclear localization. Proc Natl Acad Sci U S A 1988; 85: 7831-5.

[44]   Telang NT, Suto A, Wong GY, Osborne MP, Bradlow HL. Induction by estrogen metabolite 16 alpha-hydroxyestrone of genotoxic damage and aberrant proliferation in mouse mammary epithelial cells. J Natl Cancer Inst 1992; 84: 634-8.

[45]   de Villiers EM. Relationship between steroid hormone contraceptives and HPV, cervical intraepithelial neoplasia and cervical carcinoma. Int J Cancer 2003; 103: 705-8.

[46]   Gruber CJ, Tschugguel W, Schneeberger C, Huber JC. Production and actions of estrogens. N Engl J Med 2002; 346: 340-52.

[47]   Wang H, Eriksson H, Sahlin L. Estrogen receptors alpha and beta in the female reproductive tract of the rat during the estrous cycle. Biol Reprod 2000; 63: 1331-40.

[48]   Remoue F, Jacobs N, Miot V, Boniver J, Delvenne P. High intraepithelial expression of estrogen and progesterone receptors in the transformation zone of the uterine cervix. Am J Obstet Gynecol 2003; 189: 1660-5.

[49]   Shew ML, McGlennen R, Zaidi N, Westerheim M, Ireland M, Anderson S. Oestrogen receptor transcripts associated with cervical human papillomavirus infection. Sex Transm Infect 2002; 78: 210-4.

[50]   Au WW, Abdou-Salama S, Al-Hendy A. Inhibition of growth of cervical cancer cells using a dominant negative estrogen receptor gene. Gynecol Oncol 2007; 104: 276-80.

[51]   Heo MY, Salama SA, Khatoon N, Al-Hendy A, Au WW. Abrogation of estrogen receptor signaling augments cytotoxicity of anticancer drugs on CaSki cervical cancer cells. Anticancer Res 2008; 28: 2181-7.

[52]   Chen GG, Zeng Q, Tse GM. Estrogen and its receptors in cancer. Med Res Rev 2008; 28: 954-74.

[53]   Cho NL, Javid SH, Carothers AM, Redston M, Bertagnolli MM. Estrogen receptors alpha and beta are inhibitory modifiers of Apc-dependent tumorigenesis in the proximal colon of Min/+ mice. Cancer Res 2007; 67: 2366-72.

[54]   Ricke WA, Wang Y, Cunha GR. Steroid hormones and carcinogenesis of the prostate: the role of estrogens. Differentiation 2007; 75: 871-82.

[55]   Chung SH, Wiedmeyer K, Shai A, Korach KS, Lambert PF. Requirement for estrogen receptor alpha in a mouse model for human papillomavirus-associated cervical cancer. Cancer Res 2008; 68: 9928-34.

[56]   Mitrani-Rosenbaum S, Tsvieli R, Tur-Kaspa R. Oestrogen stimulates differential transcription of human papillomavirus type 16 in SiHa cervical carcinoma cells. J Gen Virol 1989; 70: 2227-32.

[57]   Kim CJ, Um SJ, Kim TY, *et al.* Regulation of cell growth and HPV genes by exogenous estrogen in cervical cancer cells. Int J Gynecol Cancer 2000; 10: 157-64.

[58]   Chen YH, Huang LH, Chen TM. Differential effects of progestins and estrogens on long control regions of human papillomavirus types 16 and 18. Biochem Biophys Res Commun 1996; 224: 651-9.

[59]   Vogt PK, Bos TJ. jun: oncogene and transcription factor. Adv Cancer Res 1990; 55: 1-35.

[60]   Weisz A, Rosales R. Identification of an estrogen response element upstream of the human c-fos gene that binds the estrogen receptor and the AP-1 transcription factor. Nucleic Acids Res 1990; 18: 5097-106.

[61]   Weisz A, Cicatiello L, Persico E, Scalona M, Bresciani F. Estrogen stimulates transcription of c-jun protooncogene. Mol Endocrinol 1990; 4: 1041-50.

[62]   Thierry F, Spyrou G, Yaniv M, Howley P. Two AP1 sites binding JunB are essential for human papillomavirus type 18 transcription in keratinocytes. J Virol 1992; 66: 3740-8.

[63]   Nurnberg W, Artuc M, Vorbrueggen G, *et al.* Nuclear proto-oncogene products transactivate the human papillomavirus type 16 promoter. Br J Cancer 1995; 71: 1018-24.

[64]   Paech K, Webb P, Kuiper GG, *et al.* Differential ligand activation of estrogen receptors ERalpha and ERbeta at AP1 sites. Science 1997; 277: 1508-10.

[65]   Wang WM, Chung MH, Huang SM. Regulation of nuclear receptor activities by two human papillomavirus type 18 oncoproteins, E6 and E7. Biochem Biophys Res Commun 2003; 303: 932-9.

[66]   Webster K, Taylor A, Gaston K. Oestrogen and progesterone increase the levels of apoptosis induced by the human papillomavirus type 16 E2 and E7 proteins. J Gen Virol 2001; 82: 201-13.

[67]   Webster K, Parish J, Pandya M, Stern PL, Clarke AR, Gaston K. The human papillomavirus (HPV) 16 E2 protein induces apoptosis in the absence of other HPV proteins and *via* a p53-dependent pathway. J Biol Chem 2000; 275: 87-94.

[68]   Sanchez-Perez AM, Soriano S, Clarke AR, Gaston K. Disruption of the human papillomavirus type 16 E2 gene protects cervical carcinoma cells from E2F-induced apoptosis. J Gen Virol 1997; 78: 3009-18.

[69]   Chen D, Carter TH, Auborn KJ. Apoptosis in cervical cancer cells: implications for adjunct anti-estrogen therapy for cervical cancer. Anticancer Res 2004; 24: 2649-56.

[70]   Wang Q, Li X, Wang L, Feng YH, Zeng R, Gorodeski G. Antiapoptotic effects of estrogen in normal and cancer human cervical epithelial cells. Endocrinology 2004; 145: 5568-79.

[71]   Ruutu M, Wahlroos N, Syrjanen K, Johansson B, Syrjanen S. Effects of 17beta-estradiol and progesterone on transcription of human papillomavirus 16 E6/E7 oncogenes in CaSki and SiHa cell lines. Int J Gynecol Cancer 2006; 16: 1261-8.

[72]   Comerford SA, Maika SD, Laimins LA, Messing A, Elsasser HP, Hammer RE. E6 and E7 expression from the HPV 18 LCR: development of genital hyperplasia and neoplasia in transgenic mice. Oncogene 1995; 10: 587-97.

[73]   Cid A, Auewarakul P, Garcia-Carranca A, Ovseiovich R, Gaissert H, Gissmann L. Cell-type-specific activity of the human papillomavirus type 18 upstream regulatory region in transgenic mice and its modulation by tetradecanoyl phorbol acetate and glucocorticoids. J Virol 1993; 67: 6742-52.

[74]   Michelin D, Gissmann L, Street D, *et al.* Regulation of human papillomavirus type 18 *in vivo*: effects of estrogen and progesterone in transgenic mice. Gynecol Oncol 1997; 66: 202-8.

[75]   Park JS, Rhyu JW, Kim CJ, *et al.* Neoplastic change of squamo-columnar junction in uterine cervix and vaginal epithelium by exogenous estrogen in hpv-18 URR E6/E7 transgenic mice. Gynecol Oncol 2003; 89: 360-8.

[76]   Arbeit J, Munger K, Howley PM, Hanahan D. Progressive squamous epithelial neoplasia in K14-Human papillomavirus type 16 transgenic mice. J. Virol 1994; 68:4358-4368.

[77]   Arbeit JM, Howley PM, Hanahan D. Chronic estrogen-induced cervical and vaginal squamous carcinogenesis in human papillomavirus type 16 transgenic mice. Proc Natl Acad Sci USA 1996; 93: 2930-5.

[78]   Elson DA, Riley RR, Lacey A, Thordarson G, Talamantes FJ, Arbeit JM. Sensitivity of the cervical transformation zone to estrogen-induced squamous carcinogenesis. Cancer Res 2000; 60: 1267-75.

[79]   Brake T, Lambert PF. Estrogen contributes to the onset, persistence, and malignant progression of cervical cancer in a human papillomavirus-transgenic mouse model. Proc Natl Acad Sci USA 2005; 102: 2490-5.

[80]   Balsitis S, Dick F, Dyson N, Lambert PF. Critical roles for non-pRb targets of human papillomavirus type 16 E7 in cervical carcinogenesis. Cancer Res 2006; 66: 9393-400.

[81]   Woodworth CD. HPV innate immunity. Front Biosci 2002; 7: d2058-71.

[82]   Mendoza-Villanueva D, Diaz-Chavez J, Uribe-Figueroa L, *et al.* Gene expression profile of cervical and skin tissues from human papillomavirus type 16 E6 transgenic mice. BMC Cancer 2008; 8: 347.

[83]   Hughes RG, Norval M, Howie SE. Expression of major histocompatibility class II antigens by Langerhans' cells in cervical intraepithelial neoplasia. J Clin Pathol 1988; 41: 253-9.

[84]   Frazer IH. Interaction of human papillomaviruses with the host immune system: a well evolved relationship. Virology 2009; 384: 410-4.

[85]   Kaushic C, Frauendorf E, Rossoll RM, Richardson JM., Wira CR. Influence of the estrous cycle on the presence and distribution of immune cells in the rat reproductive tract. Am J Reprod Immunol 1998; 39: 209-16.

[86]   Wira CR, Rossoll RM. Antigen-presenting cells in the female reproductive tract: influence of sex hormones on antigen presentation in the vagina. Immunology 1995; 84: 505-8.

[87]   Prabhala RH, Wira CR. Sex hormone and IL-6 regulation of antigen presentation in the female reproductive tract mucosal tissues. J Immunol 1995; 155: 5566-73.

[88]   Sporn MB, Dunlop NM, Newton DL, Smith JM. Prevention of chemical carcinogenesis by vitamin A and its synthetic analogs(retinoids). Fed Proc 1976; 35: 1332-8.

[89]   Chambon P. The nuclear receptor superfamily: a personal retrospect on the first two decades. Mol Endocrinol 2005; 19: 1418-28.

[90]   Kastner P, Mark M, Chambon P . Nonsteroid nuclear receptors: what are genetic studies telling us about their role in real life? Cell 1995; 83: 859-69.

[91]   Niederreither K, Abu-Abed S, Schuhbaur B, Petkovich M, Chambon P, Dollé P. Genetic evidence that oxidative derivatives of retinoic acid are not involved in retinoid signaling during mouse development. Nat Genet 2002; 31: 84-8.

[92]   Robinson-Rechavi M, Escriva Garcia H, Laudet V. The nuclear receptor superfamily. J Cell Sci 2003; 116: 585-6.

[93]   Giguere V, Ong ES, Segui P, Evans RM. Identification of a receptor for the morphogen retinoic acid. Nature 1987; 330: 624-9.

[94]   Benbrook D, Lernhardt E, Pfahl M. A new retinoic acid receptor identified from a hepatocellular carcinoma. Nature 1988; 333: 669-72.

[95]   Krust A, Kastner P, Petkovich M, Zelent A, Chambon P. A third human retinoic acid receptor, hRAR-gamma. Proc Natl Acad Sci USA 1989; 86: 5310-4.

[96]   Mangelsdorf DJ, Borgmeyer U, Heyman RA, *et al.* Characterization of three RXR genes that mediate the action of 9-cis retinoic acid. Genes Dev 1992; 6: 329-44.

[97]   Heyman RA, Mangelsdorf DJ, Dyck JA, *et al.* 9-cis retinoic acid is a high affinity ligand for the retinoid X receptor. Cell 1992; 68: 397-406.

[98]   Allenby G, Bocquel MT, Saunders M, *et al.* Retinoic acid receptors and retinoid X receptors: interactions with endogenous retinoic acids. Proc Natl Acad Sci USA 1993; 90: 30-34.

[99]   Mangelsdorf DJ, Evans RM. The RXR heterodimers and orphan receptors. Cell 1995; 83: 841-50.

[100] Kastner P, Mark M, Ghyselinck N, *et al.* Genetic evidence that the retinoid signal is transduced by heterodimeric RXR/RAR functional units during mouse development. Development 1997; 124: 313-26.

[101] Mark M, Ghyselinck NB, Wendling O, Dupé V, Mascrez B, Kastner P, Chambon P. A genetic dissection of the retinoid signalling pathway in the mouse. Proc Nutr Soc 1999; 58: 609-13.

[102] Zhang XK, Lehmann J, Hoffmann B, *et al.* Homodimer formation of retinoid X receptor induced by 9-cis retinoic acid. Nature 1992; 358: 587-91.

[103] Leid M, Kastner P, Chambon P. Multiplicity generates diversity in the retinoic acid signalling pathways. Trends Biochem Sci 1992; 17: 427-33.

[104] Hu X, Lazar MA. Transcriptional repression by nuclear hormone receptors. Trends Endocrinol Metab 2000;11: 6-10.

[105] Aranda A, Pascual A. Nuclear hormone receptors and gene expression. Physiol Rev 2001; 81: 1269-304.

[106] Privalsky ML. Regulation of SMRT and N-CoR corepressor function. Curr Top Microbiol Immunol 2001; 254: 117-36.

[107] McKenna NJ, O'Malley BW. Combinatorial control of gene expression by nuclear receptors and coregulators. Cell 2002; 108: 465-74.

[108] Darwiche N, Celli G, De Luca LM. Specificity of retinoid receptor gene expression in mouse cervical epithelia. Endocrinology 1994; 134: 2018-25.

[109] Li M, Indra AK, Warot X, *et al.* Skin abnormalities generated by temporally controlled RXRa mutations in mouse epidermis. Nature 2000; 407: 633-6.

[110] Metzger D, Indra AK, Li M, *et al.* Targeted conditional somatic mutagenesis in the mouse: Temporally-controlled knock out of retinoid receptors in epidermal keratinocytes. Methods Enzymol 2003; 364: 379-408.

[111] Chapellier B, Mark M, Bastien J, *et al.* A conditional floxed (loxP-flanked) allele for the retinoic acid receptor beta (RARbeta) gene. Genesis 2002; 32: 91-4.

[112] Ocadiz-Delgado, R, Castaneda-Saucedo E, Indra AK, Hernandez-Pando R, Gariglio P. Impaired cervical homeostasis upon selective ablation of RXRalpha in epithelialcells. Genesis 2008; 46: 19-28.

[113] Zhou Q, Stetler-Stevenson M, Steeg PS. Inhibition of cyclin D expression in human breast carcinoma cells by retinoids *in vitro*. Oncogene 1997; 15: 107-15.

[114] Seewaldt VL, Kim JH, Parker MB, Dietze EC, Srinivasan KV, Caldwell LE. Dysregulated expression of cyclin D1 in normal human mammary epithelial cells inhibits all-transretinoic acid-mediated G0G1 phase arrest and differentiation. Exp Cell Res 1999; 249: 70-85.

[115] Sah JF, Eckert RL, Chandraratna RA, Rorke EA. Retinoids suppress epidermal growth factor-associated cell proliferation by inhibiting epidermal growth factor receptor dependent ERK1/2/activation. J Biol Chem 2002; 277: 9728-35.

[116] Arany I, Ember IA, Tyring SK. All-trans-retinoic acid activates caspase-1 in a dose- dependent manner in cervical squamous carcinoma cells. Anticancer Res 2003; 23: 471-3.

[117] Altucci L, Gronemeyer H. The promise of retinoids to fight againts cancer. Natur Rev Cancer 2001; 1: 181-93.

[118] Clarke N, Jimenez-Lara AM, Voltz E, Gronemeyer H. Tumor suppressor IRF-1 mediateds retinoid and interferon anti-cancer signaling to death ligand TRAIL. EMBO J 2004; 23: 3051-60.

[119] Mascrez B, Mark M, Dierich A, Ghyselinck NB, Kastner P. Chambon P. The RXRα ligand-dependent activation function 2 (AF-2) is important for mouse development. Development 1998; 125: 4691-701.

[120] Sucov HM, Dyson E, Gumeringer CL, Price J, Chien KR, Evans RM. RXR alpha mutant mice establish a genetic basis for vitamin A signaling in heart morphogenesis. Genes Dev 1994; 8: 1007-18.

[121] Nagy L, Thomazy VA, Heyman RA, Davies PJ. Retinoid induced apoptosis in normal and neoplastic tissues, Cell Death Differ 1998; 5: 11-19.

[122] Chambon PA. Decade of molecular biology of retinoic acid receptors. FASEB J 1996;10: 940-54.

[123] Nagpal S, Zelent A, Chambon P. RAR-beta 4, a retinoic acid receptor isoform is generated from RAR-beta 2 by alternative splicing and usage of a CUG initiator codon. Proc Natl Acad Sci USA 1992; 89: 2718-22.

[124] Sommer KM, Chen LI, Treuting PM, Smith LT, Swisshelm K. Elevated retinoic acid receptor beta(4) protein in human breast tumor cells with nuclear and cytoplasmic localization. Proc Natl Acad Sci USA 1999; 96: 8651-6.

[125] Gebert JF, Moghal N, Frangioni JV, Sugarbaker DJ, Neel B G. High frequency of retinoic acid receptor beta abnormalities in human lung cancer. Oncogene 1991; 6: 1859-68.

[126] Xu XC, Ro JY, Lee JS, Shin DM, Hong WK, Lotan R. Differential expression of nuclear retinoid receptors in normal, premalignant, and malignant head and neck tissues. Cancer Res 1994; 54: 3580-7.

[127] Swisshelm K, Ryan K, Lee X, Tsou HC, Peacocke M, Sager R. Down-regulation of retinoic acid receptor beta in mammary carcinoma cell lines and its up-regulation in senescing normal mammary epithelial cells. Cell Growth Differ 1994; 5: 133-41.

[128] Crowe DL, Hu L, Gudas LJ, Rheinwald JG. Variable expression of retinoic acid receptor (RAR beta) mRNA in human oral and epidermal keratinocytes; relation to keratin 19 expression and keratinization potential. Differentiation 1991; 48: 199-208.

[129] Geisen C, Denk C, Gremm B, *et al.* High-level expression of the retinoic acid receptor β gene in normal cells of the uterine cervix is regulated by the retinoic acid receptor α and is abnormally down-regulated in cervical carcinoma cells. Cancer Res 1997; 57: 1460-7.

[130] Xu X, Mitchell M, Silva E, Jetten A, Lotan R. Decreased expression of retinoid acid receptors, transforming growth factor β, involucrin, and cornifin in cervical intraepithelial neoplasia. Clin Cancer Res 1999; 5: 1503-8.

[131] Houle B, Rochette-Egly C, Bradley WE. Tumor-suppressive effect of the retinoic acid receptor beta in human epidermoid lung cancer cells. Proc Natl Acad Sci USA 1993; 90: 985-9.

[132] Liu Y, Lee MO, Wang HG, *et al.* Retinoic acid receptor beta mediates the growth-inhibitory effect of retinoic acid by promoting apoptosis in human breast cancer cells. Mol Cell Biol 1996; 16: 1138-49.

[133] Si SP, Lee X, Tsou HC, Buchsbaum R, Tibaduiza E, Peacocke M. RAR beta 2-mediated growth inhibition in HeLa cells. Exp Cell Res 1996; 223: 102-11.

[134] Bérard J, Laboune F, Mukuna M, Massé S, Kothary R, Bradley WE. Lung tumors in mice expressing an antisense RARbeta2 transgene. FASEB J 1996; 10: 1091-7.

[135] Kaiser A, Herbst H, Fisher G, *et al.* Retinoic acid receptor beta regulates growth and differentiation in human pancreatic carcinoma cells. Gastroenterology 1997; 113 (3): 920-9.

[136] Faria TN, Mendelsohn C, Chambon P, Gudas LJ. The targeted disruption of both alleles of RARbeta(2) in F9 cells results in the loss of retinoic acid-associated growth arrest. J Biol Chem 1999; 274: 26783-8.

[137] Lin F, Xiao D, Kolluri SK, Zhang X. Unique anti-activator protein-1 activity of retinoic acid receptor beta. Cancer Res 2000; 60: 3271-80.

[138] Toulouse A, Morin J, Dion PA, Houle B, Bradley WE. RARbeta2 specificity in mediating RA inhibition of growth of lung cancer-derived cells. Lung Cancer 2000; 28: 127-37.

[139] Geisen C, Denk C, Küpper J, Schwarz E. Growth inhibition of cervical cancer cells by the human retinoic acid receptor β gene. Int. J Cancer 2000; 85: 289-95.

[140] Ivanova T, Petrenko A, Gritsko T, *et al.* Methylation and silencing of the retinoic acid receptor-beta 2 gene in cervical cancer. BMC Cancer 2002; 2: 4.

[141] Virmani AK, Rathi A, Zöchbauer-Müller S, *et al.* Promoter methylation and silencing of the retinoic acid receptor-beta gene in lung carcinomas. J Natl Cancer Inst 2000; 92: 1303-7.

[142] Youssef EM, Lotan D, Issa JP, *et al.* Hypermethylation of the retinoic acid receptor-beta(2) gene in head and neck carcinogenesis. Clin Cancer Res 2004; 10: 1733-42.

[143] Suh YA, Lee HY, Virmani A, *et al.* Loss of retinoic acid receptor beta gene expression is linked to aberrant histone H3 acetylation in lung cancer cell lines. Cancer Res 2002; 62: 3945-9.

[144] Wilson CL, Heppner KJ, Labosky PA Hogan BLM. Matrisian LM. Intestinal tumorigenesis is suppressed in mice lacking the metalloproteinase matrilysin. Proc Natl Acad Sci USA 1997; 94: 1402-7.

[145] Huang C, Ma W, Dawson MI, Rincon M, Flavell RA, Dong Z. Blocking activator protein-1 activity, but not activating retinoic acid response element, is required for the antitumor promotion effect of retinoic acid. Proc Natl Acad Sci USA 1997; 5826-30.

[146] De-Castro J, Soto U, van Riggelen J, Schwarz E, Hausen HZ, Rosl F. Ectopic expression of nonliganded retinoic acid receptor beta abrogates AP-1 activity by selective degradation of c-Jun in cervical carcinoma cells. J Biol Chem 2004; 279: 45408-16.

[147] De-Castro J, Göckel-Krzikalla E, Rösl F. Retinoic acid receptor beta silences human papillomavirus-18 oncogene expression by induction of de novo methylation and heterochromatinization of the viral control region. J Biol Chem 2007; 282: 28520-9.

[148] Shaulian E, Karin M. AP-1 in cell proliferation and survival. Oncogene 2001; 20: 2390-400.

[149] Suzukawa K, Colburn NH. AP-1 transrepressing retinoic acid does not deplete coactivators or AP-1 monomers but may target specific Jun or Fos containing dimers. Oncogene 2002; 21: 2181-90.

[150] Zhou XF, Shen XQ, Shemshedini L. Ligand-activated retinoic acid receptor inhibits AP-1 transactivation by disrupting c-Jun/c-Fos dimerization. Mol Endocrinol 1999; 13: 276-85.

[151] Kamei Y, Xu L, Heinzel T, *et al* A CBP integrator complex mediates transcriptional activation and AP-1 inhibition by nuclear receptors. Cell 1996; 85: 403-414.

[152] Lee HY, Walsh GL, Dawson MI, Hong WK, Kurie JM. All-trans-retinoic acid inhibits Jun N-terminal kinase-dependent signaling pathways. J Biol Chem 1998; 273: 7066-71.

CHAPTER 3

Oncogenes and Tumor Suppressor Genes

Patricio Gariglio[*]

Departamento de Genética y Biología Molecular, Centro de Investigaciones y de Estudios Avanzados IPN, México

Abstract: Randomly occurring mutations of oncogenes and genetic or epigenetic alterations of tumor suppressor genes control many important cellular processes, such as proliferation and apoptosis, involved in human cancer. These genes, as well as those encoding enzymes participating in DNA repair, telomere elongation, inflammation and angiogenesis are the major players during multi-step carcinogenesis. A very important characteristic of oncogenes is that they are active genes that cooperate to induce a transformed phenotype. There are many experimental examples supporting this cooperation, including oncogene transfection studies in cell lines and transgenic mice containing activated oncogenes. These systems and those indicating loss of function in tumor suppressor genes have been models of gene collaboration and multi-step transformation. Alterations disrupting the balance between growth-promoting and growth-inhibiting pathways can lead to cancer, but these alterations can explain only part of the human cancer pathogenesis. The complex mechanisms for regulating apoptosis and the eukaryotic cell cycle are prime targets for oncogenic and tumor suppressor mutations. Only the mutations striking the cancer stem cell population can be transmitted to descendant cells due to their unlimited proliferative potential. It seems that the widespread destabilization of cancer stem cell genomes occurs quite early in multi-step tumor progression. All these findings help molecular oncologists to prevent, diagnose and treat human cancer in more specific ways.

Keywords: Cancer, mutations, oncogenes, genetic alterations, epigenetic alterations, tumor suppressor genes, proliferation, apoptosis, multistep carcinogenesis, transformed phenotype, gene cooperation, transgenic mice, eukaryotic cell cycle, cancer stem cell, tumor progression, molecular oncology.

INTRODUCTION

A. ONCOGENES

Tumor progression is driven by a sequence of randomly occurring mutations and epigenetic alterations of DNA that affect the genes controlling cell proliferation, survival, and other traits associated with the malignant cell phenotype. These genes are basically oncogenes and tumor suppressor genes, as well as those that encode telomerase, enzymes involved in DNA repair and inflammation (Evan Nature 2001) [1] (Leder IMM 1994) [2] (Bishop MO 1996) [3] (Murray CC 1993) [4] (Harley COGD 1995) [5] (Weinberg BC 2007) [6]. The genes and proteins that are implicated in the causation of human cancer can be numbered in the hundreds; thus, it is not possible to describe in this short review all these genes. Even a few genes are difficult to describe considering the huge number of articles related to their structure and functions (Table 1). The characterization of RNA and DNA tumor viruses provided a simple and powerful theory to understand human cancer. Since a few genes from tumor viruses succeeded in transforming normal chicken and rodent cells into tumor cells, it was thought that these viruses might also transform human cells. However, most types of human cancer are unrelated to viruses and do not contain viral sequences; only a few commonly occurring tumor types (such as liver carcinomas and cervical carcinomas) are clearly linked to specific viral agents (zur Hausen JNCI 2000) [7] (Levrero Oncogene 2006) [8] (Colombo JH 1999) [9] (Koike Oncology 2002) [10].Tumor virus research proved to be critical in uncovering the cellular genes that are responsible for the cancer cell phenotype. The discovery of a large number of cellular cancer-causing genes (oncogenes and tumor suppressor genes) is consequence of early research efforts to find a viral origin for human malignant tumors.

A viable hypothesis, independent of viral oncogenes, was that physical or chemical agents induce cancer through their ability to mutate critical growth-controlling genes in the genomes of specific cells. Candidates were the

*Address correspondence to Patricio Gariglio: Departamento de Genética y Biología Molecular, Centro de Investigaciones y de Estudios Avanzados IPN, México; E-mail: vidal@cinvestav.mx

protooncogenes discovered in normal cells by their similarity to oncogenes found in the genomes of rapidly transforming retroviruses. Thus, mutated protooncogenes might function as active oncogenes driving malignant growth. A strategy for finding cellular oncogenes in various types of chemically transformed cells was to transfect DNA (to introduce DNA) of malignant cells into normal recipient cells, and then determining whether the recipient cells (NIH3T3 cell line) became transformed (originated foci of transformants). Thus, DNA extracted from tumor cells obtained from mouse fibroblasts of the C3H10T1/2 cell line, previously treated with the potent carcinogen and mutagen 3-methylcholanthrene (3-MC), was transfected into cultures of NIH3T3 recipient cells, generating many foci; the cells obtained from these foci were tumorigenic, suggesting that the donor tumor DNA contained oncogenes. Later, it was shown that DNAs extracted from cell lines derived from lung, colon or bladder carcinomas were capable of transforming recipient NIH3T3 cells. It was soon observed that oncogenes discovered in human tumor cell lines are related to those carried by transforming retroviruses. For example, a DNA probe derived from the H-ras oncogene present in Harvey rat sarcoma virus hybridized with the oncogene detected by transfection of DNA purified from human bladder carcinoma cells (Barbacid ARB 1987) [11] (Cooper CPB 1987) [12] (Parada Nature 1982) [13].

Table 1: Number of articles on frequently studied genes in molecular oncology

	Year		Accumulated (Total)		
	1990	1999	1999	2002	2009
myc	788	902	11 320	13 331	19 798
ras	998	1 918	17 770	22 105	37 166
bcl-2	61	1 564	6 348	10 256	29 389
p53	226	3 385	17 605	25 256	48 518
rb	375	615	9 230	10 928	14 422
			>60 000	>80 000	>140 000

Conversion, or activation, of a protooncogene into an oncogene generally involves a gain-of-function mutation and at least four mechanisms can produce oncogenes from the corresponding protooncogenes: (a) amplification of a DNA segment including a proto-oncogene, so that numerous copies exist, leading to overproduction of the encoded protein; (b) chromosomal translocation that brings a growth-regulatory gene under the control of a different promoter that causes inappropriate expression of the gene; (c) point mutation (*i.e.*, change in a single base pair) in a protooncogene that results in a hyperactive or constitutively active protein product; (d) chromosomal translocation that fuses two genes together to produce a hybrid gene encoding a chimeric protein whose activity, unlike that of the parent proteins, often is constitutive. The first two mechanisms generate oncogenes whose protein products are identical with the normal proteins; in contrast, the other two mechanisms generate oncoproteins that differ from the normal protooncogenic proteins. For example, the myc oncogene (derived from avian myelocytomatosis virus, AMV) can be created by at least three distinct mechanisms: (a) in some human tumors, expression of the myc gene is driven by its own natural promoter but the copy number is elevated (gene amplification) and an increase in Myc protein is observed, as in the HL60 human promyelocytic leukemia cell line. Proteins of the Myc family (c-Myc, N-Myc, L-Myc) possess potent growth-promoting powers acting as transcription factors (Adhikary NRMCB 2005) [14] (Knoepfler CR 2007) [15] (Peter Oncogene 2006) [16], and drive uncontrolled cell proliferation when present at excessive levels (Fig. **1**); (b) insertional mutagenesis mechanism causes the expression of the c-myc protooncogene to be placed under the transcriptional control of an Avian Leucosis Virus (ALV) integrated as a provirus nearby in the chromosomal DNA; the resulting constitutive overexpression of c-myc mRNA and c-Myc protein leads to excessive cellular proliferation; (c) metaphase chromosome spreads of Burkitt's lymphoma (BL) cells almost invariably carry chromosomal translocations. In BL, a region from chromosome 2, 14 or 22 is fused to a section of chromosome 8, where c-myc is placed. On the other side of the fusion site, the promoters from any one of three distinct immunoglobulin genes were found; these translocations separate the myc gene from its promoter and replace it for a highly active immunoglobulin promoter. Once myc expression is activated by the antibody gene promoters it becomes a potent oncogene and this stimulates lymphoid cell proliferation in which these promoters are highly active. In addition to these three mechanisms, frequent mutations have been observed in amplified or translocated c-myc oncogenes.

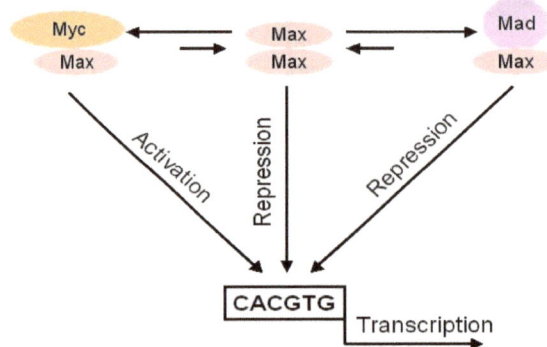

Figure 1: Transcriptional regulation induced by the Max/Max homodimer and Myc/Max heterodimer. Intracellular Max protein level is constant during the different cell cycle phases and Max/Max homodimers are transcriptional inhibitors. When a growth factor increases the intracellular Myc concentration, the formation of Myc/Max heterodimers is increased, activating expression of important genes involved in cellular proliferation and apoptosis.

Elevated levels of cyclin D1, one of the three D-type cyclins, for example, are found in many human cancers.

In certain tumors of antibody-producing B lymphocytes, for instance, the cyclin D1 gene is translocated such that its transcription is under control of an antibody-gene enhancer, causing elevated cyclin D1 production throughout the cell cycle, irrespective of extracellular signals. That cyclin D1 can function as an oncoprotein was shown by studies with transgenic mice in which the cyclin D1 gene was placed under control of an enhancer specific for mammary ductal cells. Initially the ductal cells underwent hyperproliferation, and eventually breast tumors developed in these transgenic mice. Amplification of the cyclin D1 gene and concomitant overproduction of the cyclin D1 protein is common in human breast cancer; the extra cyclin D1 helps to drive cells through the cell cycle.

Similarly to the c-myc protooncogene, or to the cyclin D1 gene, the erbB2/neu/HER2 gene also presented amplification in many breast cancers; elevated expression of this homolog of the erbB gene (discovered in the genome of avian erythroblastosis virus) is found in the majority of human carcinomas. The inverse correlation found between erbB2/HER2/neu, expression levels and long-term patient survival suggested that this gene is causally involved in driving the malignant growth of breast cancer cells (in about 30% of breast cancers). In addition to gene amplification (as observed for c-myc and erbB2/neu/HER2), protooncogenes are activated by point mutations; for example, the critical difference between the human bladder carcinoma H-ras oncogene and its protooncogene was localized to a subgenic fragment of 350 base pairs. The two DNA fragments differed at a single nucleotide (G in the protooncogene → T in the oncogene) affecting the 12th codon of the H-ras reading frame; this changed the normally present glycine-encoding codon to one specifying valine. The effects of this aminoacid substitution on the function of the H-ras protein is enormous: Ras proteins bind GDP in their inactive state and GTP in their active, signal-emitting state (Fig. **2**). The inactive Ras-GDP complex is stimulated by GEF (Guanine Exchange Factor) to release its GDP and acquire GTP, activating Ras for a short period due to the GTPase activity intrinsic to normal Ras proteins. This GTPase activity is strongly stimulated by GAPs (GTPase Activating Proteins). Aminoacid substitutions caused by oncogenic point mutations inactivate the Ras intrinsic GTPase activity, maintaining the active signal-emitting complex for extremely longer periods of time. A detailed study of the structure of the Ras proteins (K-Ras, H-Ras and N-Ras) indicated that aminoacid residues in position 12, 13 and 61 of these proteins are located around the cavity in the Ras protein conforming the GTPase catalytic active site. Mutations (substitutions) of these three aminoacids compromise the ability of GAPs to trigger hydrolysis of the GTP bound by Ras (Malumbres NRC 2003) [17].

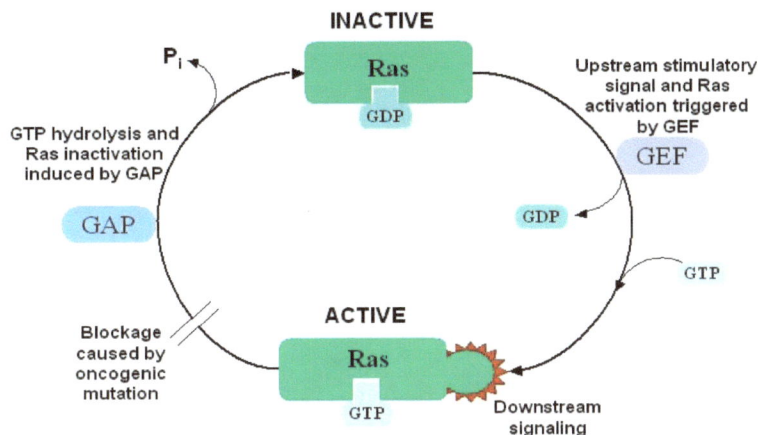

Figure 2: The Ras signaling cycle. Ras proteins operate as binary switches, binding GDP in the inactive state (top) and GTP in their active, signal emitting state (bottom). The inactive GDP-Ras complex is stimulated by a GEF (Guanine Nucleotide Exchange Factor) to release its GDP and acquire a GTP, placing Ras in its active signaling configuration for a short period due to a GTPase activity intrinsic of Ras which is strongly stimulated by GAPs (GTPase-Activating Proteins). Oncogenic, mutated Ras proteins block this cycle by inactivating the intrinsic GTPase activity of Ras, trapping Ras in its activated, signal-emitting state.

Thus, it is easy to understand why point mutations affecting few aminoacid residues are present in the ras oncogenes found in human tumors; the vast majority of point mutations striking ras protooncogenes will yield mutant Ras proteins with unmodified activity or that have lost (rather than gain) the ability to emit growth-stimulatory signals. More than 20% of human tumors carried point mutations in the GTPase active site of one of the three ras genes (K-ras, H-ras and N-ras) present in the mammalian genome. In each of these tumors, the point mutation was present in one of the mentioned three specific codons in the reading frame of a ras gene. Interestingly, the H-ras oncogene carried by Harvey Sarcoma virus not only is strongly deregulated by the viral transcription promoter, but it contains a point mutation like that discovered in the bladder carcinoma. In conclusion, many of the oncogenes discovered in avian and mammalian retroviruses could be found in a mutated activated state in human tumor cells. An important characteristic of oncogenes is their ability to promote growth stimulatory signals and to block apoptosis. For example, signals transmitted by Ras-GTP increase the activity of Raf, a serine/treonine kinase, followed by MEK1/MEK2 kinases and ERK1/ERK2 kinases (known as MAPKs). These ERKs finally lead to the stimulation of transcription factors, including AP1 (an heterodimeric complex formed by two oncoproteins: Fos and Jun). The activation of the phosphatidyl inositol 3 kinase/protein kinase B (P13K/PKB) pathway inhibits apoptosis in many cell lines (Figs. **3** and **4**). For instance, it was demonstrated that PKB can inhibit epithelial cell apoptosis (Khwaja Blodd 1999) [18] as well as fibroblast apoptosis induced by c-Myc overexpression (Kauffmann-Zeh Nature 1997) [19]. It is possible that Bad (del Peso Science 1997) [20] and NFκB are PKB substrates involved in this antiapoptotic effect (Figs. **3** and **4**). Of interest is the observation that PKB can phosphorylate and inactivate IKK (a repressor of NFκB); this leads to activation of the antiapoptotic transcription factor NFκB (Ozes Nature 1999) [21].

Another very important antiapoptotic protein is Bcl-2; the expression of the bcl-2 gene is abundant in several types of malignant tumors as well as in many cell lines. This oncogenic protein inhibits the release of proapoptotic factors from the mitochondria (Rsujimoto FEBSL 2000) [22] such as cytochrome c and Aif (Apoptosis-inducing factor); these factors activate a series of proteases called caspases, which play a crucial role in apoptosis; the resistance to apoptosis might be related to changes in the redox potential of the cell towards more reduced states. These redox changes induced by Bcl-2 have suggested therapeutic strategies (Cortazzo CR 1996) [23].

On the other hand, in the great majority of cases of Chronic Myelogenous Leukemia (CML) a translocation causes the fusion of two different reading frames; the reciprocal chromosomal translocation between human chromosomes 9 and 22, which carry the abl and bcr genes, respectively, results in the formation of fused, hybrid genes that encode hybrid Bcr-Abl proteins. The weak kinase activity of the Abl protein is largely increased in the fusion oncoprotein, causing it to emit deregulated growth-promoting signals. Many other quite distinct translocations have been reported in human cancer that also result in the formation of active hybrid oncoproteins.

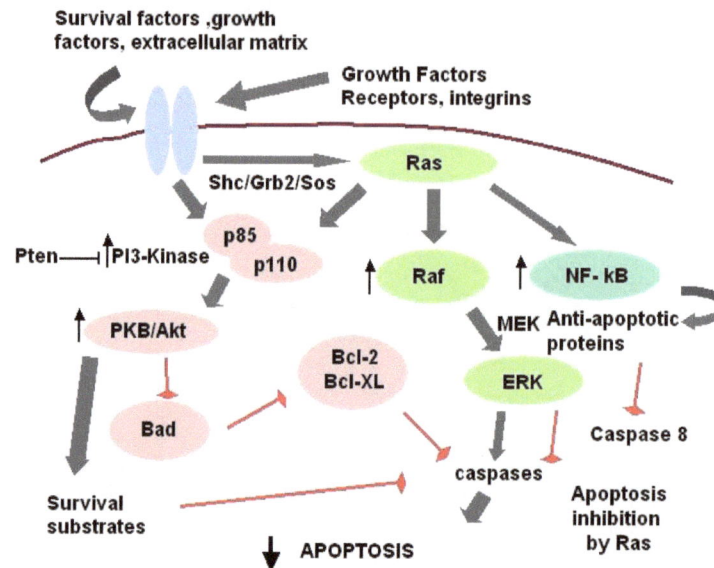

Figure 3: Apoptosis regulation induced by Ras oncoprotein. Ras activation frequently leads to inactivation of proteases belonging to the caspase family and to apoptosis inhibition in certain susceptible cells. The scheme shows three of the most studied antiapoptotic pathways: that of Pkb/Akt, the Raf-Erk pathway and that of NFκB. In certain cells and under certain conditions, the Raf-Erk pathway can stimulate apoptosis. Phosphorylation inactivates Bad proteins, inducing the activation of antiapoptotic proteins such as Bcl-2 and Bcl-XL. Thus, Bad inactivation leads to apoptosis inhibition. The activation of transcription factor NFκB increase the expression of antiapoptotic proteins.

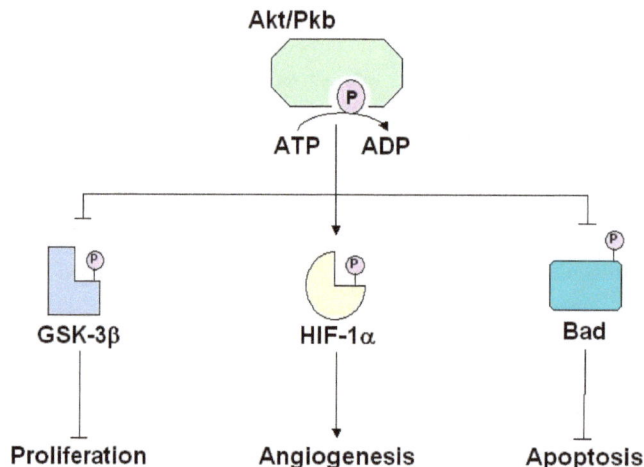

Figure 4: Pleiotropic actions of Akt/Pkb. The Akt/Pkb kinase (a serine/threonine kinase) can influence a wide variety of biological processes through phosphorylation of major control proteins. Thus, it can inactivate the antiproliferative power of GSK-3β (see later), and the proapoptotic action of Bad, which normally inhibits antiapoptotic Bcl-2 or Bcl-XL proteins. In its phosphorylated form, Bad is inactivated and can not inhibit Bcl-2 or Bcl-XL.

The formation of several human carcinomas involves activation of plasma membrane receptors, as for example, the receptor for Epidermal Growth Factor (EGFr); in these tumors, this receptor lacks most of its extracellular domain but send growth-stimulatory signals into cells, even in the absence of any EGF, acting as a potent oncogenic protein (Schlessinger Cell 2002) [24]. The discovery of oncogenes such as erbB (i, e., the EGF receptor) and sis (which encodes an altered form of platelet-derived growth factor, PDGF) revealed the intimate connections between growth factor signaling and the mechanisms of cell transformation, suggesting that malignant transformation results from hyperactivation of the mitogenic signaling pathways and in particular of growth factor receptors (Bishop MO 1996) [3] (Weinberg BC 2007) [6] (Lo HW 2006) [25]. Growth factors bind to receptor ectodomains inducing dimerization of both the ectodomains and the cytoplasmic domains of these receptors (Figs. **5** and **7**). This enables the cytoplasmic domains to activate their Tyrosine Kinases (TK), enzymes that transfer phosphate groups to tyrosine residues of various proteins (Fig. **7**). The cytoplasmic domains of these receptors (TKR or Tyrosine Kinase Receptors) are structurally and functionally related to the Src oncoprotein and are capable to transphosphorylate the cytoplasmic domain of the other monomer. This yields phosphorylated cytoplasmic tails of receptor molecules that allow signaling to proceed. Hyperactive signaling by these receptors is encountered in many types of human cancer cells. Often, the receptors are overexpressed or mutated, resulting in ligand-independent signaling. Interestingly, the TGF-β receptors are superficially similar to the RTKs, in that they have a ligand-binding ectodomain and a signal-emitting kinase domain in their cytoplasmic portion (Fig. **5**).

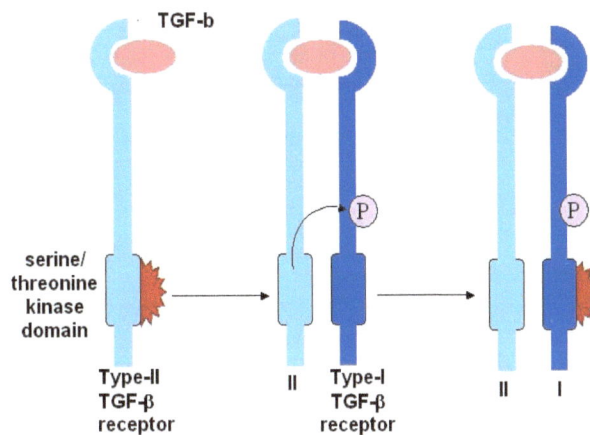

Figure 5: Structure of the TGF-β receptor. The structure of this receptor is similar to that of tyrosine kinase receptors because both types of receptors signal through cytoplasmic kinase domains. However, the kinase domains of TGF-β receptors are serine/threonine specific. When mutated, the TGF-β receptor, or components of this pathway act as oncogenic proteins.

However, these receptors form heterodimers and the kinases of the TGF-β receptors are serine/threonine kinases signaling through a much different mechanism (de Caestecker JNCI 2000) [26] (Massague JC 2000) [27] (Wrana Cell 1992) [28] (Attisano COCB 2000) [29] (Pietenpol PNAS 1990) [30] (Chen PNAS 2001) [31] (Seoane NCB 2001) [32] even more important, in their active state they block cellular growth acting as tumor suppressors. The Notch, Patch-Smoothened, and Frizzled receptor classes use a diversity of signal-transducing mechanisms to release signals into the cytoplasm. For example, growth factors of the Wnt class activate receptors of the Frizzled family, which are complex receptors that weave back and forth through the plasma membrane multiple times. In the absence of ligand binding, a complex of Axin and Apc allows Glycogen Synthase Kinase-3β (GSK-3β) to phosphorylate β-catenin (Fig. **6**).

This marks β-catenin for rapid destruction by proteolysis. However, when a Wnt ligand binds to a Frizzled receptor, acting *via* the Dishevelled protein, causes inhibition of GSK-3β. This spares β-catenin, which acting as an oncogenic protein may accumulate and promote cell proliferation. Aberrant signaling by these receptors play a key role in the pathogenesis of many types of human cancers. Another class of receptors, the integrins, sense cellular contacts with the Extracellular Matrix (ECM); having bound components of the ECM, the heterodimeric integrin receptors (composed of an α plus a β subunit) transduce signals into cells that stimulate proliferation and suppress apoptosis. It has been reported that an important attribute of transformed cells is their ability to grow in an anchorage-independent fashion, *i.e.*, to proliferate without attachment to a solid substrate. This behavior contrasts with that of normal cells, which require attachment in order to proliferate. Indeed, in the absence of such attachment, many types of normal cells will activate a version of their death program (apoptosis) that is often termed anoikis. One possible connection between Ras and the tyrosine kinase receptors came from the discovery that an activated ras oncogene causes many types of cells to produce and release growth factors, such as Transforming Growth Factor-α (TGF-α), an EGF-like growth factor that was found to be released by a variety of oncogene-transformed cells. Like EGF, TFG-α binds to and activates the EGF receptor (Fig. 7).

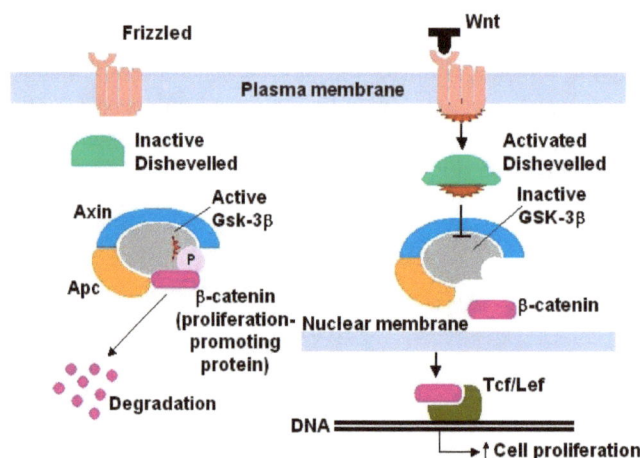

Figure 6: Signaling by the frizzled receptors. In the absence of wnt (left) a complex of Apc and Axin allows Glycogen Synthase Kinase-3β (GSK-3β) to phosphorylate β-catenin inducing its proteolysis. When wnt ligand binds a frizzled receptor, the activated receptor, acting *via* the Disheveled protein causes phosphorylation and inhibition of GSK-3β. This spares β-catenin which accumulates, induces the expression of several genes and promotes cell proliferation.

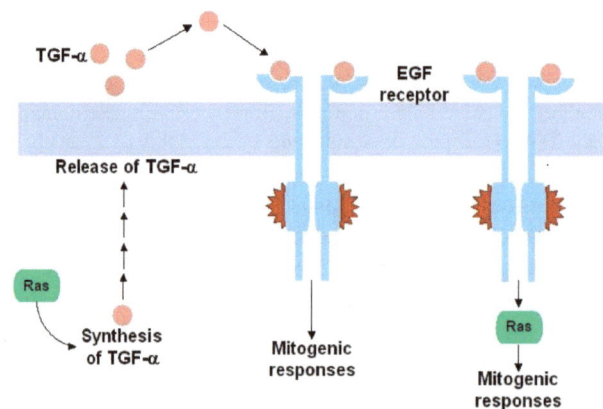

Figure 7: Two mechanisms of Ras transformation. Ras-transformed cells release several growth factors, such as TGF-α. Once secreted, TGF-α might act in an autocrine fashion (left) to activate a receptor, as the EGF receptor, promoting cell proliferation. Ras can also operate downstream of growth factor receptors such as the EGF receptor (right), promoting mitosis.

This suggested that once released by a ras-transformed cell, TGF-α might function in an autocrine manner to activate EGF receptors displayed on the surface of that cell. This, in turn, would evoke a series of responses quite similar to those created by a mutant, constitutively activated EGF receptor. Thus, Ras appeared to operate upstream of a growth factor receptor; however, this autocrine scheme was able to explain only a small part of ras function, since this oncogene was found to be able to transform cells that lacked receptors for the growth factors that it induced. In addition, it has been reported that ligand binding of growth factor receptors led rapidly to activation of Ras suggesting a direct intracellular signaling between ligand-activated growth factor receptors and Ras proteins. Detailed biological characterization of human tumor cells overexpressing certain growth factor receptors also suggested another dimension of complexity. In the case of human breast cancers, overexpression of the HER2/Neu receptor was found to be correlated with a large array of phenotypes displayed by the associated cancer cells (Yarden Oncology 2001) [33]. Those cells expressing elevated levels of this protein showed increased rates of DNA synthesis, better anchorage-independent growth, greater efficiency in forming tumors when implanted into host mice (*i.e.*, tumorigenicity), greater tendency to metastasize, and less dependence on estrogen for their growth. Hence, these receptor proteins were acting pleiotropically to confer a number of distinct changes on cancer cells. Such action seemed to be incompatible with a simple linear signaling cascade operating downstream of activated receptors. Instead, it appeared more likely that a number of distinct downstream signaling pathways were radiating out from these receptors, each involved in evoking a distinct cancer cell phenotype (Weinberg BC 2007) [6].

Genes that are present in normal configuration and at normal copy number can be transcribed at very high levels in human cancer cells due to deregulated transcription factors such as AP1 (Eferl NRC 2003) [34]. On the other hand, only about 50% of amplified genes in cancer cell genomes will show corresponding increases in their mRNAs. Thus, the somatic mutations that cause protooncogene activation can be divided into those that caused changes in the structure of encoded proteins and those that increase the expression levels of these proteins (due to promoter activation or to deregulated transcription factors).

Another important characteristic of oncogenes is that they cooperate to induce a transformed phenotype. There are many experimental examples supporting this cooperation; for example, when a myc oncogene was introduced together with an H-ras oncogene into rat embryo fibroblasts, the cells responded by becoming morphologically transformed and tumorigenic; neither of these oncogenes, on its own, could create such transformed cells (Parada Nature 1982) [13]. The ras oncogene could also collaborate with the SV40 large T oncogene, with the polyoma large T oncogene or with a mutant p53 gene in cell transformation. Conversely, myc could collaborate with the polyoma middle T oncogene, with src or with raf oncogene to transform and produce tumorigenic cells; it could also collaborate with bcl-2. Interestingly. Myc is basically a nuclear protein that strongly stimulates proliferation and weakly favors apoptosis (Prendergast Oncogene 1999) [35] the Bcl-2 protein is cytoplasmic and as we have previously mentioned, a strong apoptosis inhibitor (Rsujimoto FEBSL 2000) [22] (Ekert CDD 1999) [36] (Reed Oncogene 1998) [37]. The role of Myc in stem cell and cancer biology as well as in the amplification of proliferation and apoptosis pathways (it amplifies the intrinsic mitochondrial pathway and it triggers the death receptor pathways) has been recently reviewed (Meyer NRC 2008) [38] (Hoffman Oncogene 2008) [39] (Eilers GD 2008) [40] (Bueno CC 2008) [41] (Prochownik CMM 2008) [42] . Many efforts have directed cancer cells to self-destruct with proapoptotic receptor agonists (Ashkenazi NRDD 2008)[43], as well as with Bcl-2 antagonists (Lessene NRDD 2008) [44]. In addition, the role of the Bcl-2 oncogenic protein in autophagy is becoming increasingly clear (Heath-Engel Oncogene 2008) [45] (Yip Oncogene 2008) [46].

Transgenic mice provide models of oncogene collaboration and multi-step transformation. The ability to create transgenic mice, made possible to determine whether oncogenes are able to collaborate *in vivo* as well as *in vitro*. Mice were created to bore either the MMTV-ras or the MMTV-myc transgene in their germ line. The MMTV (Mouse Mammary Tumor Virus) transcriptional promoter ensured expression of the transgene largely in the mammary glands. Mice of these two transgenic strains were bred to create double-transgenic mice carrying both transgenes. The incidence of mammary carcinomas in mice carrying either the MMTV-myc or MMTV-ras transgenes in their germ lines was followed over many months. Double-transgenic mice contracted tumors at a greatly accelerated rate and at high frequency compared with mice inheriting only one of the transgenes. Therefore, the two oncogenic transgenes could collaborate *in vivo* to generate tumors, corroborating the conclusions of the *in vitro* experiments described earlier. Interestingly, even with two mutant oncogenes expressed in the great majority of mammary cells from early in development, tumors did not appear in these mice soon after birth, but instead were seen with great delay. Hence, the concomitant expression of two powerful oncogenes was still not sufficient to fully transform mouse mammary epithelial cells; instead, these cells clearly required at least one additional somatic mutation, before they would proliferate like cancer cells. A hint about the identity of this third event has come from careful analysis of rat cells that have been transformed *in vitro* by the ras + myc protocol; sooner or later, such cells usually acquire a mutation or methylation event that leads to inactivation of the p53 tumor suppressor pathway. In human cells, five different regulatory pathways need to be altered experimentally before these cells can generate a tumor in immunocompromised mice.

The role of mutant cellular genes in cancer pathogenesis eclipsed for some years the observation that certain human cancers are likely caused by infectious agents (mainly viruses and bacteria). Now the importance of infections in human cancer pathogenesis is clear; we can presently estimate that approximately 20% of the global cancer incidence can be linked to infections (zur Hausen Biochem 2008) [47]. This includes not only viral infections (*e.g.* Epstein-Barr virus, human herpes virus type 8, high risk human papillomavirus types, hepatitis B and C viruses, human T-lymphotropic retrovirus), but also bacterial (*Helicobacter pylori*) and some parasitic infections. In some cases, the infectious agent introduce oncogenes into cells, contributing to carcinogenesis mainly by increasing cellular proliferation and inhibiting apoptotic pathways; in other instances, infection causes chronic tissue damage and associated inflammation. It is presently known that cellular oncogenes and their functions can explain only part of the human cancer pathogenesis and that other genetic elements are involved in cancer development; the discovery of cellular oncogenes was a very good beginning and further work related mainly with tumor suppressor genes (antigrowth genes or antioncogenes), with epigenetic regulation of these genes and with DNA repair systems (involving caretaker genes) will give us a more complete picture of human carcinogenesis.

B. TUMOR SUPPRESSOR GENES

Mutations that disrupt the balance between growth-promoting and growth-inhibiting pathways can lead to cancer. The complex mechanisms for regulating the eukaryotic cell cycle are prime targets for oncogenic and tumor suppressor mutations. Both positive- and negative-acting proteins precisely control the entry of cells into and their progression through the cell cycle, which consists of four main phases: G1, S, G2, and mitosis. This regulatory system assures the proper coordination of cellular growth during G1 and G2, DNA synthesis during the S phase, and chromosome segregation and cell division during mitosis. In addition, cells that have sustained damage to their DNA normally are arrested before their DNA is replicated or in G2 before chromosome segregation. This arrest allows time for the DNA damage to be repaired; alternatively, the arrested cells commit suicide *via* programmed cell death (or apoptosis) or stop dividing. The whole cell-cycle control system functions to prevent cells from becoming cancerous. As might be expected, mutations in this system often lead to abnormal development or contribute to cancer. Once a cell progresses past a certain point in late G1, called the restriction point, it becomes irreversibly committed to entering the S phase and replicating its DNA.

1. Retinoblastoma Protein (Rb)

This tumor suppressor protein, together with D-type-cyclins and Cyclin-Dependent Kinases (CDKs) are important elements of the control system that regulate passage through the restriction point (R) (Fig. **8**).

The expression of D-type cyclin genes is induced by many extracellular growth factors, or mitogens (Liu MCB 1995) [48] (Filmus Oncogene 1994) [49]. These cyclins assemble with their partners CDK4 and CDK6 to generate catalytically active cyclin-CDK complexes, whose kinase activity promotes progression past the restriction point. Mitogen withdrawal prior to passage through the restriction point leads to accumulation of the tumor suppressor proteins known as p16 (Serrano Cell 1997) [50]. Like p15, p16 binds specifically to CDK4 and CDK6, thereby inhibiting their kinase activity and causing G1 arrest. Under normal circumstances, phosphorylation of Rb protein is initiated midway through G1 by active cyclin D-CDK4 and cyclin D-CDK6 complexes. Unphosphorylated Rb binds to and sequesters E2F transcription factors in the cytoplasm.

These factors stimulate transcription of genes encoding proteins required for DNA synthesis. Rb phosphorylation is completed by other cyclin-CDK complexes in late G1, allowing release and activation of E2F transcription factors and G1→S progression (Lundberg MCB 1998) [51]. The complete phosphorylation of Rb and its dissociation from E2F irreversibly commits the cell to DNA synthesis. Most tumors contain an oncogenic mutation that causes overproduction or loss of one of the components of this pathway such that the cells are propelled into the S phase in the absence of the proper extracellular growth signals.

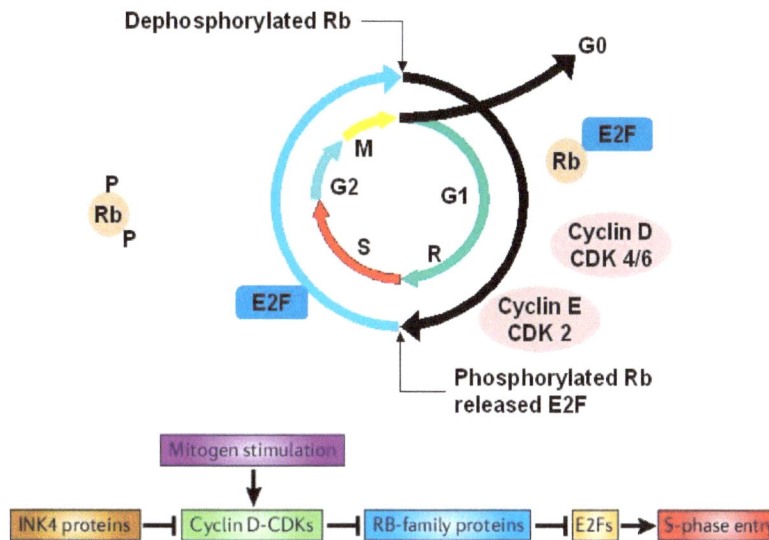

Figure 8: Dephosphorylated Rb blocks the cell cycle. The phosphorylation state of Rb is closely coordinated with the advance of the cell cycle. As cells pass through the M/G1 transition Rb protein is dephosphorylated and binds transcription factor E2F; when they progress through G1, cyclin D-CDK 4/6 causes Rb hypophosphorylation. After the restriction point (R), cyclin E-CDK2 heavily phosphorylates Rb/E2F complexes and E2F is released. This released transcription factor can now activate genes required for cell proliferation.

The proteins that function as cyclin-CDK inhibitors (such as p15 or p16) play an important role in regulating the cell cycle. In particular, loss-of-function mutations that prevent p16 from inhibiting cyclin D-CDK4/6 kinase activity are common in several human cancers; loss of p16 mimics overproduction of cyclin D1, leading to Rb hyperphosphorylation and release of active E2F transcription factor (DeGregori PNAS 1997) [52] (Polager TCB 2008) [53]. Thus, as mentioned, p16 normally acts as a tumor suppressor. Although the p16 gene is deleted in some human cancers, in others the p16 sequence is normal, but it is inactivated by hypermethylation of its promoter region, which prevents transcription.

Inactivating mutations in both rb alleles lead to childhood retinoblastoma, a relatively rare type of cancer. However, loss of rb gene function also is found in more common cancers that arise later in life (*e.g.*, carcinomas of lung, breast, and bladder). These tissues, unlike retinal tissue, most likely produce other proteins (*e.g.*, p107 and p130, both structurally related to Rb) whose function is redundant with that of Rb, and thus loss of Rb is not so critical for preventing cancer (Sun JCB 2007) [54]. One way or another, Rb functions are eventually shut down. In addition to inactivating mutations, Rb function can be eliminated by the binding of viral oncoproteins, such as E7, encoded by high risk human papillomavirus (HR-HPVs).

Tumors with inactivating mutations in Rb generally produce normal levels of cyclin D1 and functional p16 protein. Conversely, tumor cells that overproduce cyclin D1 or have lost p16 function generally retain wild-type Rb. Thus loss of only one component of this regulatory pathway for controlling passage through the restriction point is all that is necessary to subvert normal growth control and set the stage for cancer.

2. Chromatin Structure Remodeling

Besides mutations, tumor-suppressor genes can also be silenced by repressive chromatin structures. In recent years the importance of multiprotein chromatin-remodeling complexes, such as the SWI/SNF complex, in transcriptional control has become increasingly clear. These large and diverse complexes have at their core an ATP-dependent helicase and often control histone modification and chromatin remodeling. By causing changes in the positions or structures of nucleosomes, SWI/SNF complexes make genes accessible or inaccessible to DNA-binding proteins that control transcription. If a gene is normally activated or repressed by SWI/SNF-mediated chromatin changes, mutations in the genes encoding the SWI or SNF proteins will cause changes in expression of the target gene. The target genes regulated by SWI/SNF and similar complexes are only partially known, but they include some growth-regulating genes such as E2F; studies with transgenic mice suggest that SWI/SNF plays a role in repressing the E2F genes. Loss of function of the components of the SWI/SNF complex increases the proliferative effects of E2F indicating that SWI/SNF normally inhibits the function of this important transcription factor. Thus loss of SWI/SNF function, just like loss of Rb function, can lead to overgrowth and perhaps cancer. Indeed, in mice, Rb protein recruits SWI/SNF proteins to repress transcription of the E2F gene. Rb represses genes *via* this transcriptional effect on E2F and by recruitment of histone deacetylases and histone methyltransferases (Siddiqui MCB 2003) [55] (Ferreira Oncogene 2001) [56] (Yoshimoto ECR 2006) [57] (Vandel MCB 2001) [58] (Brehm Nature 1998) [59]. Interestingly, microarray studies after SNF5 elimination showed gene-expression similarity of mouse and human tumors indicating that the loss of SNF5 leads to heightened expression of cell cycle genes including many regulated by E2F. In mice, the loss of SNF5 leads to derepression of the E2F gene, and the simultaneous loss of p53 causes the E2F to be fully active in promoting the G1 →S cell cycle transition. With chromatin-remodeling complexes involved in so many aspects of transcriptional control, it is expected that SWI/SNF and similar complexes will be linked to many cancers. In humans, mutations in *Brg1,* which encodes the SWI/SNF catalytic subunit, have been found in prostate, lung and breast tumors. Components of the SWI/SNF complex also have been found to associate with BRCA-1, the nuclear protein that helps suppress human breast cancer. BRCA-1 is involved in the repair of double-strand DNA breaks and in transcriptional control, so the SWI/SNF complex may assist BRCA-1 in these functions (Zhang Oncogene 2009) [60].

3. p53

This is a very important tumor suppressor gene; loss of p53 induces genome instability abolishing the DNA-damage checkpoint (Cox Bioessays 1995) [61] (Levine Nature 1991) [62] (Lee Cell 1995) [63]. Cells with functional p53 become arrested in G1 when exposed to DNA-damaging irradiation, whereas cells lacking functional p53 are not arrested; when the p53 G1 checkpoint control does not operate properly, damaged DNA can replicate, perpetuating mutations. (Deng Cell 1995) [64] (Bunz Science 1998) [65]. Loss-of-function mutations in the p53 gene occur in more than 50 percent of human cancers (Joerger ARB 2008) [66]. Unlike other cell-cycle proteins, p53 is present at very low levels in normal cells because it is extremely unstable and rapidly degraded. Mice lacking p53 are largely viable and healthy, except for a predisposition to develop multiple types of tumors. In normal mice, the amount of p53 protein is heightened due to post-transcriptional responses observed in stressful situations, such as ultraviolet or γ irradiation, heat, and low oxygen. DNA damage by γ irradiation or by other stresses somehow leads to the activation of Atm or Atr, serine kinases that phosphorylate and thereby stabilize p53, leading to a marked increase in its concentration; the stabilized p53 activates transcription of the gene encoding $p21^{CIP}$, which binds to and inhibits mammalian G1 cyclin-CDK complexes (Figs. **9** and **10**). As a result, cells with damaged DNA are arrested in G1, allowing time for DNA repair by several mechanisms or the cells permanently arrest, *i.e.*, become senescent. In addition to its role in the G1→S transition, p53-induced production of $p21^{CIP}$ results in the inhibition of CDK1, which in turn blocks the cyclin B-CDK1 complex that is required for entry into mitosis, thus causing cells to arrest in G2. Directly or indirectly, p53 also represses expression of the genes encoding cyclin B and topoisomerase II, which also are required for the G2 →mitosis transition. Thus, if DNA is damaged following its replication, p53-induced G2 arrest will prevent its transmission to daughter cells.

This tumor suppressor protein is also stabilized after oncogenic stress and transcriptional activation of Arf (Fig. **10**); the tumor suppressor protein Arf sequesters the oncogenic protein Mdm2 leading to p53 accumulation.

The active form of p53 is a tetramer of four identical subunits. A missense point mutation in one of the two p53 alleles in a cell can abrogate almost all p53 activity because virtually all the oligomers will contain at least one defective subunit, and it has been determined that such oligomers have reduced ability to activate transcription. Oncogenic p53 mutations thus act as dominant negatives, with mutations in a single allele causing a loss of function. In addition, tumor cells still sometimes lose the remaining functional allele (Loss of Heterozygosity or LOH). In contrast, loss-of-function mutations in other tumor-suppressor genes (*e.g.*, rb) are recessive because the encoded proteins function as monomers and mutations of a single allele has little functional consequence.

Under stressful conditions, the Atm kinase also phosphorylates and activates Chk2, a protein kinase that phosphorylates the oncoprotein phosphatase Cdc25A, marking it for ubiquitin-mediated destruction (Galaktionov Nature 1996) [67].

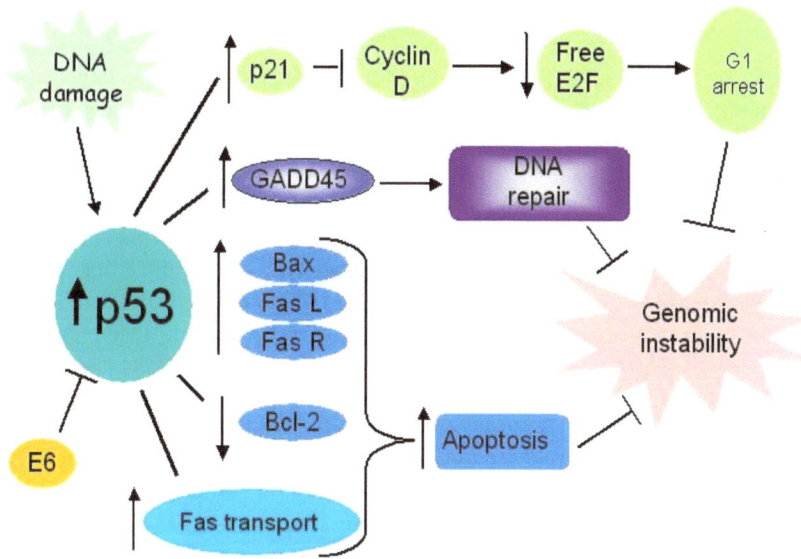

Figure 9: Properties of p53 tumor suppressor protein. The antioncogenic p53 protein induces apoptosis after severe DNA damage. Acting as transcription factor activates expression of several proteins involved in cell cycle arrest (p21), repair of DNA damage (GADD45) or apoptosis induction (Bax, FasL, Fas/CD95). In addition, p53 inhibits antiapoptotic Bcl-2 expression and facilitates CD95/Fas transport to the cellular membrane, leading to apoptosis induction. Inactivated p53 (mutated or complexed to oncogenic proteins such as Mdm2 or E6) cause apoptosis reduction and genomic instability, which increase neoplasia development.

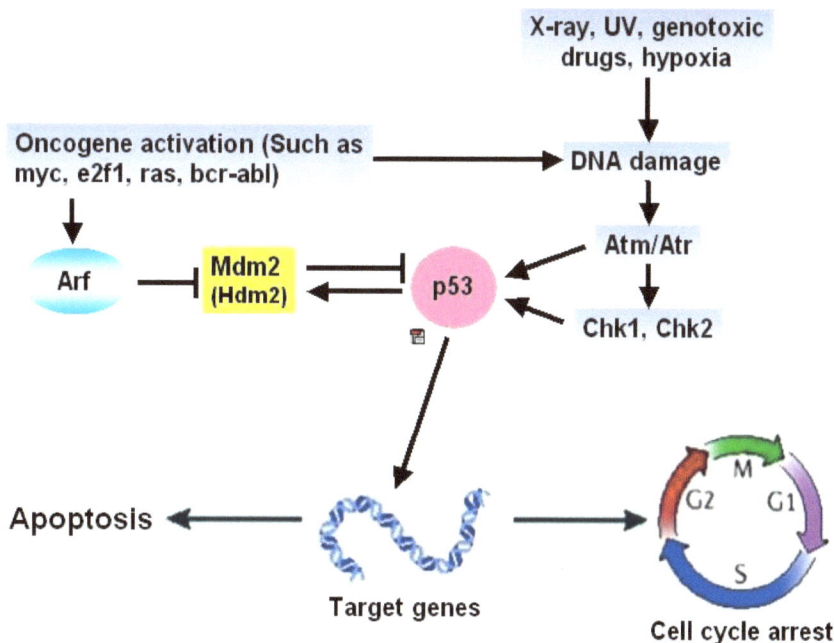

Figure 10: Deregulated growth signals and DNA damage cause p53 stabilization. Several monitoring systems send alarm signals to p53. For example, this tumor suppressor protein can be stabilized after oncogenic stress (activation of Myc, Ras or Bcr-Abl) and transcriptional activation of the tumor suppressor protein Arf, which sequesters the oncogenic protein Mdm2 inducing the accumulation of p53. In addition, p53 can be directly phosphorylated and stabilized by several kinases such as Atm/Atr or Chk1/Chk2.

This phosphatase normally removes the inhibitory phosphate from Cdk2, a prerequisite for cells to enter the S phase. Decreased levels of Cdc25A thus block progression into and through the S phase. Thus, loss-of-function mutations in the atm or chk2 genes have some of the effects of p53 mutations.

As previously mentioned (Fig. **10**), the activity of p53 normally is kept low by a protein called Mdm2. When Mdm2 is bound to p53, it inhibits the transcription-activating ability of p53 and catalyzes the addition of ubiquitin molecules, thus targeting p53 for proteasomal degradation. Phosphorylation of p53 by Atm or Atr displaces bound Mdm2 from p53, thereby stabilizing this important tumor suppressor protein. At the same time the Atm kinase can phosphorylate Mdm2 in a way that causes its functional inactivation; as a consequence of this phosphorylation of both p53 and Mdm2, p53 is not ubiquitylated and escapes destruction, and p53 concentration in the cell increases rapidly. Because the mdm2 gene is itself transcriptionally activated by p53, Mdm2 functions in an autoregulatory feedback loop with p53, perhaps normally preventing excess p53 function (Bond Cell 2004) [68]. The mdm2 oncogene is amplified in many human tumors that contain a normal p53 gene (Momand Cell 1992) [69]. Even though functional p53 is produced by such tumor cells, the elevated Mdm2 levels reduce the p53 concentration enough to abolish the p53-induced G1 arrest in response to irradiation, suggesting that the p53 pathway is always defective in human malignant tumors. The activity of p53 is also inhibited by E6 oncoproteins encoded by HR-HPVs (Tommasino Bioessays 1995) [70]. The activity of p53 is not limited to inducing cell-cycle arrest; in addition to this important activity, this tumor suppressor protein stimulates production of proapoptotic proteins, such as Fas L, Fas R or Bax (Wang Anticancer 1999) [71] (Arrowsmith CDD 1999) [72] (May Oncogene 1999) [73]. Senescence and apoptosis may in fact be the most important means through which p53 prevents tumor growth (Bunz Science 1998) [65] (Schmitt Cell 2002) [74] (Ho CDD 2003) [75] (Murphy CC 2004) [76] (Innocente PNAS 1999) [77]. It was also found that p53 induces production of DNA-repair enzymes.

Recent research on p53 is mainly directed towards tailored cancer therapies. For example, it has been reported that some small molecules are selective inhibitors of the p53-Mdm2 interaction and therefore they show therapeutic potential (Patel EOID 2008) [78] (Vazquez NRDD 2008) [79]. Additionally, p53-based strategies involving inhibition of MDM2-mediated p53 ubiquitylation and restoration of DNA-binding activity of mutant p53 protein, as well as combination therapies simultaneously targeting p53 and NFκB pathways (Karin NRC 2002) [80] will greatly improve cancer therapy (Dey NTDD 2008) [81].

4. The Pten Gene

The phosphatase encoded by this gene dephosphorylates phosphatidylinositol 3,4,5-trisphosphate, a second messenger that functions activating protein kinase B. Cells lacking Pten phosphatase have elevated levels of phosphatidylinositol 3,4,5-trisphosphate and active protein kinase B, which promotes cell survival and prevents apoptosis by several pathways. Thus Pten acts as a pro-apoptotic tumor suppressor protein by decreasing the anti-apoptotic effect of protein kinase B (Fig. **3**).

5. The Apc Gene

It is well known that the great majority (>95%) of colon cancers appear to be sporadic, that is, occurs randomly without any apparent predisposition (different to those caused by a heritable genetic susceptibility). (Miyoshi HMD 1992) [82] (Smith PNAS 1993) [83] (Powel Nature 1992) [84].

The cloning of the apc gene led, after many years of research, to a reasonably clear view of how this gene and its encoded Apc protein are able to control cell proliferation within the colon. During colon carcinogenesis, the only type of mutations that can lead subsequently to the development of a cancer are those mutations that block both the out-migration of colonic epithelial cells from the crypts and the cell death that follows soon thereafter; any additional mutant alleles acquired subsequently by their progeny in genes that induce a neoplastic growth state will similarly be retained in the crypts. In the molecular mechanism controlling this out-migration of enterocytes from the colonic crypt β-catenin plays an important role. As previously described, when Wnts bind cell surface receptors, cytoplasmic β-catenin is saved from destruction, accumulates, and migrates to the nucleus, where it binds a group of DNA-binding proteins termed variously Tcf or Lef (Fig. **6**) (Korinek Science 1997) [85] (Morin Science 1997) [86] (Aberle EMBOJ 1997) [87] (Behrens Nature 1996) [88] (Nelson Science 2004) [89]. The resulting heterodimeric transcription factor attracts other nuclear proteins, forming multi-protein complexes that activate expression of a series of target genes programming (in the case of enterocytes) the stem-cell phenotype. In the context of the colonic crypt, enterocyte stem cells encounter Wnt factors released by stromal cells near the bottom of the crypt, which keep β-catenin levels high in the enterocytes. Indeed, these cells are held in a stem cell-like state by the high levels of intracellular β-catenin. However, as some of the progeny of these stem cells begin their upward migration, they no longer experience Wnt signaling, and intracellular β-catenin levels fall. As a consequence, these cells lose their stem cell phenotype, exit the cell cycle, and differentiate into functional enterocytes. The levels of β-catenin in the cytosol are negatively controlled by Apc, the product of the adenomatous polyposis coli gene; in cells at the bottom of the normal crypts, the apc gene is not expressed at detectable levels and β-catenin is present at high levels (Korinek Science 1997) [85] (Aberle EMBOJ 1997) [87]. However, as cells begin their upward migration out of the crypts, the level of Apc expression in these cells increases greatly and, in the absence of Wnts, this protein drives down the intracellular levels of β-catenin. The inverse expression is explained nicely by the known molecular mechanism of Apc, a large protein of 2843 amino acid residues. Together with two scaffolding proteins termed axin and conductin, Apc forms, as mentioned, a multiprotein complex that enables GSK-3β to phosphorylate four amino-terminal residues of β-catenin (Fig. **6**); the phosphorylation then leads to the degradation of β-catenin *via* the ubiquitin-proteasome pathway. In sum, Apc is essential for triggering the degradation of β-catenin, and in its absence β-catenin levels accumulate to high levels within cells (Aberle EMBOJ 1997) [87] (Rubinfeld Science 1996) [90] (Jeanes Oncogene 2008) [91]. Many human colon mutations in apc cause premature termination of the Apc protein, thereby removing domains that are important for its ability to associate with β-catenin and axin and for the resulting degradation of β-catenin. The accumulation of β-catenin is the most important consequence of Apc inactivation, which can be observed in about 90% of sporadic colon carcinomas. The remaining minority (approximately 10%) of sporadic colon carcinomas carry wild-type apc alleles, but either the apc gene promoter is hypermethylated and rendered inactive, or the gene encoding β-catenin carries point mutations, and the resulting mutant β-catenin molecules lose the amino acid residues that are normally phosphorylated by GSK-3β. Since they cannot be phosphorylated, these mutant β-catenin molecules escape degradation and accumulate. When β-catenin accumulates in enterocyte precursors they retain a stem cell-like phenotype, which precludes them from migrating out of the crypts. This leads to the accumulation of large numbers of relatively undifferentiated cells in a colonic crypt, which eventually form adenomatous polyps and can later sustain further mutations (such as K-ras) originating more advanced polyps and carcinomas. The first of these mutations invariably involves inactivation of Apc function. In addition to cytoplasmic Apc functions, cells lacking Apc function have been found to exhibit a marked increase in chromosomal instability, which results in increases and decreases in chromosome number, usually because of inappropriate segregation of chromosomes during mitosis. The aneuploidy that results from these chromosomal segregation defects alters the relative numbers of critical growth-promoting and growth inhibiting genes, which obviously contributes to tumorigenesis.

6. Nf1

The Nf1 gene was cloned in 1990; the genetic behavior of the nf1 gene parallels closely that of the rb gene. At the cellular level, the originally heterozygous configuration of this gene (Nf1$^{+/-}$) is converted to a homozygous state (Nf1$^{-/-}$) in tumor cells through loss of heterozygosity. As is the case with the rb gene, *de novo* mutations usually occur during spermatogenesis in the fathers of afflicted patients. Once the cloned gene was sequenced, it became possible to assign a function to neurofibromin, the nf1-encoded protein; it showed extensive sequence relatedness to a protein, termed Ira, that functions as a GTPase-Activating Protein (GAP) for yeast Ras, as well as to two mammalian Ras-GAP proteins (Ballester Cell 1990) [92]. Like most if not all eukaryotes, yeast cells use Ras proteins to regulate important aspects of their metabolism and proliferation. Detailed genetic analyses had already shown that in yeast, the positive signaling functions of Ras are countered by the Ira protein. By provoking Ras to activate its intrinsic GTPase activity, Ira forces Ras to convert itself from its activated GTP-bound form to its inactive, GDP-bound form (Fig. **2**), precisely the same function carried out by the mammalian Ras-GAP proteins. Interaction of Ras with Nf1 can increase the GTPase activity of Ras more than 1000-fold. Indeed, a Ras-GAP may inactivate Ras before the latter has had a chance to stimulate its downstream effectors. Nf1 is expressed widely throughout the body, with especially high levels found in the adult peripheral and central nervous systems. When cells first experience growth factor stimulation, they may degrade Nf1, enabling Ras signaling to proceed without interference by Nf1. However, after about 1 hour Nf1 levels return to normal, and this protein inhibits further Ras signaling in a negative-feedback control. Ras proteins are predicted to exist in their activated, GTP-bound state for longer-than-normal periods of times in neuroectodermal cells lacking Nf1 function. In fact, in the cells of neurofibromas, which are genetically Nf1$^{-/-}$, elevated levels of activated Ras and Ras effector proteins can be found producing a similar effect to that observed with mutant ras oncogenes.

As we have seen, the formation of a tumor is a complex process that usually proceeds in multi-steps over a period of decades. As tumor progression advances, tumor genomes often become increasingly unstable; cancer cells progress to ever more malignant states due to mutations in oncogenes and tumor suppressor genes as well as epigenetic regulation of cancer related genes (Shelton COMT 2008) [93] (Gronbaek BCPT 2008) [94] (Gopalakrishnan MR 2008) [95]. As previously mentioned, five distinct cellular regulatory circuits need to be altered experimentally before human cells can grow as tumor cells in immunocompromised mice. These changes involve: (1) The mitogenic signaling pathway controlled by Ras. (2) The cell cycle checkpoint controlled by Rb. (3) The alarm and apoptosis pathway controlled by p53. (4) The telomerere maintenance pathway controlled by hTERT. (5) The signaling pathway controlled by protein phosphatase 2A (Weinberg BC 2007) [6].

Interestingly, tumors are composed of minority and majority cell populations that show vast differences in their tumorigenicity (Singh CR 2003) [96] as well as in antigenic markers due to their different states of differentiation. The genetic evolution associated with multi-step tumor progression may occur in relatively small subpopulations of cancer cells, the minority tumor stem cells, rather than in the much larger population of neoplastic transit-amplifying cells. This means that only the mutations striking the cancer stem cell population can be transmitted to descendant cells due to their unlimited proliferative potential (Malanchi COO 2009) [97] (Ischenko CMC 2008) [98] (Ambler JP 2009) [99]. It seems that widespread destabilization of cell genomes occurs quite early in multi-step tumor progression; tumor cell genomes often become more mutable as tumor progression advances probably due to mutations of components of the DNA repair apparatus, suggesting that this particular property of tumor stem cells should be considered in tailored cancer therapy.

Nonmutagenic (nongenotoxic) agents, including those favoring cell proliferation, make important contributions to tumorigenesis. Toxic and mitogenic agents (such as estrogens) can act as human tumor promoters. Cytotoxic agents can function as tumor promoters simply by causing the proliferation of the cells that have survived the toxic effects of these agents. Relatively few human tumor promoters act through purely cytotoxic or mitogenic mechanisms, instead the great majority seems to drive clonal expansion through mechanisms involving inflammation. Anti-inflammatory drugs, such as aspirin, function to reduce the incidence of several human carcinomas; this effect could be due to the observed inhibition of cyclooxygenase-2 (Cox-2) by aspirin. Cox-2 is inducible in many tissues in response to inflammatory stimuli and is likely to be important in the early stages of carcinoma progression (Singh MRMC 2008) [100] (Reddy CPD 2007) [101] (Surh CCDT 2007) [102]. For example, Cox-2 expression is high in early pre-malignant breast tumors (Howe BCR 2007) [103] Harris SB 2007) [104]. Thus, inflammation in a variety of epithelial tissues functions as a tumor promoter that can lead to carcinomas; this can collaborate with an oncogene or an altered tumor suppressor gene in a way that resembles the collaboration between two oncogenes until the time when the descendants of initiated tumor cells acquire additional oncogenes and therefore no longer need to depend on the reversible effects of tumor promoters for their continued proliferation and survival. The recognition that chronic inflammation and infections are two important sources of tumor promotion has profound implications in diagnosis as well as in therapy and in general for reducing cancer incidence.

CONCLUSION

In conclusion, oncogenes and tumor suppressor genes play a major role during the early steps of carcinogenesis. Nonmutagenic agents make also important contributions to multi-step carcinogenesis. The properties of cancer related genes, such as oncogenes and tumor suppressor genes, are strongly influencing our view of malignant cell functioning and improving prevention, diagnosis and therapy of this disease.

ACKNOWLEDGEMENTS

I would like to thank Elizabeth Alvarez Ríos, Enrique García Villa and Gabriela T. Mora Macías for the elaboration of this manuscript. I also thank CONACYT for financial support.

REFERENCES

[1]   Evan GI, Vousden KH. Proliferation, cell cycle and apoptosis in cancer. Nature 2001; 411(6835): 342-8.

[2]   Leder P, Clayton DA. Rubenstein E. Introduction to Molecular Medicine (New York Scientific American Inc 1994.

[3]   Bishop JM, Weinberg RA. Molecular Oncology New York Scientific American Inc 1996.

[4]   Murray AW, Hunt T. The Cell Cycle: An Introduction (New York WH Freeman) 1993.

[5]   Harley CB, Villeponteau B. Telomeres and telomerase in aging and cancer. Curr Opin Genet Dev 1995; 5: 249-55.

[6]   Weinberg R. The Biology of Cancer. Garland Science New York 2007.

[7]   zur Hausen H. Papillomaviruses causing cancer: evasion from host-cell control in early events in carcinogenesis. J Natl Cancer Inst 2000; 92(9): 690-8.

[8]   Levrero M. Viral hepatitis and liver cancer: the case of hepatitis C. Oncogene 2006; 25(27): 3834-47. Review.

[9]   Colombo M. Natural history and pathogenesis of hepatitis C virus related hepatocellular carcinoma. J Hepatol 1999; 31 Suppl 1: 25-30. Review.

[10]   Koike K, Tsutsumi T, Fujie H, Shintani Y, Kyoji M. Molecular mechanism of viral hepatocarcinogenesis. Oncology 2002; 62 Suppl 1: 29-37. Review.

[11]   Barbacid M. Ras Genes. Annu Rev Biochem 1987; 56: 779-827.

[12]   Cooper GM. Cellular oncogenes and cancer. Clin Physiol Biochem 1987; 5(3-4): 122-9.

[13]   Parada LF, Tabin CJ, Shih C, Weinberg RA. Human EJ bladder carcinoma oncogene is homologue of Harvey sarcoma virus ras gene. Nature 1982; 297(5866): 474-8.

[14]   Adhikary S, Eilers M. Transcriptional regulation and transformation by Myc proteins. Nat Rev Mol Cell Biol 2005; 6(8): 635-45. Review.

[15]   Knoepfler PS. Myc goes global: new tricks for an old oncogene. Cancer Res 2007; 67(11): 5061-3. Review.

[16]   Peter M, Rosty C, Couturier J, Radvanyi F, Teshima H, Sastre-Garau X. MYC activation associated with the integration of HPV DNA at the MYC locus in genital tumors. Oncogene 2006; 25(44): 5985-93.

[17]   Malumbres M, Barbacid M. Ras oncogenes; the first thirty years. Nat Rev Cancer 2003; 3: 459-65.

[18]   Khwaja A, Tatton L. Caspase-mediated proteolysis and activation of protein kinase C delta plays a central role in neutrophil apoptosis. Blood 1999; 94(1): 291-301.

[19]   Kauffmann-Zeh A, Rodriguez-Viciana P, Ulrich E, *et al.* Suppression of c-Myc-induced apoptosis by Ras signalling through PI(3)K and PKB. Nature 1997; 385(6616): 544-8.

[20]   del Peso L, González-García M, Page C, Herrera R, Nuñez G. Interleukin-3-induced phosphorylation of BAD through the protein kinase Akt. Science 1997; 278(5338): 687-9.

[21]   Ozes ON, Mayo LD, Gustin JA, Pfeffer SR, Pfeffer LM, Donner DB. NF-kappaB activation by tumour necrosis factor requires the Akt serine-threonine kinase. Nature 1999; 401(6748): 82-5.

[22]   Rsujimoto, Shimizu S. Bcl-2 family: life-or-death switch. FEBS Lett 2000; 466: 6-10.

[23]   Cortazzo M, Schor NF. Potentiation of enediyne-induced apoptosis and differentiation by Bcl-2. Cancer Res 1996; 56: 1199-203.

[24]   Schelessinger J. Ligand-induced receptor-mediated dimerization and activation of EGF receptor. Cell 2002; 110: 669-72.

[25]   Lo HW, Hung MC. Nuclear EGFR signalling network in cancers: linking EGFR pathway to cell cycle progression, nitric oxide pathway and patient survival. Br J Cancer 2006; 94(2): 184-8. Review.

[26]   de Caestecker MP, Piek E, Roberts AB. Role of transforming growth factor-beta signaling in cancer. J Natl Cancer Inst 2000; 92(17): 1388-402.

[27]   Massagué J, Blain SW, Lo RS. TGFbeta signalling in growth control, cancer, and heritable disorders. Cell 2000; 103: 295-309.

[28]   Wrana JL, Attisano L, Carcamo J, *et al.* TGF beta signals through a heteromeric protein kinase receptor complex. Cell 1992; 71: 1003-14.

[29]   Attisano L, Wrana JL. Smads as transcriptional co-modulators. Curr Opi Cell Biol 2000; 12: 235-43.

[30]   Pietenpol JA, Holt JT, Stein RW, Moses HL. Transforming growth factor beta 1 suppression of c-myc gene transcription: role in inhibition of keratinocyte proliferation. Proc Natl Acad Sci USA 1990; 87: 3758-62.

[31]   Chen CR, Kang Y, Massagué J. Defective repression of c-myc in breast cancer cells: a loss at the core of the transforming growth factor beta growth arrest program. Proc Natl Acad Sci USA 2001; 98: 992-9.

[32]   Seoane J, Pouponnot C, Staller P, Schader M, Eilers M, Massagué J. TGFbeta influences Myc, Miz-1 and Smad to control the CDK inhibitor p15INK4b. Nat Cell Biol 2001; 3: 400-8.

[33]   Yarden Y. Biology of HER2 and its importance in breast cancer. Oncology 2001; 2: 1-13. Review.

[34]   Eferl R, Wagner EF. AP-1: a double-edged sword in tumorigenesis. Nat Rev Cancer 2003; 3(11): 859-68.

[35]   Prendergast GC. Mechanisms of apoptosis by c-Myc. Oncogene 1999; 18: 2967-87.

[36]   Ekert PG, Silke J, Vaux DL. Caspase inhibitors. Cell Death Differ 1999; 6: 1081-6.

[37]   Reed J. Bcl-2 family proteins. Oncogene 1998; 17: 3225-36.

[38]   Meyer N, Penn LZ. Reflecting on 25 years with MYC Nat Rev Cancer 2008; 8(12): 976-90.

[39]   Hoffman B, Liebermann DA. apoptotic signalling by c-Myc. Oncogene 2008; 27(50): 6462-72.

[40]   Eilers M, Eisenman RN. Myc's broad reach. Genes 2008; 22(20): 2755-66.

[41]   Bueno MJ, de Castro IP, Malumbres M. Control of cell proliferation pathways by microRNAs. Cell Cycle 2008; 3143- 8.

[42]   Prochownik EV. C-Myc: linking transformation and genomic instability. Curr Mol Med 2008; 8(6): 446-58.

[43]   Ashkenazi A. Directing cancer cells to self-destruct with pro apoptotic receptor agonists. Nat Rev Drug Discov 2008; 1001- 2.

[44]   Lessene G, Czabotar PE. BCL-2 family antagonists for cancer therapy. Nat Rev Drug Discov 2008; 989-1000.

[45]   Heath-Engel HM, Chang NC, Shore GC. The endoplasmic reticulum in apoptosis and autophagy: role of the BCL-2 protein family. Oncogene 2008; 6419-33.

[46]   Yip KW, Reed JC. Bcl-2 family proteins and cancer. Oncogene 2008; 27(50): 6398-406.

[47]   Zur Hausen H. Papillomaviruses-to Vaccination and Beyond. Biochemistry 2008; 73: (5)498-503.

[48]   Liu JJ, Chao JR, Jiang MC, Ng SY, Yen JJ, Yang-Yen HF. Ras transformation results in an elevated level of cyclin D1 and acceleration of G1 progression in NIH 3T3 cells. Mol Cell Biol 1995; 15(7): 3654-63.

[49]   Filmus J, Robles AI, Shi W, Wong MJ, Colombo LL, Conti CJ. Induction of cyclin D1 overexpression by activated ras Oncogene 1994; 9: 3627-33.

[50]   Serrano M, Lin AW, McCurrach ME, Beach D, Lowe SW. Oncogenic ras provokes premature cell senescence associated with accumulation of p53 and p161NK4a. Cell 1997; 88: 593-602.

[51]   Lundberg AS, Weinberg RA. Functional inactivation of the retinoblastoma protein requires sequential modification by at least two distinct cyclin-cdk complexes. Mol Cell Biol 1998; 18: 753-61.

[52]   DeGregori J, Leone G, Miron A, Jakoi L, Nevins JR. Distinct roles for E2F proteins in cell growth control and apoptosis. Proc Natl Acad Sci USA 1997; 94(14):7245-50.

[53]   Polager S, Ginsberg D. E2F is at the crossroads of life and death. Trends Cell Biol 2008; 528-35.

[54]   Sun A, Bagella L, Tutton S, Romano G, Giordano A. From G0 to S phase: a view of the roles played by the retinoblastoma (Rb) family members in the Rb-E2F pathway. J Cell Biochem 2007; 102(6):1400-4. Review.

[55]   Siddiqui H, Solomon DA, Gunawardena RW, Wang Y, Knudsen ES. Histone deacetylation of RB-responsive promoters: requisite for specific gene repression but dispensable for cell cycle inhibition. Mol Cell Biol 2003; 23(21): 7719-31.

[56]   Ferreira R, Naguibneva I, Pritchard LL, Ait-Si-Ali S, Harel-Bellan A. The Rb/chromatin connection and epigenetic control: opinion. Oncogene 2001; 20(24):3128-33. Review.

[57]   Yoshimoto T, Boehm M, Olive M, et al. The arginine methyltransferase PRMT2 binds RB and regulates E2F function. Exp Cell Res 2006; 312(11): 2040-53.

[58]   Vandel L, Nicolas E, Vaute O, Ferreira R, Ait-Si-Ali S, Trouche D. Transcriptional repression by the retinoblastoma protein through the recruitment of a histone methyltransferase. Mol Cell Biol 2001; 21(19): 6484-94.

[59]   Brehm A, Miska EA, McCance DJ, Reid JL, Bannister AJ, Kouzarides T. Retinoblastoma protein recruits histone deacetylase to repress transcription. Nature 1998; 391(6667): 597-601.

[60]   Zhang B, Chambers KJ, Leprince D, Faller DV, Wang S. Requirement for chromatin-remodeling complex in novel tumor suppressor HICI-mediated transcriptional repression and growth control. Oncogene 2009; 28(5): 651-61.

[61]   Cox LS, Lane DP. Tumour suppressors, kinases and clamps: how p53 regulates the cell cycle in response to DNA damage. Bioessays 1995; 17: 501-8.

[62]   Levine AJ, Momand J, Finlay C.A. The p53 tumour suppressor gene. Nature 1991; 351: 453-6.

[63]   Lee S, Elenbaas B, Levine A, Griffith J. p53 in its 14 kDa C-terminal domain recognize primary DNA damage in the form of insertion/deletion mismatches. Cell 1995; 81: 1013-20.

[64]   Deng C, Zhang P, Harper JW, Elledge SJ, Leder P. Mice lacking p21CIP1/WAF1 undergo normal development, but are defective in G1 checkpoint control. Cell 1995; 82(4): 675-84.

[65]   Bunz F, Dutriaux A, Lengauer C, et al. Requirement for p53 and p21 to sustain G2 arrest after DNA damage. Science 1998; 282(5393): 1497-501.

[66]   Joerger AC, Fersht AR. Structural biology of the tumor suppressor p53. Annu Rev Biochem 2008; 77: 557-82. Review.

[67]   Galaktionov K, Chen X, Beach D. Cdc25 cell-cycle phosphatase as a target of c-myc. Nature 1996; 82: 511-7.

[68]   Bond GL, Hu W, Bond EE, et al. A single nucleotide polymorphism in the MDM2 promoter attenuates the p53 tumor suppressor pathway and accelerates tumor formation in humans. Cell 2004; 119(5): 591-602.

[69] Momand J, Zambetti GP, Olson DC, George D, Levine AJ. The mdm-2 oncogene product forms a complex with the p53 protein and inhibits p53-mediated transactivation. Cell 1992; 69(7): 1237-45.

[70] Tommasino M, Crawford L. Human papillomavirus E6 and E7: proteins which deregulate the cell cycle. Bioessays 1995; 17: 509-18.

[71] Wang XW. Role of p53 and apoptosis in carcinogenesis. Anticancer Res 1999; 19: 4759-771.

[72] Arrowsmith CH. Structure and function in the p53 family. Cell Death Differ 1999; 6: 1169-73.

[73] May P, May E. Twenty years of p53 research: structural and functional aspects of the p53 protein. Oncogene 1999; 18: 7621-36.

[74] Schmitt CA, Fridman JS, Yang M, *et al.* A senescence program controlled by p53 and p16INK4a contributes to the outcome of cancer therapy. Cell 2002; 109(3): 335-46.

[75] Ho J, Benchimol S. Transcriptional repression mediated by the p53 tumour suppressor. Cell Death Differ 2003; 10(4): 404-8. Review.

[76] Murphy ME, Leu JI, George DL. p53 moves to mitochondria: a turn on the path to apoptosis. Cell Cycle 2004; 3(7): 836-9. Review.

[77] Innocente SA, Abrahamson JL, Cogswell JP, Lee JM. p53 regulates a G2 checkpoint through cyclin B1. Proc Natl Acad Sci USA 1999; 96(5): 2147-52.

[78] Patel S, Player MR. Small-molecule inhibitors of the p53-HDM2 interaction for the treatment of cancer. Expert Opin Investig Drugs 2008: 1865-82.

[79] Vazquez A, Bond EE, Levine AJ, Bond GL. The genetics of the p53 pathway, apoptosis and cancer therapy. Nat Rev Drug Discov 2008: 979-87.

[80] Karin M, Cao Y, Greten FR, Li ZW. NFκB in cancer: from innocent bystander to major culprit. Nat Rev Can 2002: 2: 301-10.

[81] Dey A, Tergaonkar V, Lane DP. Double-edged swords as cancer therapeutics: simultaneously targeting p53 and NF kappaB pathways. Nat Rev Drug Discov 2008: 1031-40.

[82] Miyoshi H, Nagase H, Ando A, *et al.* Somatic Mutations Of The Apc Gene in colorectal tumors: mutation cluster region in the APC gene. Hum Mol Genet 1992; 1: 229-33.

[83] Smith KJ, Johnson KA, Bryan TM, *et al.* The Apc Gene Product In Normal And Tumor Cells. Proc Natl Acad Sci 1993; 90: 2846-50.

[84] Powell SM, Zilz N, Beazer-Barclay Y, *et al.* Apc Mutations Occur Early During Colorectal Tumorigenesis. Nature 1992; 359: 235-7.

[85] Korinek V, Barker N, Morin PJ, *et al.* Constitutive Transcriptional Activation By A Beta-Catenin-Tcf Complex In Apc-/- Colon Carcinoma. Science 1997; 275: 1784-7.

[86] Morin PJ, Sparks, Korinek V, *et al.* Activation of beta-catenin-Tcf signaling in colon cancer by mutations in beta-catenin or APC. Science 1997; 275: 1787-90.

[87] Aberle H, Bauer A, Stappert J, Kispert A, Kemler R. betacatenin is a target for the ubiquitin-proteasome pathway. EMBO J 1997; 16: 3797-804.

[88] Behrens J, Von Kries JP, Kuhl M, *et al.* Functional interaction of betacatenin with the transcription factor LEF-1. Nature 1996; 382: 638-42.

[89] Nelson WJ, Nusse R. Convergence of Wnt, beta-catenin and cadherin pathways. Science 2004:1483-7

[90] Rubinfeld B, Albert P, Porfiri E, Fiol C, Munemitsu S, Polakis P. Binding of GSK3beta to the APC-beta-catenin complex and regulation of complex assembly. Science 1996; 272: 1023-6.

[91] Jeanes A, Gottardi CJ, Yap AS. Caherins and cancer: how does cadherin dysfunction promote tumor progression? Oncogene 2008; 27(55): 6920-9.

[92] Ballester R, Marchuk D, Boguski M, *et al.* The NF1 locus encodes a protein functionally related to mammalian GAP and yeast IRA proteins. Cell 1990; 63: 851-9.

[93] Shelton BP, Misso NL, Shaw OM, Arthaningtyas E, Bhoola KD. Epigentic regulation of human epithelial cell cancers. Curr Opin Mol Ther 2008: 568-8.

[94] Gronbaek K, Treppendahl M, Asmar F, Gulberg P. Epigenetic changes in cancer as potential targets for prophylaxis and maintenance therapy. Basic Clin Pharmacol Toxicol 2008: 389-96.

[95] Gopalakrishnan S, Van Emburgh BO, Robertson KD. DNA methylation in development and human disease. Mutat Res 2008; 647(1-2): 30-8.

[96] Singh SK, Clarke ID, Terasaki M, *et al.* Identification of a cancer stem cell in human brain tumors. Cancer Res 2003; 63(18): 5821-8.

[97] Malanchi I, Huelsken J. Cancer stem cells: never Wnt away from the niche. Curr Opin Oncol 2009:41-6.

[98] Ischenko I, Seeliger H, Schaffer M, Jauch KW, Bruns CJ. Cancer stem cells: how can we target them? Curr Med Chem 2008: 3171-84.

[99] Ambler CA, Maatta A. Epidermal stem cells: location, potential and contribution to cancer. J. Pathol 2009; 217(2): 206-16.

[100] Singh P, Mittal A. Current status of COX-2 inhibitors. Mini Rev Med Chem 2008; 8(1):73-90.

[101] Reddy RN, Mutyala R, Aparoy P, Reddanna P, Reddy MR. Computer aided drug design approaches to develop cyclooxygenase based novel anti-inflammatory and anti-cancer drugs. Curr Pharm Des 2007; 13(34): 3505-17.

[102] Surh YJ, Kundu JK. Cancer preventive phytochemicals as speed breakers in inflammatory signaling involved in aberrant COX-2 expression. Curr Cancer Drug Targets 2007; 7(5): 447-58.

[103] Howe LR. Inflammation and breast cancer. Cyclooxygenase/ prostaglandin signaling and breast cancer. Breast Cancer Res 2007; 9(4): 210-7.

[104] Harris RE. Cyclooxygenase-2 (cox-2) and the inflammogenesis of cancer. Subcell Biochem 2007; 42: 93-126.

CHAPTER 4

Epigenetics of Cancer

Claudia M. García-Cuellar[1,*] and Alfonso Dueñas-González[1,2]

[1]*Subdirección de Investigación Básica, Instituto Nacional de Cancerología, Mexico City, Mexico and* [2]*Unidad de Investigación Biomédica en Cáncer, Instituto Nacional de Cancerología/Instituto de Investigaciones Biomédicas (INCan/IIB), Universidad Nacional Autónoma de México (UNAM). Mexico City, Mexico*

Abstract: In most cancers, a number of epigenetic alterations occur during all stages of carcinogenesis. These include global DNA hypomethylation, hypermethylation of key tumor suppressor genes, and histone modifications. Unlike genetic alterations, which are almost impossible to reverse, epigenetic aberrations are potentially reversible, allowing the malignant cell population to revert to a more normal state. With the advent of numerous drugs that target specific enzymes involved in the epigenetic regulation of gene expression, the utilization of epigenetic targets is emerging as an effective and valuable approach to chemotherapy. This revision is an overview of general epigenetic aspects involved in cancer and the potential utilization of drugs with effects in epigenetic targets that could be useful in cancer therapy.

Keywords: Epigenetics, chromatin, DNA methylation, histone modifications, histone deacetylases epigenetic therapy, Hydralazine.

INTRODUCTION

Cancer is defined as a heterogeneous group of cellular disorders, with marked and different biological characteristics in which abnormal cells divide without control and are able to invade other tissues. Advances in cancer clinical and basic research have identified the participation of genetic changes in tumor development, as well the characterization of some epigenetic alterations. The identification of epigenetic modification that occurs in almost all cancer types represents a popular point of view that is emerging in the understanding of tumor biology. The scenario of epigenetic alteration in pathologies such as cancer, and the knowledge related to the interconnection of different factors that conform the network of diverse molecular participants in the carcinogenic mechanism have allowed for the creation of specific deregulation profiles associated with each cancer type. This has had an important impact on the development of new therapies that could modify epigenetic alterations in cancerous cells.

Since its discovery in 1983, the epigenetics of human cancer has been in the shadows of human cancer genetics, but today, it is the epicenter of modern medicine because it can help explain the relationship between an individual's genetic background, the environment, aging, and disease. It can do so because the epigenetic state varies among tissues and throughout a lifetime, whereas the DNA sequence remains essentially the same [1]. The observation that cancer cells suffer profound alterations in the DNA methylation profile, with functional consequences in the activity of key genes, together with the recognition that epigenetic alterations might be as important as genetic defects in the origin of cancers, has started a new era in cancer research [2]. It is now clear that epigenetic alterations are as important, if not more important than the genetic ones. Therefore, there is an urgent need to have a more comprehensive characterization of the epigenetic changes that occur in cancer cells to maximize the potential of therapeutic approaches targeting the epigenome The epigenome is modulated at several distinct levels that can involve chemical modifications to DNA, such as methylation, nucleosome remodeling, or covalent post-transcriptional modifications in the proteins that are closely associated with DNA (the histones, which form the cores of chromatin packaging and provide a scaffold for the chromatin structure) or incorporation of histone variants; a prominent role for non-coding RNAs (nc-RNA) is also emerging [3]. Clearly, the regulation of the chromatin structure is a complex and dynamic process and there is still very much to study and understand. It is well known

*Address correspondence to Claudia M. García-Cuellar:** Instituto Nacional de Cancerología, Subdirección de Investigación Básica, San Fernando No. 22, Tlalpan, 14080 Mexico City, Mexico; Tel: (+52-55) 5628-0462; Fax: (+52-55) 5628-0432; E-mail: claudia.garciac@salud.gob.mx

Javier Camacho (Ed)

that genes are more than their sequences, and in this context, epigenetics is typically defined as the study of mitotically and/or meiotically heritable variations in gene expression that are not due to changes in DNA sequence [4]. Each cell type has it own epigenetic signature, the epigenome. The genome and the epigenome together determine the phenotype, and hence, the function of diverse biological properties can be affected by epigenetic mechanisms. Functionally, epigenetic marks act to regulate gene expression and function as a memory imprint of past or current expression. Epigenetic changes are crucial for the development and differentiation of the various cell types in an organism, as well as for normal cellular processes, such as X-chromosome inactivation in female mammals; however, the epigenetic state can become disrupted by environmental influences, such as toxic compounds, toxins, nutrients, and drugs, or during aging, all of which can affect specific gene expression patterns. The importance of epigenetic changes in the development of a wide range of complexes, often age-related diseases including cancer and other diseases, is increasingly being appreciated [5].

CHROMATIN ORGANIZATION AND EPIGENETIC CONTROL OF NUCLEAR ARCHITECTURE

Chromatin is the physiologically relevant substrate for all genetic and epigenetic processes inside the nuclei of eukaryotic cells. Dynamic changes in the local and global organization of chromatin are emerging as key regulators of genomic function. Indeed, a multitude of signals from outside and inside the cell converge on this gigantic signaling platform. Numerous post-translational modifications of histones, the main protein components of chromatin, have been documented and analyzed in detail. These 'marks' appear to crucially mediate the functional activity of the genome in response to upstream signaling pathways. Different layers of crosstalk between several components of this complex regulatory system are emerging [6]. The increasing scientific amount of data obtained in recent years also shows that our DNA, chromosomes, and nuclear structure are not a random event occurring in the cell. There is a delicate superstructure of large chromatin domains, chromosomal territories, and sub-nuclear compartments that require reliable, yet, at the same time, dynamic caretakers. Perhaps the most direct indication of the role of nuclear architecture in gene function is in the disease state, which is often characterized by altered gene expression patterns associated with aberrant nuclear morphologies, or vice versa. An immediate example is cancer. Many cancer cell types exhibit gross alterations of the nuclear architecture in the form of spatial organization changes, chromatin and chromosome domain textures, nuclear size and shape alterations, and changes in the number and size of nucleoli. In fact, morphological abnormalities of the nuclear compartments are used as key diagnostic features for many cancer types [7]. The mammalian genome is organized and packaged into chromatin, a highly compact and structured complex of DNA and proteins that can adopt different tridimensional conformations depending on the nuclear context and biochemical modifications present both in DNA and histones [8]. A simplified view of chromatin recognizes two basic states: an open, transcriptionally competent euchromatin and a more condensed, transcriptionally silent heterochromatin. Besides those structural regions of the genome that present constitutive chromatin (essentially found at centromeres), other genomic regions can undergo transitions between a more open conformation and a more compact, facultative heterochromatin; these transitions are vital to set the different transcription patterns [8]. The nucleosome is the basic unit of chromatin [9]. In detail, its structure is 147 base pairs of double stranded DNA wrapped around the surface of an octamer of histone proteins consisting of a central $(H3-H4)_2$ tetramer that is flanked on either side by two H2A-H2B dimmers [10, 11]. Epigenetic marks, such as DNA methylation [12] and histone modifications [13], are excellent candidates to assume this critical role (Fig. **1**). A tight association between nucleosomes and DNA results in chromatin condensation, with consequent suppression of gene expression [14]. Acetylation of lysine residues in external tails of histones H3 and/or H4 tends to reduce the interaction between DNA and nucleosomes, which, in turn, allows for the access of various transcription factors to the DNA [15]. Histone tail acetylation of lysine residues is carried out by histone acetyltransferases (HATs) [16], whereas histone deacetylases (HDACs) have the ability to remove the acetyl group from lysine residues [16]. The effect of histone tails methylation enhances the binding affinity of the nucleosome for DNA, which is an anionic macromolecule [17, 18]. This results in a tighter association between nucleosomes and genomic DNA, which has a propensity to confer a non-permissive configuration for gene expression [19-21]. However, histone tails methylation does not always suppress transcription. In fact, histone tails methylation can have differential effects on gene expression, depending on the position of the methylated lysine residue [16]. For instance, methylation of lysine 9 in histone H3 (H3-K9) and/or lysine 27 in histone H3 (H3-K27) is associated with a suppression of transcriptional activity, whereas methylation of H3-K4 has a correlation with activation of transcription [21]. Histone tails methylation is removed by a histone demethylase (LSD1, alias BHC110 or p110) [22, 23]. Polycomb Group (PcG) proteins, which were initially described to play an essential role in long-term gene silencing in Drosophila, have also been shown to be involved in gene silencing in mammalian cancer cells. PcG proteins are classified into two groups, Polycomb Repressive Complex 2 (PRC2), which is involved in the initiation of gene repression, and Polycomb Repressive Complex 1 (PRC1), which acts as a "maintenance" complex. EZH2 (Enhancer of Zeste homolog 2), a member of PRC2, catalyses the addition of methyl groups to H3K27 (H3K27 trimethylation). EZH2 also interacts with DNMTs and is essential for DNA methylation of EZH2-target promoters, suggesting that there is a direct link between PcG-mediated gene repression and DNA methylation [24-26].

Epigenetic modifications affect the arrangement in gene expression through two main mechanisms: methylation of CpG rich islands present in the genomic DNA [27, 28] and methylation and/or acetylation of histones H3 and H4 [29, 30]. The methylation of cytosine residues in CpG motifs can silence a promoter by displacing transcription factors and consequently, RNA polymerase II complexes [27]. To date, four types of DNA methyltransferases (DNMT) have been identified: DNMT1, DNMT3a, DNMT3b, and DNMT3L [31]. Histones H3 and H4 methylation and/or acetylation occur in lysine or arginine residues in the amino terminus of histonic tails [32]. DNA methylation and histone H3 and H4 methylation and/or acetylation induce chromatin remodeling. Histones form nucleosomes, which are wrapped by chromosomal DNA.

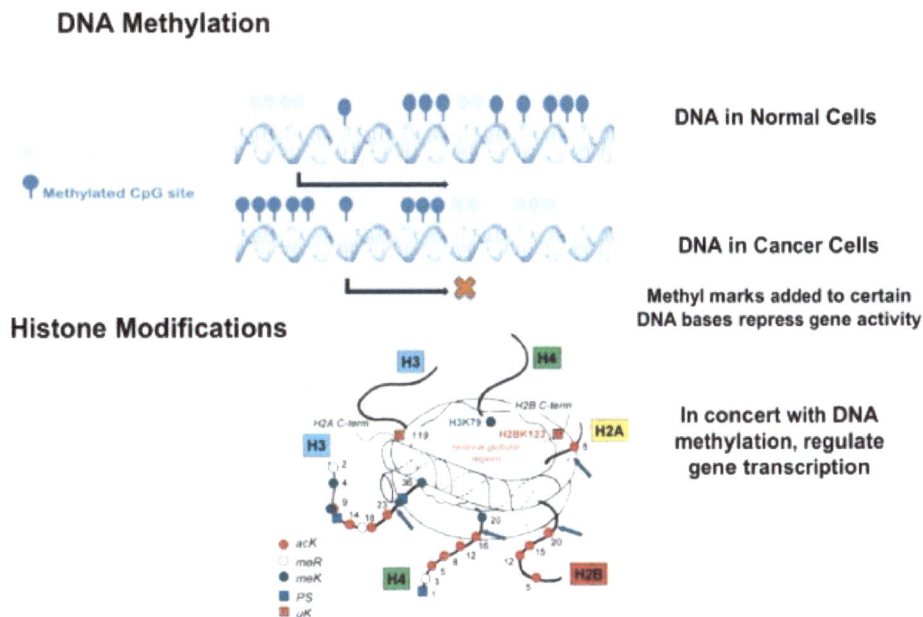

Figure 1: The main components of the epigenetic code

DNA METHYLATION

DNA methylation was the first epigenetic alteration to be observed in cancer cells [33]. Their involvement in cancer has become one of the hottest topics in cancer research. A major breakthrough in the field within the last ten years has been the recognition of the key role of chromatin as a mediator between DNA methylation and transcriptional silencing of genes relevant to cancer [2]. Considerable efforts have been expended in the area of DNA methylation during recent decades. Neoplasia is known to be epigenetically characterized by global DNA demethylation as well-localized hypomethylation and hypermethylation of specific genes [34]. Cytosine methylation at CpG dinucleotides is the most common modification of eukaryotic genomes. In vertebrates, methylation occurs globally throughout the genome, with the exception of CpG islands (CG-rich regions of DNA stretchings). Over the past 20 years, an increasing number of cancers have been found to be associated with aberrant patterns of methylation, in particular, global genomic hypomethylation [35] and localized hypermethylation in normally unmethylated CpG islands [36].

DNA HYPOMETHYLATION IN TUMORS

Global and focal hypomethylation is an important characteristic of neoplasias. The low level of DNA methylation in tumors, as compared with the level of DNA methylation in their normal-tissue counterparts, was one of the first epigenetic alterations to be found in human cancer [37]. During the development of a neoplasm, the degree of hypomethylation of genomic DNA increases as the lesion progresses from a benign proliferation of cells to an invasive cancer. It is clear that the genome-wide loss of 5-methylcytosine is a molecular hallmark associated with the acquisition of a transformed phenotype [38]. Observed levels of hypomethylation vary widely within and between different cancer types, as can the timing of demethylation in relation to disease stage and grade. DNA hypomethylation can be indicative of the early stage of disease for some cancer types or of later stage disease, poor prognosis, and heightened malignancy in others [34]. Global hypomethylation appears to be an early event for colon and breast cancer, as well as for chronic lymphocytic leukemia [34]. For colon cancer, hypomethylation can also be observed in the healthy tissue adjacent to tumors, suggesting a role in the initiation of the disease [39]. For other cancers, including hepatocellular carcinoma, the degree of hypomethylation increases with stage or histological grade [40]. Thus, the relative timing of global demethylation and its role during cancer initiation and progression may differ between cancer types. Gene-specific hypomethylation occurs frequently in a range of cancers, including cancers of the colon [41, 42] and breast cancer [43]. Demethylation of specific genes often correlates well with increased transcription levels [44]. Few studies have investigated an association of focal demethylation with global hypomethylation [45-47]. There are three proposed mechanisms to explain the contribution of DNA hypomethylation to the development of a cancer cell: generation of chromosomal activity, reactivation of transposable elements, and loss of imprinting [48]; however, the importance of this change for human tumorigenesis remains as an open question.

HYPERMETHYLATION IN TUMOURS

Aberrant promoter hypermethylation is a prevalent phenomenon in human cancers. Tumor suppressor genes are often hypermethylated due to the increased activity or deregulation of DNMTs. Increasing evidence also reveals that viral genes are one of the key players in regulating DNA methylation. The importance of epigenetic processes in the development of cancer is clear. The study of epigenetics is therefore bound to contribute to the improvement of human health. Aberrations in DNA methylation, post-translational modifications of histones, chromatin remodeling, and microRNAs patterns are the main epigenetic alterations, and these are associated with tumorigenesis. Epigenetic technologies in cancer studies are helping to increase the number of cancer candidate genes and allow us to examine changes in 5-methylcytosine DNA and histone modifications at a genome-wide level. In fact, epigenetic genes in cancer affect all the various cellular pathways contributing to the neoplastic phenotype. They are being explored as biomarkers in clinical use for early detection of disease, tumor classification and response to treatment with classical chemotherapy agents, target compounds, and epigenetic drugs. Encouraging results have been obtained with histone deacetylase and DNA methyltransferase inhibitors, leading the US Food and Drug Administration to approve several of them for the treatment of hematological malignancies and lymphoproliferative disorders, such as myelodysplastic syndrome and cutaneous lymphoma. However, many tasks remain, such as the clinical validation of epigenetic biomarkers to allow the accurate prediction of the outcome of cancer patients and their potential chemosensitivity to current pharmacological treatments. The observation that cancer cells suffer profound alterations in the DNA methylation profile, with functional consequences in the activity of key genes, together with the recognition that epigenetic alterations might be as important as genetic defects in the origin of cancers, has started a new era in cancer research. In just a few years, key discoveries have abruptly changed our vision of the determinants of cancer. Breakthroughs in the cancer epigenetics field include the finding of a tumor-type specificity of genes that suffer epigenetic deregulation at both DNA methylation and histone modifications, the interconnection between different epigenetic marks, the identification of mechanisms of targeting of epigenetic alterations, including the participation of Polycomb group (PcG) proteins, and the involvement of small RNAs, which regulate hundreds of target genes. All of these findings have multiple implications. First, they shed light on the mechanistic insights by which epigenetic defects complement genetic alterations in the development and progression of cancer. Second, epigenetic alterations appear to play a prominent role in the initiation of cancer. In addition, because epigenetic changes are reversible, enzymes involved in their maintenance stand as targets for a variety of compounds for therapy.

HISTONE COVALENT MODIFICATIONS

Core histone proteins are evolutionarily conserved and consist mainly of flexible amino-terminal tails protruding outward from the nucleosome and globular carboxy-terminal domains making up the nucleosome scaffold. Histones function as acceptors for a variety of post-translational modifications [6]. Distinct histone amino-terminal tails and globular domains are subject to a vast array modifications, such as methylation of arginine (R), methylation, acetylation, ubiquitination, ADP-ribosylation, and sumoilation of lysines (K). Phosphorylation of serines (S) and threonines (T) can generate synergistic or antagonistic interaction affinities for chromatin-associated proteins, which, in turn, dictate dynamic transitions between transcriptionally active or transcriptionally silent chromatin states [49]. Extra complexity comes partly from the fact that methylation on lysines of arginines may be one of three different forms: mono-, di-, or trimethyl for lysines, and mono- or di- (asymmetric or symmetric) for arginines. This vast array of modifications gives enormous potential for functional responses, but it must be remembered that not all modifications will be on the same histone at the same time. The timing of the appearance of a modification will depend on the signaling conditions within the cell [50]. The combinatorial nature of histone amino-terminal modifications thus reveals a "histone code" that considerably extends the information potential of the genetic code [51]. The histone code influences higher-order chromatin structures by affecting contacts between different histones and between histones and DNA [52]. Specific histone modifications are responsible for the compartmentalization of the genome into distinct domains, such as transcriptionally silent heterochromatin and transcriptionally active euchromatin. The ability of the histone code to dictate the chromatin environment allows it to regulate nuclear processes, such as replication, transcription, DNA repair, and chromosome condensation [50]. These patterns can be altered by multiple extracellular and intracellular stimuli, and chromatin itself has been proposed to serve as a signaling platform and to function as a genomic integrator of various signaling pathways [53].

HISTONE LYSINE ACETYLATION

Histone acetylation is a modification in highly dynamic histones and consisting in the transfer of an acetyl group from acetyl-CoA to the ε-NH$_2$ of the amino acid side chain of lysine residues, and is usually carried out by a variety of histone acetyltransferase (HATs) complexes. The initial functional hypothesis of the role of a hyperacetylation state was that this state provides a more open chromatin structure correlating with gene transcription. This was supported by the physicochemical environment produced due to reduced ionic interaction of the positively charged histone tails with the negatively charged DNA backbone and reduced internucleosomal interactions [54]. Therefore, inhibitors of histone deacetylases (HDACs) are considered as candidate drugs for cancer therapy. Histone deacetylase inhibitors alter histone acetylation and chromatin structures, which modulates gene expression, as well as promoting the acetylation of non-histone proteins [55]. Broadly, acetylation of histones is linked to transcriptional activation, and histone acetylation is able to recruit many bromodomain-containing transcriptional co-activators and mediators. Histone acetylation is also linked to other cellular functions, including DNA replication and repair and chromatin assembly [56]. Therefore, it is not surprising that many of the enzymes responsible for acetylation of histones at different residues were first known as transcriptional co-activators and later as enzymes. Most histone acetyltransferases take part in huge multiprotein complexes involved in locus targeting, thus providing chromosomal domain specificity in addition to the substrate specificity displayed by each individual acetyltransferase. The opposing effects of HATs and HDACs govern the acetylating status of chromatin. Disturbance of this balance through the disruption of HAT or HDAC activity can lead to cancer [56]. There are three main families of HATs: the Gcn5-related N-acetyltransferase (GNAT) family, the MOZ/YBF2/SAS2/TIP60 (MYST) family, and the CBP/p300 family. These HATs, forming multisubunit complexes, acetylate, with poor specificity, multiple lysine sites in the core histones and primarily promote active transcription. They also acetylate several non-histone proteins, such as p53, pRb and E2F, and modulate their transcriptional activities on target genes [50]. HDACs remove the acetyl groups from histone lysine tails and are thought to facilitate transcriptional repression by decreasing the level of histone acetylation. Like HATs, HDACs also have non-histone targets, such as p53, E2F, and TFIIF [57]. The 18 HDACs identified to date can be categorized into four classes: class I (HDAC1-3, HDAC8), class II (HDAC4-7, 9-10), class III (sirtuin 1-7) and class IV.

HISTONE METHYLATION

Nucleosomal histones can be methylated *in vivo* at multiple residues and defined methylation patterns are related to distinct functional readouts of chromosomal DNA. Histone methylation has emerged as an important post-translational modification involved in transcriptional regulation and genome integrity. Recent progress in determining the cis and trans determinants of this process revealed multiple roles for histone methylation in epigenetic memory of active and silent states [58]. The analysis of imprinted, X-linked, and heterochromatic sequences disclosed mechanistic similarities for heritable transcriptional repression, pointing to a common mode of action. Moreover, the view of histone methylation as a stable modification has recently been challenged by studies revealing a number of pathways that are capable of removing histone methylation [59, 60]. Thus, in addition to having great *in vivo* complexity, this modification appears more dynamic than was previously thought. Three distinct classes of histone demethylases have now been recognized. The first class includes PADI4 (petidylarginine deiminase 4), which functions by converting a methyl-lysine to citrulline. The second class includes LSD1 (lysine-specific demethylase 1), which can reverse histone H3K4 and H3K9 modifications by an oxidative demethylation reaction. The third class of demethylases, and the largest so far, includes Jumonji C (JmjC) domain, containing histone demethylases (JHDMs), which, unlike LSD1, are capable of demethylating all three methylated states (mono-, di-and tri-methylated lysine). So far, JHDMs have been shown to demethylate H3K36 (JHDM1), H3K9 (JHDM2A) and H3K9/K27 (JHDM3 and JMJD2A-D) [61].

HISTONE SERINE PHOSPHORYLATION

In addition to regulating transcription, chromatin remodeling also regulates many non-transcriptional cellular processes, including DNA-damage repair, cell cycle checkpoints, chromosomal stability, and apoptosis, mechanisms with connections to oncogenesis. Evidences indicate that histone serine phosphorylation is a crucial event in the DNA damage repair regulation, chromosome stability, and apoptosis [56, 62]. DNA damage repair is one of the most important mechanisms for maintaining the genome and preventing tumorigenesis [63]; the phosphorylation at serine 139 in the C-terminal H2A.X, a variant of the H2A histone, has been shown to play important roles in DNA double strand break (DSB) repair and tumor suppression. DSBs stalled replication forks and led to rapid H2A.X phosphorylation (γ-H2A.X) in chromatin regions, flanking these DSBs mediated by the phosphatidylinositol 3-kinase-like kinases (ATM, ATR, and DNA-PK), and defects in these kinases usually result in cancer predisposition [63, 64]. Increased aneuploidy has been linked to high tumor grade, advanced stage of cancer, and poor prognosis. Aberrant expression of HP1 proteins, a highly conserved family of eukaryotic proteins that bind to methylated histone H3 lysine 9 (H3K9) and are required for heterochromatic gene silencing [65], can lead to aneuploidy. Aurora-kinase-B phosphorylation of H3 serine 10 might act as a "phos-methyl switch," resulting in dissociation of HP1 from heterochromatin while maintaining H3K9 methylation during mitosis [56]. Thus, dynamic phosphorylation of H3 serine 10 by Aurora kinase B during mitosis plays an integral part in maintaining chromosome stability [66].

AN EPIGENETIC ROLE FOR RNA

RNA can also be regarded as an epigenetic component involved in chromatin regulation. The interference RNA (RNAi) pathway is also linked to chromatin structure; disruption of components of the RNAi machinery affects the formation of heterochromatin. Whether these processes can be directly linked to cancer remains to be determined [67]. However, in the case of micro RNA (miRNA), the link is strong [68]. MicroRNAs (miRNAs) have an important role in cancer and metastasis and are also regulated by epigenetic mechanisms in malignancies [69]. By virtue of having multiple targets, a microRNA (miRNA) can have variable effects on oncogenesis by acting as tumor suppressor or oncogene in a context-dependent manner. Genome-wide epigenetic changes that occur in various cancers affect the transcription of many genes. Since the transcriptional regulation of miRNAs remains an unexplored field, it is still unknown how epigenetic changes will affect the regulation of miRNAs. Many miRNAs are intron-bound within the body of a protein-coding gene. Any change to the transcription of the gene affects the transcription and genesis of the resident miRNA [70]. Micro RNAs affect the expression of genes linked to the cell cycle (*e.g.*, down-regulation of E2F1), and expression of miRNAs is altered in cancer cells [71]. Furthermore, miRNA profiling has proved to be a very useful aid for classifying different cancer types [71].

EPIGENETIC ALTERATIONS IN TUMOURS

Many studies have explored the mosaic patterns of DNA methylation and histone modification in cancer cells on a gene-by-gene basis. Recent studies indicate that epigenetic alterations might initiate the expansion of pre-malignant cells during the early stages of tumorigenesis. During the earliest steps of development of principal tumor types, such as colon [72-74], lung [75-78], and prostate [79] tumors, early epigenetic changes that occur in these cells might determine the subsequent genetic changes and thereby foster progression of these clones [80]. The most frequent genes that undergo aberrant CpG island methylation in human cancer, including stomach [81], colon [82], liver [83], cervix [84], breast [85], prostate [86], and hematologic malignancies [87], among others, are included in Table **1**. These genes affect cellular pathways such as cell cycle, p53 network, APC/β-catenin/E-cadherin pathways, DNA repair, hormonal response, cytokine signaling, and apoptotic and detoxifier pathways, among others, and have relevant consequences altering the expression on their regulated genes [88-90].

CLINIC IMPLICATIONS FOR EPIGENETICS

The initiation and progression of cancer is controlled by both genetic and epigenetic events. Unlike genetic alterations, which are almost impossible to reverse, epigenetic aberrations are potentially reversible, allowing the malignant cell population to revert to a more normal state. With the use of numerous drugs that target specific enzymes involved in the epigenetic regulation of gene expression, the utilization of epigenetic targets is emerging as an effective and valuable approach to chemotherapy [91]. A better understanding of tumor host biology has led to improvements in the multidisciplinary management of cancer, and traditional pathologic evaluation is being complemented by more sophisticated genomic approaches.

Table 1: Selected list of genes with CpG hypermethylation in human cancer

Gene	Function	Tumor Profile	Consequences
p16^{ink4a}	Cyclin-dependent kinase inhibitor	Multiple type	Entrance in cell cycle
p14^{ARF}	MDM2 inhibitor	Colon, stomach, kidney	Degradation of p53
hMLH1	DNA mismatch repair	Colon, endometrium, stomach	Frameshift mutations
GSTP1	Conjugation to glutathione	Prostate, breast, kidney	Adduct accumulation
BRCA1	DNA repair, transcription	Breast, ovary	Double-strand breaks
ER	Estrogen receptor	Breast	Hormone insensitivity
PR	Progesterone receptor	Breast	Hormone insensitivity
AR	Androgen receptor	Prostate	Hormone insensitivity
RAR2	Retinoic acid receptor	Colon, lung, head and neck	Vitamin insensitivity
Rb	Cell cycle inhibitor	Retinoblastoma	Entrance in cell cycle
CDH1	Cell cycle, adhesion	Breast, stomach, leukemia	Dissemination
APC	Inhibitor of catenin	Aerodigestive tract	Activation of catenin route
COX2	Cyclooxigenase	Colon, stomach	Anti-inflammatory resistance
SOCS1	Inhibitor of JAK/STAT	Liver, myeloma	JAK2 activation
DAPK	Pro-apoptotic	Breast	Resistance to apoptosis

A number of genomic biomarkers have been developed for clinical use, and increasingly, pharmacokinetic end points are being incorporated into clinical trial design. When an individual is diagnosed with cancer, prognostic or predictive information is most useful when coupled with targeted therapeutic approaches. The immediate challenge is to learn how to use the molecular characteristics of an individual and their tumor to improve detection and treatment, and ultimately, to prevent the development of cancer. Over the last two decades, preclinical and clinical research has implicated epigenetic alterations in the pathogenesis and progression of cancer. Epigenetic changes, involving both DNA methylation and alterations in chromatin structure, are associated with the inhibition of transcription of key cell regulatory genes that, under normal conditions, control the cell cycle and initiate apoptotic cell death in neoplastic cells. Drugs have been developed with functional effects, including DNA hypomethylation and histone acetylation, that serve to restore the normal transcription of cell regulatory genes (*e.g.*, tumor suppressor genes) [92-97].

EPIGENETIC THERAPY

Like many other tumors, breast carcinomas exhibit a number of epigenetic alterations that lead to the silencing of over 100 individual genes [85]. For instances, BRCA1 is commonly found silenced by promoter hypermethylation in sporadic breast and ovarian cancer [98]. Another example of a genetically and epigenetically regulated gene is cyclin-dependent kinase inhibitor 2A, responsible for maintaining the retinoblastoma protein in an active and non-phosphorylated state in the cyclin D-Rb pathway. Its silencing leads to loss of cell cycle control [99]. The fact that transcriptional silencing of tumor suppressor genes by DNA methylation and histone deacetylation are two key events in tumor progression led to the formulation of so-called epigenetic drugs for the treatment of cancer. Currently, epigenetic drugs essentially fall in two categories: inhibitors of DNMT to remove aberrant patterns of DNA methylation [100], and inhibitors of HDACs (classes I, II, and IV), which are termed HDACi [101]. There are a vast number of preclinical studies testing the antitumor activity of these inhibitors either alone or in combination, as there is a marked synergy between DNMTi and HDACi to reactivate the expression of tumor suppressor genes [102-104]. An example of epigenetic enzymes that are approved or in evaluation as therapeutic targets are listed in Table **2**.

Table 2: Epigenetic enzymes approved or in evaluation as therapeutic targets

DNA Methylation
DNMT1, DNMT3A, DNMT3B, MBDPs
Histone Acetylation
HDACs Class I, II
HDACs Class III (Sirtuins)
Histone Methylation
G9a (H3K9 methylation)
EZH (H3K27 methylation)
Histone Demethylation
LSD1

Currently, there are two FDA-approved DNA methylation inhibitors for the treatment of myelodysplastic syndrome, 5-azacitidine and its analog 2′-deoxy-5-azacytidine. However, it is still undefined whether the activity of these agents, developed as classic cytotoxics, is due to their demethylating or cytotoxic activity. In fact, recent data provides evidence that the inhibition of proliferation of human cancer cells by 2′-deoxy-5-azacytidine is due to DNA damage as knocking-out DNMTs does not have antiproliferative effect [105]. Moreover, these agents are chemically unstable, carcinogenic, highly myelosuppressive, and exhibit poor activity against solid tumors [106] and marked myelosuppression when combined with cisplatin [107, 108]. Therefore, there is a high need for discovering DNA methylation inhibitors which could be used in solid tumors. Likewise, HDAC inhibitors are being assayed at present in solid tumors; to date, only one agent of this class –vorinostat- has been approved for cutaneous-T-cell lymphoma [109]. In Box 2, several epigenetic agents approved or in evaluation are shown. Although it is well-known that breast cancer exhibits a number of tumor suppressor genes silenced by methylation and that breast tumors may exhibit a methylator phenotype by the over-expression of DNMTs enzymes [110], no clinical trials of 5-azacitidine and its analog 2′-deoxy-5-azacytidine to exploit their demethylating activity have been performed in breast cancer. Likewise, early clinical studies of vorinostat in solid tumors are scarce, but so far, the antitumor activity of this HDACi against head and neck, ovarian, lung, and breast cancer has been limited or none at all [111]. This is intriguing, at least for breast cancer, which is a tumor that over-expresses HDACs [112, 113]. The activity of vorinostat and other HDACs is noticeable in preclinical studies of breast cancer [114].

Clinical Development of Epigenetic Therapy with Hydralazine and Valproate

In our research group, we are doing the preclinical and clinical development of an epigenetic therapy combination with a non-nucleoside DNA methylation inhibitor–hydralazine (Hyd) and the widely used antiepileptic magnesium valproate (MgV) as HDACi. The results of this development have been recently updated in a recent publication [97]. Concerning breast cancer, we have reported the results of a proof-of-principle single arm study of this therapy in locally advanced disease associated with doxorubicin-cyclophosphamide chemotherapy in a neoadjuvant setting. Patients were treated with a daily dose of a slow-release formulation of Hyd tablets containing either 182 mg for rapid-acetylators or 83 mg for slow-acetylators, and MgV tablets of 700 mg at a dose of 30 mg/Kb t.i.d. from day 7 until the last day of the fourth chemotherapy cycle. Sixteen patients were included. All patients were evaluated for clinical response and toxicity, and 14 patients were evaluated for pathological response. There were 5 (31%) clinical CR and 8 (50%) PR, for an overall RR of 81% and no one progressed. Among pathological responses, one (6.6%) had CR; however, in 70% of cases, the residual disease was <3 cm; 33% of cases had pathological negative lymph nodes, and no case had extranodal extension. The treatment was well-tolerated. The pharmacodynamic evaluation showed reduction in the 5^mC content from peripheral blood cells DNA as well as a reduction in HDAC activity. These effects were achieved at a mean concentration VPA of 87.5µg/mL. Microarray analysis in three patients revealed that the number of genes up- or down-regulated by at least a 3-fold difference was 1,091 and 89, respectively (GEO GSE6304) [115].

In another phase II, single-arm study, Hyd and MgV were added to the same schedule of chemotherapy on which patients were progressing. Primary sites included cervix (3), breast (3), lung (1), testis (1), and ovarian (7) carcinomas schedules comprised of cisplatin, carboplatin, paclitaxel, vinorelbine, gemcitabine, pemetrexed, topotecan, doxorubicin, cyclophosphamide, and anastrozol. Among 17 patients evaluable for toxicity and 15 for response, a clinical benefit was observed in 12 (80%) patients: four PR, and eight SD. The most significant toxicity was hematological [116]. In a third phase II study, the combination of MgV and Hyd was added to standard cisplatin chemoradiation in FIGO stage IIIB cervical cancer patients. Out of 18 patients evaluable for response, all had a clinical CR at the end of external radiation and no side-effects other than increased but manageable myelotoxicity. In this study, 10 pairs of tumor samples before and after MgV-Hyd could be analyzed for expression arrays. There were 964 significant up-regulated genes with a false discovery rate <5% (GEO Submissions (GSE8604) belonging to multiple pathways, including ribosomal proteins, oxidative phosphorylation, and MAPK signaling; focal adhesion, cell cycle, antigen processing and presentation, proteasome, apoptosis, PI3K signaling, Wnt signaling, calcium signaling, TGF-beta signaling, and ubiquitin-mediated proteolysis among others). A genome-wide screen for promoter methylation in these samples found 122 genes that became demethylated (and re-expressed) after treatment (manuscript in preparation). Currently, we are performing three randomized, placebo-controlled phase III trials in cervical, ovarian, and breast cancer. The preliminary analysis of the trial that started first (metastatic or recurrent cervical cancer) shows statistically significant differences in favor of the experimental arm (cisplatin-topotecan-Hyd-MgV) (cisplatin-topotecan-placebo, in control arm) in the progression-free survival which was the main endpoint of the study (ClinicalTrials.gov Identifier NCT00532818). With these results, we are looking for approval of TRANSKRIP R/L by the COFEPRIS (FDA equivalent) for its use with chemotherapy for metastatic, recurrent, or persistent cervical cancer.

Nevertheless, the clinical development of epigenetically targeted agents is considered to be in its infancy, as no predictive factors for response have consistently been found. Surrogate markers, such as global histone hyperacetylation, and global DNA methylation are still imperfect regarding their ability to predict response. In addition, the multiple layers of epigenetic regulation and the increasing number of epigenetic players coming to the scene in malignant tumors make it imperative to have a more comprehensive characterization of the epigenetic changes that occur in breast cancer cells to maximize the potential of epigenetic therapy.

Epigenetic Therapy: Beyond DNA Methylation and Class I-II-IV HDAC Inhibitors

There are other epigenetic players, which have a definitive role in the pathogenesis of cancer, such as inhibitors of the class III HDAC, also termed sirtuins. In contrast to class I/II/IV HDACi, the inhibitors of class III HDACs are much less validated as anticancer agents and, in general, less developed on the pharmacological side. Sirtuins play an important role in many cellular processes, such as gene silencing, regulation of transcription factors [*i.e.*, the tumor suppressor and sequence-specific DNA-binding transcription factor p53, the p53-related p73, p300 histone acetyltransferase (HAT), E2F1, NF-κB, and others], fatty acid metabolism, cell cycle regulation, and lifespan extension [117-120]. In particular, SIRT1-promoted deacetylation of p53 and p73, as well as E2F1, represses the expression of target genes inhibiting apoptosis, whereas deacetylation of BCL-6 increases its oncogenic activity [121, 122]. In addition, the anticancer action of SIRT inhibitors have been also reported to act *via* reactivation of methylated genes without evident DNA demethylation at the promoters level Pruitt *et al.*, 2006, #41835}. These findings, joined to the report that SIRT1 is upregulated in human lung cancer, prostate cancer, leukemia and breast cancer [123-126], highlight the potential anticancer use of SIRTi. Nicotinamide has been reported as an inhibitor of sirtuins [127].

Inhibitors of Histone Methylation

Histone Methyltransferases, such as EZH2, are able to silence genes that delay cell growth [128, 129]. Thus, HKMTs seem to be a valuable target for anticancer therapy. BIX-01294 was discovered through a HTS performed with 125,000 molecules, and selectively inhibits the G9a-mediated H3K9me2 (IC50 = 1.7 μM) *in vitro* and *in vivo*, giving significant reduction of promoter-proximal H3K9me2 marks in mouse ES cells and fibroblasts [130]. Although G9a has not directly been involved in tumorigenesis, treatment of cancer cells with DNMT and HDAC inhibitors, results in transcriptional stimulation that correlate with the removal of H3K9me2 — but not H3K9me3 — at the promoters of several tumor suppressor genes [131]. In addition, small interfering RNA (siRNA)-mediated knockdown of G9A and DNMT1 led to increased MASPIN expression in breast cancer cell line MDA-MB-231, to levels that were supra-additive, verifying the importance of these enzymes in maintaining multiple layers of epigenetic repression in breast tumor cells further supporting an important role for H3 K9 methylation in the aberrant repression of tumor suppressor genes in human cancer [132]. Thereby, G9a inhibitors may, in the future, find application in the cancer field [130].6

On the other hand, the S-adenosylhomocysteine hydrolase inhibitor 3-Deazaneplanocin A (DZNep) induces efficient apoptotic cell death in cancer cells, but not in normal cells by effectively depleting cellular levels of PRC2 components EZH2, SUZ12, and EED and inhibited associated H3K27 (but not H3K9 methylation). By integrating RNAi, genome-wide expression analysis, and ChIP, a prominent set of genes selectively repressed by PRC2 in breast cancer that can be reactivated by DZNep was identified. It has further shown the preferential reactivation of a set of these genes by DZNep, including a novel apoptosis effector, FBXO32, which contributes to DZNep-induced apoptosis in breast cancer cells. These results demonstrate the unique feature of DZNep as a novel chromatin remodeling compound and suggest that pharmacologic reversal of PRC2-mediated gene repression by DZNep may constitute a novel approach for cancer therapy [133]. Lysine-specific histone demethylase 1 (LSD1) is a FAD-dependent enzyme that catalyzes the oxidative removal of one or two methyl groups from H3K4. LSD1 takes part in a transcriptional repressor complex, with the repressor protein CoREST and HDAC1 or HDAC2, leading to gene silencing [134]. LSD1 has been found upregulated in certain high-risk tumors [56, 135], thus, the development of LSD1 inhibitors may represent a significant weapon against cancer. To date, tranylcypromine, which is a well-known anti-MAO agent, has been described as LSD1 inhibitor [136, 137], however, no data are available about their effects in cancer. Recent data, however, points out the potential anticancer actions of LSD1 inhibitors. Polyamine analogues are potent inhibitors of LSD1 and by doing this in human colon carcinoma cells lead to the re-expression of multiple, aberrantly silenced genes important in the development of colon cancer. Furthermore, it has been demonstrated by ChIP analysis that the reexpression is concurrent with increased H3K4me2 and acetyl-H3K9 marks, and decreased H3K9me1 and H3K9me2 repressive marks. Thus, LSD1 inhibitors define important new agents for reversing aberrant repression of gene transcription (71) [138].

Targeted Cancer Therapy

Currently, there are successful examples of this newer drug discovery approach. Most of the target-specific agents only provide small gains in symptom control and/or survival, whereas others have consistently failed in the clinical testing. There is, however, a characteristic shared by these agents: their high cost. This is expected as drug discovery and development are generally carried out within the commercial, rather than the academic realm. An alternative drug development strategy is the exploitation of established drugs that have already been approved for treatment of non-cancerous diseases and whose cancer target has already been discovered. This strategy is also denominated drug repurposing. More and more companies are scanning the existing pharmacopoeia for repositioning candidates, and the number of repositioning success stories is increasing. In a recent review (submitted), we provided noteworthy examples of known drugs whose potential anticancer activities have been highlighted in order to encourage further research on these known drugs as a means to foster their translation into clinical trials utilizing the more limited public-sector resources. If these drug types eventually result in being effective, it follows that they could be much more affordable for cancer patients.

CONCLUDING REMARKS AND FUTURE DIRECTIONS

Epigenetic alterations are at least as, if not more, important than genetic defects for the development and progression of malignant diseases. In most cancers, a number of epigenetic alterations occur during all stages of carcinogenesis.

These include global DNA hypomethylation, hypermethylation of key tumor suppressor genes, and histone modifications. From the diagnostic point of view, because epigenetic abnormalities occur very early in the carcinogenic process, the methylation aberrations can potentially be exploited as molecular markers for early detection. Assesment of hypermethylated genes in the primary tumor or in serum DNA may serve as a prognostic factor or as a means of predicting response to radiation, chemotherapy, and transcriptional agents in the therapeutic field. Transcriptional therapy is a very promising form of cancer treatment that is being extensively evaluated. An increasing recognition of the role of epigenetic changes in carcinogenesis presents a fresh challenge, as alterations in DNA methylation, histone modification, and microRNA in response to environmental exposures demand a new generation of exposure biomarkers. The overall importance of this area of research is brought into sharp focus by the large prospective cohort studies which need accurate exposure measurement in order to shed light on the complex gene behavior and environment interactions underlying common chronic disorders including cancer. Interventions and policy changes have been mounted to reduce risks from several important environmental carcinogens. Several new and promising biomarkers are now becoming available for epidemiologic studies, thanks to the development of high-throughput technologies and theoretical advances in biology. These include toxicogenomics, alterations in gene methylation and gene expression, proteomics, and metabonomics, which allow large-scale studies, including discovery-oriented, as well as hypothesis-testing investigations. However, most of these newer biomarkers have not been adequately validated, and their role in the causal paradigm is not clear. There is a need for their systematic validation using principles and criteria established over the past several decades in molecular cancer epidemiology

ACKNOWLEDGEMENT

Claudia M. García-Cuellar was partially supported by "Parker B. Francis fellowship" from Francis Fellowship Program of Francis family foundation USA.

REFERENCES

[1]   Feinberg AP. Epigenetics at the epicenter of modern medicine. JAMA 2008; 299: 1345-50.

[2]   Ballestar E, Esteller M. Chapter 9 epigenetic gene regulation in cancer. Adv Genet 2008; 61: 247-67.

[3]   Altucci L, Stunnenberg HG. Time for epigenetics. Int J Biochem Cell Biol 2009; 41: 2-3.

[4]   Delcuve GP, Rastegar M, Davie JR. Epigenetic control. J Cell Physiol 2009; 219: 243-50

[5]   Kargul J, Laurent GJ. Epigenetics and human disease. Int J Biochem Cell Biol 2009; 41: 1.

[6]   Fischle W, Wang Y, Allis CD. Histone and chromatin cross-talk. Curr Opin Cell Biol 2003; 15: 172-83.

[7]   Zink D, Fischer AH, Nickerson JA. Nuclear structure in cancer cells. Nat Rev Cancer 2004; 4: 677-87.

[8]   Espada J, Esteller M. Epigenetic control of nuclear architecture. Cell Mol Life Sci 2007; 64: 449-57.

[9]   Kornberg RD, Klug A. The nucleosome. Sci Am 1981; 244: 52-64.

[10] Luger K, Mader AW, Richmond RK, Sargent DF, Richmond TJ. Crystal structure of the nucleosome core particle at 2.8 A resolution. Nature 1997; 389: 251-60.

[11] Park YJ, Luger K. Structure and function of nucleosome assembly proteins. Biochem Cell Biol 2006; 84: 549-558.

[12] Prokhortchouk E, Defossez PA. The cell biology of DNA methylation in mammals. Biochim Biophys Acta 2008; 1783: 2167-73.

[13] Zinner R, Albiez H, Walter J, Peters AH, Cremer T, Cremer M. Histone lysine methylation patterns in human cell types are arranged in distinct three-dimensional nuclear zones. Histochem Cell Biol 2006; 125: 3-19.

[14] Lee DY, Hayes JJ, Pruss D, Wolffe AP. A positive role for histone acetylation in transcription factor access to nucleosomal DNA. Cell 1993; 72: 73-84.

[15] Thiriet C, Hayes JJ. Functionally relevant histone-DNA interactions extend beyond the classically defined nucleosome core region. J Biol Chem 1998; 273: 21352-8.

[16] Rice JC, Allis CD. Histone methylation versus histone acetylation: new insights into epigenetic regulation. Curr Opin Cell Biol 2001; 13: 263-73.

[17] Byvoet P, Shepherd GR, Hardin JM, Noland BJ. The distribution and turnover of labeled methyl groups in histone fractions of cultured mammalian cells. Arch Biochem Biophys 1972; 148: 558-67.

[18] Baxter CS, Byvoet P. Intercalating agents as probes of the spatial relationship between chromatin components. Biochem Biophys Res Commun 1975; 63: 286-91.

[19] Nielsen SJ, Schneider R, Bauer UM, *et al.* Rb targets histone H3 methylation and HP1 to promoters. Nature 2001; 412: 561-5.

[20]   Schotta G, Lachner M, Sarma K, *et al.* A silencing pathway to induce H3-K9 and H4-K20 trimethylation at constitutive heterochromatin. Genes Dev 2004; 18: 1251-62.

[21]   Stewart MD, Li J, Wong J. Relationship between histone H3 lysine 9 methylation, transcription repression, and heterochromatin protein 1 recruitment. Mol Cell Biol 2005; 25: 2525-38.

[22]   Paik WK, Kim S. Enzymatic demethylation of calf thymus histones. Biochem Biophys Res Commun 1973;51:781-788.

[23]   Shi Y, Lan F, Matson C, *et al.* Histone demethylation mediated by the nuclear amine oxidase homolog LSD1. Cell 2004; 119: 941-53.

[24]   Cao R, Wang L, Wang H *et al.* Role of histone H3 lysine 27 methylation in Polycomb-group silencing. Science 2002; 298: 1039-43.

[25]   Abbosh PH, Montgomery JS, Starkey JA, *et al.* Dominant-negative histone H3 lysine 27 mutant derepresses silenced tumor suppressor genes and reverses the drug-resistant phenotype in cancer cells. Cancer Res 2006; 66: 5582-91.

[26]   Simon JA, Lange CA. Roles of the EZH2 histone methyltransferase in cancer epigenetics. Mutat Res 2008; 647: 21-9.

[27]   Romano G, Michell P, Pacilio C, Giordano A. Latest developments in gene transfer technology: achievements, perspectives, and controversies over therapeutic applications. Stem Cells 2000; 18: 19-39.

[28]   Sigalotti L, Fratta E, Coral S, *et al.* Epigenetic drugs as pleiotropic agents in cancer treatment: biomolecular aspects and clinical applications. J Cell Physiol 2007; 212: 330-44.

[29]   Jones PA, Baylin SB. The fundamental role of epigenetic events in cancer. Nat Rev Genet 2002; 3: 415-28.

[30]   Sparmann A, van Lohuizen M. Polycomb silencers control cell fate, development and cancer. Nat Rev Cancer 2006; 6: 846-56.

[31]   Chen T, Li E. Structure and function of eukaryotic DNA methyltransferases. Curr Top Dev Biol 2004; 60: 55-89.

[32]   Smith BC, Denu JM. Chemical mechanisms of histone lysine and arginine modifications Biochim Biophys Acta 2009; 1789: 45-57.

[33]   Feinberg AP, Tycko B. The history of cancer epigenetics. Nat Rev Cancer 2004; 4: 143-53.

[34]   Wilson AS, Power BE, Molloy PL. DNA hypomethylation and human diseases. Biochim Biophys Acta 2007; 1775: 138-62.

[35]   Esteller M. Epigenetics in cancer. N Engl J Med 2008; 358: 1148-59.

[36]   Laird PW, Jaenisch R. DNA methylation and cancer. Hum Mol Genet 1994; 3 Spec No: 1487-95.

[37]   Feinberg AP, Vogelstein B. Hypomethylation distinguishes genes of some human cancers from their normal counterparts. Nature 1983; 301: 89-92.

[38]   Fraga MF, Herranz M, Espada J, *et al.* A mouse skin multistage carcinogenesis model reflects the aberrant DNA methylation patterns of human tumors. Cancer Res 2004; 64: 5527-34.

[39]   Suter CM, Martin DI, Ward RL. Hypomethylation of L1 retrotransposons in colorectal cancer and adjacent normal tissue. Int J Colorectal Dis 2004; 19: 95-101.

[40]   Lin CH, Hsieh SY, Sheen IS, *et al.* Genome-wide hypomethylation in hepatocellular carcinogenesis. Cancer Res 2001; 61: 4238-43.

[41]   Frigola J, Sole X, Paz MF, *et al.* Differential DNA hypermethylation and hypomethylation signatures in colorectal cancer. Hum Mol Genet 2005; 14: 319-26.

[42]   Sato N, Maitra A, Fukushima N, *et al.* Frequent hypomethylation of multiple genes overexpressed in pancreatic ductal adenocarcinoma. Cancer Res 2003; 63: 4158-66.

[43]   Piotrowski A, Benetkiewicz M, Menzel U, *et al.* Microarray-based survey of CpG islands identifies concurrent hyper- and hypomethylation patterns in tissues derived from patients with breast cancer. Genes Chromosomes Cancer 2006; 45: 656-67.

[44]   Nishigaki M, Aoyagi K, Danjoh I, *et al.* Discovery of aberrant expression of K-RAS by cancer-linked DNA hypomethylation in gastric cancer using microarrays. Cancer Res 2005; 65: 2115-24.

[45]   Kaneda A, Tsukamoto T, Takamura-Enya T, *et al.* Frequent hypomethylation in multiple promoter CpG islands is associated with global hypomethylation, but not with frequent promoter hypermethylation. Cancer Sci 2004; 95: 58-64.

[46]   Xiao J, Chen HS, Fei R, *et al.* Expression of MAGE-A1 mRNA is associated with gene hypomethylation in hepatocarcinoma cell lines. J Gastroenterol 2005; 40: 716-21.

[47]   Fujisawa K, Maesawa C, Sato R, *et al.* Epigenetic status and aberrant expression of the maspin gene in human hepato-biliary tract carcinomas. Lab Invest 2005; 85: 214-24.

[48]   Howard G, Eiges R, Gaudet F, Jaenisch R, Eden A. Activation and transposition of endogenous retroviral elements in hypomethylation induced tumors in mice. Oncogene 2008; 27: 404-8.

[49]   Li B, Carey M, Workman JL. The role of chromatin during transcription. Cell 2007; 128: 707-19.

[50]   Kouzarides T. Chromatin modifications and their function. Cell 2007; 128: 693-705.

[51]   Jenuwein T, Allis CD. Translating the histone code. Science 2001; 293: 1074-80.

[52]   Bartova E, Krejci J, Harnicarova A, Galiova G, Kozubek S. Histone modifications and nuclear architecture: a review. J Histochem Cytochem 2008; 56: 711-21.

[53]   Cheung P, Allis CD, Sassone-Corsi P. Signaling to chromatin through histone modifications. Cell 2000; 103: 263-71.

[54]   Durrin LK, Mann RK, Kayne PS, Grunstein M. Yeast histone H4 N-terminal sequence is required for promoter activation *in vivo*. Cell 1991; 65: 1023-31.

[55]   Spange S, Wagner T, Heinzel T, Kramer OH. Acetylation of non-histone proteins modulates cellular signalling at multiple levels. Int J Biochem Cell Biol 2009; 41: 185-98.

[56]   Wang GG, Allis CD, Chi P. Chromatin remodeling and cancer, Part I: Covalent histone modifications. Trends Mol Med 2007; 13: 363-72.

[57]   Marks P, Rifkind RA, Richon VM, Breslow R, Miller T, Kelly WK. Histone deacetylases and cancer: causes and therapies. Nat Rev Cancer 2001; 1: 194-202.

[58]   Peters AH, Schubeler D. Methylation of histones: playing memory with DNA. Curr Opin Cell Biol 2005; 17: 230-8.

[59]   Whetstine JR, Nottke A, Lan F, *et al.* Reversal of histone lysine trimethylation by the JMJD2 family of histone demethylases. Cell 2006; 125: 467-81.

[60]   Yamane K, Toumazou C, Tsukada Y, *et al.* JHDM2A, a JmjC-containing H3K9 demethylase, facilitates transcription activation by androgen receptor. Cell 2006; 125: 483-95.

[61]   Marmorstein R, Trievel RC. Histone modifying enzymes: Structures, mechanisms, and specificities. Biochim Biophys Acta 2009; 1789: 58-68.

[62]   Pandita TK, Richardson C. Chromatin remodeling finds its place in the DNA double-strand break response. Nucleic Acids Res 2009

[63]   Fernandez-Capetillo O, Lee A, Nussenzweig M, Nussenzweig A. H2AX: the histone guardian of the genome. DNA Repair (Amst) 2004; 3: 959-67.

[64]   Fernandez-Capetillo O, Celeste A, Nussenzweig A. Focusing on foci: H2AX and the recruitment of DNA-damage response factors. Cell Cycle 2003; 2: 426-7.

[65]   Motamedi MR, Hong EJ, Li X, *et al.* HP1 proteins form distinct complexes and mediate heterochromatic gene silencing by nonoverlapping mechanisms. Mol Cell 2008; 32:778-90.

[66]   Hirota T, Lipp JJ, Toh BH, Peters JM. Histone H3 serine 10 phosphorylation by Aurora B causes HP1 dissociation from heterochromatin. Nature 2005; 438: 1176-80.

[67]   Teixeira FK, Heredia F, Sarazin A, *et al.* A Role for RNAi in the Selective Correction of DNA Methylation Defects. Science 2009; 323: 1600-4

[68]   Kim DH, Saetrom P, Snove OJ, Rossi JJ. MicroRNA-directed transcriptional gene silencing in mammalian cells. Proc Natl Acad Sci USA 2008; 105: 16230-5.

[69]   Lujambio A, Esteller M. How epigenetics can explain human metastasis: A new role for microRNAs. Cell Cycle 2009; 8: 377-82.

[70]   Rouhi A, Mager DL, Humphries RK, Kuchenbauer F. MiRNAs, epigenetics, and cancer. Mamm Genome 2008; 19: 517-25.

[71]   Mattick JS, Makunin IV. Non-coding RNA. Hum Mol Genet 2006; 15 Spec No 1:R17-29.

[72]   Aaltonen LA. The multistep process of colon carcinogenesis. Cytokines Mol Ther 1996; 2: 111-4.

[73]   Cruz-Correa M, Cui H, Giardiello FM, *et al.* Loss of imprinting of insulin growth factor II gene: a potential heritable biomarker for colon neoplasia predisposition. Gastroenterology 2004; 126: 964-70.

[74]   Goelz SE, Vogelstein B, Hamilton SR, Feinberg AP. Hypomethylation of DNA from benign and malignant human colon neoplasms. Science 1985; 228: 187-90.

[75]   Belinsky SA, Nikula KJ, Palmisano WA, *et al.* Aberrant methylation of p16(INK4a) is an early event in lung cancer and a potential biomarker for early diagnosis. Proc Natl Acad Sci USA 1998;95: 11891-6.

[76]   Belinsky SA. Gene-promoter hypermethylation as a biomarker in lung cancer. Nat Rev Cancer 2004; 4: 707-17.

[77]   Belinsky SA. Silencing of genes by promoter hypermethylation: key event in rodent and human lung cancer. Carcinogenesis 2005; 26: 1481-7.

[78]   Risch A, Plass C. Lung cancer epigenetics and genetics. Int J Cancer 2008; 123: 1-7.

[79]   Lee WH, Morton RA, Epstein JI, *et al.* Cytidine methylation of regulatory sequences near the pi-class glutathione S-transferase gene accompanies human prostatic carcinogenesis. Proc Natl Acad Sci USA 1994; 91: 11733-7.

[80]   Baylin SB, Ohm JE. Epigenetic gene silencing in cancer - a mechanism for early oncogenic pathway addiction? Nat Rev Cancer 2006; 6: 107-16.

[81]   Poplawski T, Tomaszewska K, Galicki M, Morawiec Z, Blasiak J. Promoter methylation of cancer-related genes in gastric carcinoma. Exp Oncol 2008; 30: 112-6.

[82]   Irizarry RA, Ladd-Acosta C, Wen B, *et al.* The human colon cancer methylome shows similar hypo- and hypermethylation at conserved tissue-specific CpG island shores. Nat Genet 2009

[83]   Gao W, Kondo Y, Shen L, *et al.* Variable DNA methylation patterns associated with progression of disease in hepatocellular carcinomas. Carcinogenesis 2008; 29: 1901-10.

[84]   Yang HJ, Liu VW, Wang Y, Tsang PC, Ngan HY. Differential DNA methylation profiles in gynecological cancers and correlation with clinico-pathological data. BMC Cancer 2006; 6: 212.

[85]   Hinshelwood RA, Clark SJ. Breast cancer epigenetics: normal human mammary epithelial cells as a model system. J Mol Med 2008; 86: 1315-28.

[86]   Chung W, Kwabi-Addo B, Ittmann M, *et al.* Identification of novel tumor markers in prostate, colon and breast cancer by unbiased methylation profiling. PLoS ONE 2008; 3:e2079.

[87]   Boultwood J, Wainscoat JS. Gene silencing by DNA methylation in haematological malignancies. Br J Haematol. 2007; 138: 3-11.

[88]   Esteller M. Cancer epigenetics: DNA methylation and chromatin alterations in human cancer. Adv Exp Med Biol 2003; 532: 39-49.

[89]   Esteller M. Aberrant DNA methylation as a cancer-inducing mechanism. Annu Rev Pharmacol Toxicol 2005; 45: 629-56.

[90]   Esteller M. Epigenetic gene silencing in cancer: the DNA hypermethylome. Hum Mol Genet. 2007;16 Spec No 1:R50-9.

[91]   Yoo CB, Jones PA. Epigenetic therapy of cancer: past, present and future. Nat Rev Drug Discov 2006; 5: 37-50.

[92]   Segura-Pacheco B, Trejo-Becerril C, Perez-Cardenas E, *et al.* Reactivation of tumor suppressor genes by the cardiovascular drugs hydralazine and procainamide and their potential use in cancer therapy. Clin Cancer Res 2003; 9: 1596-603.

[93]   Zambrano P, Segura-Pacheco B, Perez-Cardenas E, *et al.* A phase I study of hydralazine to demethylate and reactivate the expression of tumor suppressor genes. BMC Cancer 2005; 5: 44.

[94]   Segura-Pacheco B, Perez-Cardenas E, Taja-Chayeb L, *et al.* Global DNA hypermethylation-associated cancer chemotherapy resistance and its reversion with the demethylating agent hydralazine J Transl Med 2006; 4: 32.

[95]   Chavez-Blanco A, Perez-Plasencia C, Perez-Cardenas E, *et al.* Antineoplastic effects of the DNA methylation inhibitor hydralazine and the histone deacetylase inhibitor valproic acid in cancer cell lines. Cancer Cell Int 2006; 6: 2.

[96]   de la Cruz-Hernandez E, Perez-Cardenas E, Contreras-Paredes A, *et al.* The effects of DNA methylation and histone deacetylase inhibitors on human papillomavirus early gene expression in cervical cancer, an *in vitro* and clinical study. Virol J 2007; 4: 18.

[97]   Duenas-Gonzalez A, Candelaria M, Perez-Plascencia C, Perez-Cardenas E, de la Cruz-Hernandez E, Herrera LA. Valproic acid as epigenetic cancer drug: preclinical, clinical and transcriptional effects on solid tumors. Cancer Treat Rev 2008; 34: 206-22.

[98]   Esteller M, Silva JM, Dominguez G, *et al.* Promoter hypermethylation and BRCA1 inactivation in sporadic breast and ovarian tumors. J Natl Cancer Inst 2000; 92: 564-9.

[99]   Herman JG, Merlo A, Mao L, *et al.* Inactivation of the CDKN2/p16/MTS1 gene is frequently associated with aberrant DNA methylation in all common human cancers. Cancer Res 1995; 55: 4525-30.

[100] Issa JP. DNA methylation as a therapeutic target in cancer. Clin Cancer Res 2007; 13: 1634-7.

[101] Carew JS, Giles FJ, Nawrocki ST. Histone deacetylase inhibitors: mechanisms of cell death and promise in combination cancer therapy. Cancer Lett 2008; 269: 7-17.

[102] Cameron EE, Bachman KE, Myohanen S, Herman JG, Baylin SB. Synergy of demethylation and histone deacetylase inhibition in the re-expression of genes silenced in cancer. Nat Genet 1999; 21: 103-7.

[103] Luo RX, Dean DC. Chromatin remodeling and transcriptional regulation. J Natl Cancer Inst 1999; 91: 1288-94.

[104] Zhu WG, Otterson GA. The interaction of histone deacetylase inhibitors and DNA methyltransferase inhibitors in the treatment of human cancer cells. Curr Med Chem Anticancer Agents 2003; 3: 187-99.

[105] Chai G, Li L, Zhou W *et al.* HDAC inhibitors act with 5-aza-2'-deoxycytidine to inhibit cell proliferation by suppressing removal of incorporated abases in lung cancer cells. PLoS ONE 2008; 3: e2445.

[106] Aparicio A, Weber JS. Review of the clinical experience with 5-azacytidine and 5-aza-2'-deoxycytidine in solid tumors. Curr Opin Investig Drugs 2002; 3: 627-33.

[107] Schwartsmann G, Schunemann H, Gorini CN, *et al.* A phase I trial of cisplatin plus decitabine, a new DNA-hypomethylating agent, in patients with advanced solid tumors and a follow-up early phase II evaluation in patients with inoperable non-small cell lung cancer. Invest New Drugs 2000; 18: 83-91.

[108] Pohlmann P, DiLeone LP, Cancella AI, *et al.* Phase II trial of cisplatin plus decitabine, a new DNA hypomethylating agent, in patients with advanced squamous cell carcinoma of the cervix. Am J Clin Oncol 2002; 25: 496-501.

[109] Duvic M, Vu J. Vorinostat: a new oral histone deacetylase inhibitor approved for cutaneous T-cell lymphoma. Expert Opin Investig Drugs 2007; 16: 1111-20.

[110] Roll JD, Rivenbark AG, Jones WD, Coleman WB. DNMT3b overexpression contributes to a hypermethylator phenotype in human breast cancer cell lines. Mol Cancer 2008; 7: 15.

[111] Vansteenkiste J, Van Cutsem E, Dumez H, *et al.* Early phase II trial of oral vorinostat in relapsed or refractory breast, colorectal, or non-small cell lung cancer. Invest New Drugs 2008; 26: 483-8.

[112] Feng W, Lu Z, Luo RZ, *et al.* Multiple histone deacetylases repress tumor suppressor gene ARHI in breast cancer. Int J Cancer 2007; 120: 1664-8.

[113] Nakagawa M, Oda Y, Eguchi T *et al.* Expression profile of class I histone deacetylases in human cancer tissues. Oncol Rep 2007; 18: 769-74.

[114] De los Santos M, Martinez-Iglesias O, Aranda A. Anti-estrogenic actions of histone deacetylase inhibitors in MCF-7 breast cancer cells. Endocr Relat Cancer 2007; 14: 1021-8.

[115] Arce C, Perez-Plasencia C, Gonzalez-Fierro A, *et al.* A proof-of-principle study of epigenetic therapy added to neoadjuvant doxorubicin cyclophosphamide for locally advanced breast cancer PLoS ONE. 2006; 1:e98.

[116] Candelaria M, Gallardo-Rincon D, Arce C, *et al.* A phase II study of epigenetic therapy with hydralazine and magnesium valproate to overcome chemotherapy resistance in refractory solid tumors. Ann Oncol 2007; 18: 1529-38.

[117] Guarente L. Sir2 links chromatin silencing, metabolism, and aging. Genes Dev 2000; 14: 1021-6.

[118] Blander G, Guarente L. The Sir2 family of protein deacetylases. Annu Rev Biochem 2004; 73: 417-35.

[119] Lamming DW, Wood JG, Sinclair DA. Small molecules that regulate lifespan: evidence for xenohormesis. Mol Microbiol 2004; 53: 1003-9.

[120] Fraga MF, Agrelo R, Esteller M. Cross-talk between aging and cancer: the epigenetic language. Ann N Y Acad Sci 2007; 1100: 60-74.

[121] Vaziri H, Dessain SK, Ng Eaton E, *et al.* hSIR2 (SIRT1) functions as an NAD-dependent p53 deacetylase. Cell 2001; 107: 149-59.

[122] Bereshchenko OR, Gu W, Dalla-Favera R. Acetylation inactivates the transcriptional repressor BCL6. Nat Genet 2002; 32: 606-13.

[123] Ashraf N, Zino S, Macintyre A, *et al.* Altered sirtuin expression is associated with node-positive breast cancer. Br J Cancer 2006; 95: 1056-61.

[124] Bradbury CA, Khanim FL, Hayden R *et al.* Histone deacetylases in acute myeloid leukaemia show a distinctive pattern of expression that changes selectively in response to deacetylase inhibitors. Leukemia 2005; 19: 1751-9.

[125] Kuzmichev A, Margueron R, Vaquero A, *et al.* Composition and histone substrates of polycomb repressive group complexes change during cellular differentiation. Proc Natl Acad Sci USA 2005; 102: 1859-64.

[126] Yeung F, Hoberg JE, Ramsey CS, *et al.* Modulation of NF-kappaB-dependent transcription and cell survival by the SIRT1 deacetylase. EMBO J 2004; 23: 2369-80.

[127] Sanders BD, Zhao K, Slama JT, Marmorstein R. Structural basis for nicotinamide inhibition and base exchange in Sir2 enzymes. Mol Cell 2007; 25: 463-72.

[128] Kleer CG, Cao Q, Varambally S, *et al.* EZH2 is a marker of aggressive breast cancer and promotes neoplastic transformation of breast epithelial cells. Proc Natl Acad Sci USA 2003;100:11606-11611.

[129] Sellers WR, Loda M. The EZH2 polycomb transcriptional repressor--a marker or mover of metastatic prostate cancer? Cancer Cell 2002; 2: 349-50.

[130] Kubicek S, O'Sullivan RJ, August EM, *et al.* Reversal of H3K9me2 by a small-molecule inhibitor for the G9a histone methyltransferase. Mol Cell 2007; 25: 473-81.

[131] McGarvey KM, Fahrner JA, Greene E, Martens J, Jenuwein T, Baylin SB. Silenced tumor suppressor genes reactivated by DNA demethylation do not return to a fully euchromatic chromatin state. Cancer Res 2006; 66: 3541-9.

[132] Wozniak RJ, Klimecki WT, Lau SS, Feinstein Y, Futscher BW. 5-Aza-2'-deoxycytidine-mediated reductions in G9A histone methyltransferase and histone H3 K9 di-methylation levels are linked to tumor suppressor gene reactivation. Oncogene 2007; 26: 77-90.

[133] Tan J, Yang X, Zhuang L, *et al.* Pharmacologic disruption of Polycomb-repressive complex 2-mediated gene repression selectively induces apoptosis in cancer cells. Genes Dev 2007; 21: 1050-63.

[134] You A, Tong JK, Grozinger CM, Schreiber SL. CoREST is an integral component of the CoREST- human histone deacetylase complex. Proc Natl Acad Sci USA 2001; 98: 1454-8.

[135] Kahl P, Gullotti L, Heukamp LC, *et al.* Androgen receptor coactivators lysine-specific histone demethylase 1 and four and a half LIM domain protein 2 predict risk of prostate cancer recurrence. Cancer Res 2006; 66: 11341-7.

[136] Schmidt DM, McCafferty DG. trans-2-Phenylcyclopropylamine is a mechanism-based inactivator of the histone demethylase LSD1. Biochemistry 2007; 46: 4408-16.

[137] Yang M, Culhane JC, Szewczuk LM, *et al.* Structural basis for the inhibition of the LSD1 histone demethylase by the antidepressant trans-2-phenylcyclopropylamine. Biochemistry 2007; 46: 8058-65.

[138] Huang Y, Greene E, Murray Stewart T, *et al.* Inhibition of lysine-specific demethylase 1 by polyamine analogues results in reexpression of aberrantly silenced genes. Proc Natl Acad Sci USA 2007; 104: 8023-8.

CHAPTER 5

Signal Transduction Pathways in Cancer

Lucrecia Márquez-Rosado[*]

Public Health Sciences Division, Fred Hutchinson Cancer Research Center, Seattle Washington, USA

Abstract: Signal transduction has proven to occur not through linear pathways linking individual receptors to specific cellular responses, but rather, occurs through a set of interconnected pathways which form complex signaling networks. Some key pathways, such as Ras-Raf-MEK-ERK, PI3K-Akt-NF-κB, JAK-STAT, and Src are often initiated by receptor tyrosine kinases. They function as entry points for many extracellular cues, and play a critical role in recruiting the intracellular signaling cascades that orchestrate a wide range of biological processes regulating essentially all aspects of normal and malignant cell behavior. It is clear that enhanced or deregulated signaling can generate signals leading to tumor growth and metastasis. Herein, defects in the apoptotic signaling pathways, which have been recognized as a hallmark of cancer, are described with particular focus on the key players of intrinsic pathway of apoptosis.

Keywords: Cancer, tumorigenesis, signal transduction, receptor tyrosine kinases, Ras-MAPK signaling, PI3K-Akt signaling, classical NF-κB pathway, alternative NF-κB pathway, JAK-STAT signaling, FAK-Src signaling, apoptosis, Bax, Bcl-2.

INTRODUCTION

Cell signaling refers to the process involving the transmission of molecular signals by which extracellular substances can produce an intracellular response. Cells receive external signals from direct contact with other cells, direct contact with matrix molecules, and through many different growth factor receptors to regulate diverse processes essential to tumor cell development such as cell growth, differentiation, migration and apoptosis. These processes are regulated by multiple signaling pathways, and many changes that occur in cancer cells result from the activation of oncogenes and inactivation of tumor suppressor genes causing many alterations in cellular signaling machinery (Martin CC 2003) [1]. A proto-oncogene is a normal gene whose expressed proteins normally participate in signal transduction pathways. When a proto-oncogene is altered or modified by mutation it can become an oncogene. Many oncogenes encode members of signal transduction pathways causing the transformation of normal cells into cancerous tumor cells, *e.g.*, EGFR, Ras, and Bcl-2 (Zandi CS 2007) [2] (Osborne Oncologist 2004) [3]. On the other hand, tumor suppressor genes refer to those genes which encode for proteins whose normal function is to inhibit cell transformation and whose inactivation is advantageous for tumor cell growth and survival, *e.g.*, p53, Bax, and PTEN (Osborne Oncologist 2004) [3].

This chapter will discuss both inactivation of some tumor suppressor genes as well as the oncogenic activation of some proto-oncogenes associated with cancer events. Among them, the activation of receptor tyrosine kinases, which play a critical role in the control of the cell cycle, cell migration, and survival as well as cell proliferation and differentiation (Schlessinger Cell 2000) [4]. Oncogenic receptor tyrosine kinases can aberrantly activate downstream signaling molecules, such as Ras-MAPK, PI3K phosphoinositide 3-kinase (PI3K)-Akt-mTOR-NF-κB, JAK(Janus Kinase)- STATs and Src.

The Ras-Raf-MEK (mitogen-activated protein kinase)-ERK kinase (extracellular-signal-regulated kinase) pathway regulates essentially all aspects of malignant cell behaviour. Consequently, aberrant signaling caused by mutations in the Ras-Raf-MEK-ERK pathway and its upstream activators is a critical contribution to development and progression in many types of cancer. PI3K-Akt-NF-κB signaling has a well-defined role as a survival pathway by

---

*Address correspondence to Lucrecia Márquez-Rosado: Public Health Sciences Division, Fred Hutchinson Cancer Research Center, Seattle Washington, USA; E-mail: lmarquez@fhcrc.org

exerting anti-apoptotic activity, in part by preventing the release of cytochrome c from the mitochondria. Moreover, NF-κB has a critical role on the production of growth and angiogenesis factors and might directly stimulate cell-cycle progression through transcriptional activation of cell-cycle genes, especially cyclin D1 (Joyce CGFR 2001) [5]. The effects of PTEN tumor suppressor loss, which is a central negative regulator of the PI3K-Akt signaling cascade, are predominantly manifest by increased proliferation and decreased apoptosis. Thus, it is not surprising that alterations of the PTEN gene are found in various types of human cancer and that it has become one of the most frequently mutated of all tumor suppressors (Chow CL 2006) [6].

Other pathways involved in tumorigenesis include signaling by JAK-STAT and Focal adhesion kinase (FAK)-Src. The critical role of JAK-STAT in regulating cell growth and differentiation is reflected by the aberrant activation of this signaling pathway and its association in a wide variety of human cancers, especially leukemia (Hayakawa ANYAS 2006) [7]. FAK-Src promotes cell motility, cell cycle progression and cell survival. Thus, enhanced or deregulated FAK-Src can generate signals leading to tumor growth and metastasis (Mitra COCB 2006) [8].

In addition, given the central role of apoptosis for cellular homeostasis, it is no wonder that loss of fine control of apoptotic signaling is a critical component for the survival of a malignant cell. In this chapter, several of the molecular mechanisms by which cancer cells are protected from apoptosis have been mentioned.

SIGNALING THROUGH RECEPTOR TYROSINE KINASES

Functional phosphorylation of signal transduction molecules is a major activation event that leads to dramatic changes in tumor growth. Tyrosine kinases play a central role in signal transduction, acting as relay points for a complex network of interdependent signaling molecules that ultimately affect gene transcription within the nucleus. They are enzymes that transfer -phosphate groups from ATP to the hydroxyl group of tyrosine residues on signal transduction molecules (Schlessinger Cell 2000) [4]. Tyrosine kinases are primarily classified as receptor tyrosine kinases, *e.g.*, the Epidermal Growth Factor Receptor (EGFR), Platelet Derived Growth Factor Receptor (PDGFR), Fibroblast Growth Factor Receptor (FGFR), Vascular Endothelial Growth Factor Receptor (VEGFR) and the Insulin Receptor (IR), and non-receptor tyrosine kinases, *e.g.*, Src, JAK and FAK.

The receptor tyrosine kinases are transmembrane proteins that span the plasma membrane only once; their activation initiates a number of intracellular signaling pathways leading to the nucleus which contains critical genes that regulate the tumorigenesis events. Approximately 20 different receptor tyrosine kinases classes have been identified, all of which share a similar structure that includes an Extracellular Ligand-Binding domain (ELB domain), a single Transmembrane domain (TM domain), and an Intracellular Tyrosine Kinase domain (ITK domain) (Fig. **1A**). The receptor tyrosine kinases exhibit dual functions where their extracellular domains can receive and transmit information leading to activation of their intrinsic cytoplasmic kinase activity. They use ATP to catalyze phosphorylation of select tyrosine residues in target proteins. Most growth factor receptors belong to the receptor tyrosine kinase family (Blume-Jensen Nature 2001) [9], such as EGFR, PDGFR and VEGFR. They are activated by the binding of a ligand to their extracellular domain (Fig. **1B**). Ligands are extracellular signal molecules (*e.g.*, EGF, PDGF, VEGF, etc) that induce receptor dimerization and consequently protein tyrosine kinase activation. Stimulation leads to a wide array of intracellular responses such as cell cycle, proliferation, differentiation, motility and survival (Vlahovic Oncologist 2003) [10].

It is well known that receptor tyrosine kinases regulate diverse functions in normal cells; however, when they are mutated or structurally altered they become potent oncoproteins. Therefore, it is not surprising that abnormal activation of receptor tyrosine kinases has been shown to be causally involved in the development and progression of many human cancers, from pre-cancerous lesions to malignant tumors (Blume-Jensen Nature 2001) [9]. Following these observations, as shown in Fig. **1C**, there are multiple mechanisms by which oncogenic activation of receptor tyrosine kinases can occur. For instance, excess ligand expression or EGFR expression, mutations within the ELB domain, the failure of inactivation mechanisms, or transactivation through receptor dimerization caused by mutations in the transmembrane domains which stabilize the receptor tyrosine kinase dimer. (Bargmann EJ 1988) [11] (Segatto MCB 1988) [12]. The major signaling pathways emanating from receptor tyrosine kinases, such as Ras-MAPK, PI3K-Akt-NF-κB, and JAK-STAT (Fig. **1B**), will be more fully described below.

RAS-MAPK SIGNALING PATHWAY

The Ras family of small GTPases plays essential roles in controlling the activity of several crucial cellular processes including growth, differentiation, apoptosis, cytoskeletal organization and membrane trafficking. After a ligand binds to its corresponding receptor, dimerization of receptor occurs, as described previously in receptor tyrosine kinase section (Fig. **1B**).

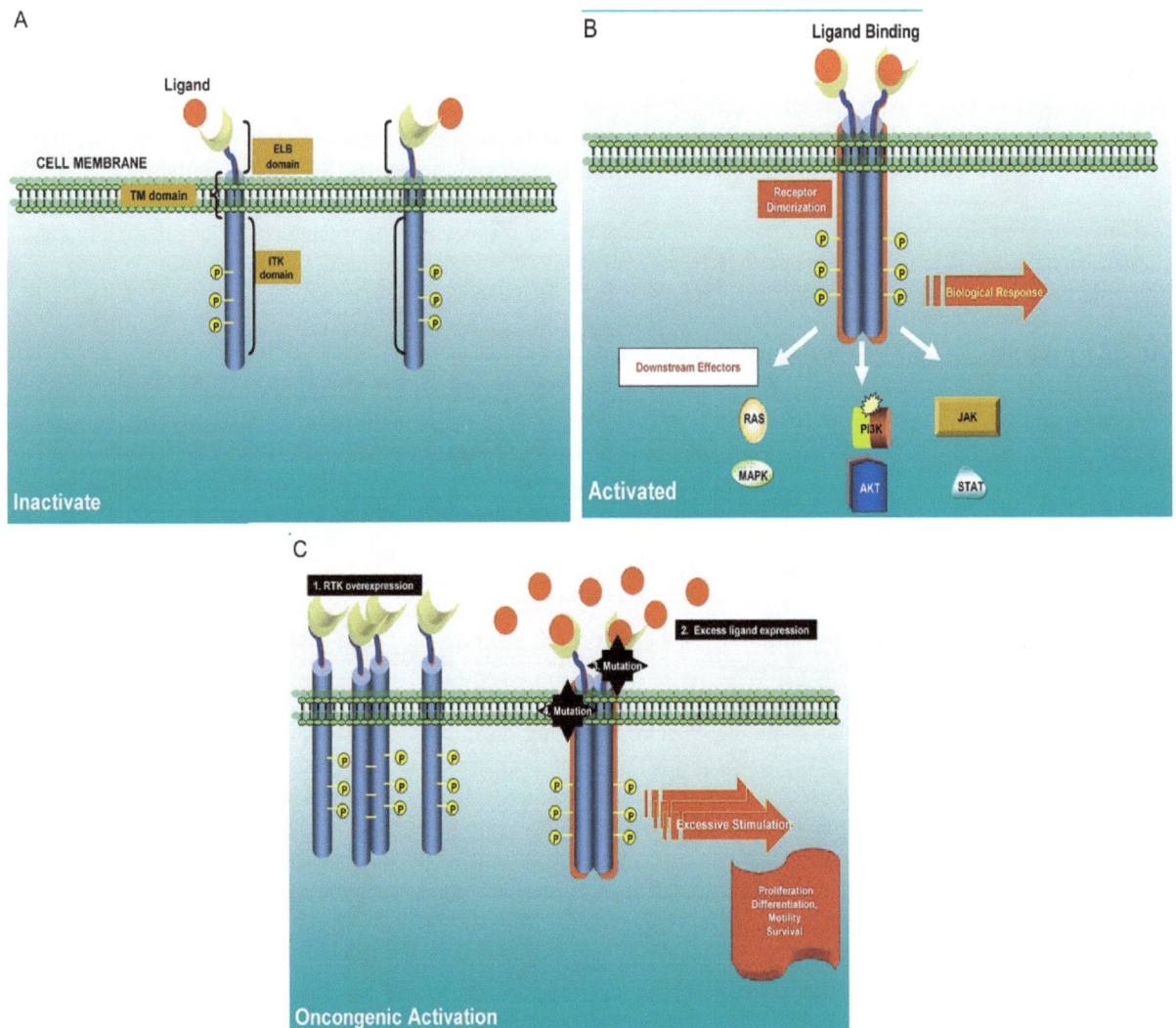

Figure 1: (A) Inactive RTK. RTK is found prior to ligand binding as an inactive monomer. The structural organization of RTK contains three major domains. LBE domain is responsible for binding of ligand and receiving the external signal, TM domain connects the extracellular and intracellular domains and spans the membrane a single time, and ITK domain mediates the biological response and transmission of intracellular signal transduction. (B) Activation of RTK. Ligand binding to the RTK induces dimerization that results in cross-autophosphorylation of key tyrosine residues in the cytoplasmic domain, which function as docking sites for downstream signal transducers. (C) Oncongenic activation of RTK. There are several mechanisms by which tyrosine kinase might acquire transforming functions such as verexpression of RTK (1), overexpression of RTK ligands (2), mutations within the ELB domain (3), mutations in TM domains (4). The result is the constitutive activation of RTK leading to excessive stimulation of other signaling proteins that regulate diverse functions. Abreviations: RTK, receptor tyrosine kinase; LBE domain, extracellular ligand-binding domain; TM domain, transmembrane domain; ITK, domain intracellular tyrosine kinase domain.

Dimerization causes the intracellular tyrosine kinase(s) to become phosphorylated, then these phosphorylated tyrosine residues serve as docking sites for various adaptor proteins such as Grb2 (Fig. **2B**). The adaptor protein Grb2 is complexed with SOS, Guanine Nucleotide Exchange Factor (GEF). The Grb2/SOS complex is recruited to an activated receptor tyrosine kinase through the binding of the Grb2 SH2 domain to specific pTyr sites of the receptor. The recruitment of the Grb2/SOS complex to the plasma membrane brings SOS into close proximity to Ras, thus allowing it to activate Ras by stimulating the exchange of GDP for GTP (Fig. **2B**). The normal activation cycle of Ras proteins depends on whether they are bound to GTP (active Ras proteins which relay signals from cell surface receptors to some effectors molecules) or GDP (inactive Ras proteins which fail to relay signals to these effectors molecules) (Campbell Oncogene 1998) [13]. Fig. **2A** illustrates the cycling of Ras between these two forms. After Ras activation, the downstream effectors of Ras are Raf kinases (the MEK-ERK pathway), PI3K and Rac-1, which in turn stimulate a signaling cascade that induces a variety of cellular responses (Fig. **2B**) (Downward NRC 2003) [14].

The multiplicity of signaling pathways emanating from Ras proteins emphasizes their critical function as regulators of cell growth. In this context, alterations in Ras signaling pathways have been found in a large number and wide variety of human tumors. Activating mutations in K-Ras and N-Ras occur in varying frequencies in different types of cancer and are invariably found at codons 12, 13 or 61 (Braun CCRes 2008) [15]. These genes encode Ras proteins that contain point mutations in the GTPase domain that reduce its activity, resulting in a constitutively active Ras protein (GTP bound conformation) due to a decreased rate of GTP hydrolysis. Ras is also activated in cancer cells by other mechanisms, including by perturbations in other signaling components, such as the receptor tyrosine kinase. In particular, EGFR is overexpressed or mutationally activated in many human cancers, and hyperactivation of EGFR tyrosine kinase activity in turn causes persistent activation of Ras and Ras-mediated signaling (Fig. **2C**). In addition, mutations in proteins which downregulate Ras have also been shown to contribute to Ras transforming potential (Tsygankova MCB 2007) [16].

The Ras-ERK MAPK signaling pathway plays a particularly important role in cell growth and differentiation. In response to a wide variety of extracellular stimuli, ERK signaling is initiated through the binding and activation of receptor tyrosine kinases, which facilitates the binding and activation of GTP to the GTPase Ras at the plasma membrane (Fig. **2B**). Ras recruits the MAP kinase kinase kinase Raf to the membrane, where it is subject to phosphorylation at multiple residues that promote its activation. Raf then activates MEK1/2, which in turn phosphorylate and activate the MAPK ERK1/2. Following activation, ERKs translocate to the nucleus and phosphorylate a variety of substrates including 90 kDa ribosomal S6 protein kinase (p90RSK), and the growth promoting transcription factors c-Myc and Elk-1 (2B) (Wada Oncogene 2004) [17].

The Ras-ERK pathway is characterized by a cascade of phosphorylation events that transduce and integrate information in response to growth factors and cellular/extracellular signals, and which play key roles in a variety of cellular responses such as cell proliferation, differentiation, migration and apoptosis. Given the role of MAPK signaling in critical biological processes, abnormalities in MAPK signaling play an important role in the development and progression of cancer. Activating mutations in the Ras-ERK module are particularly common in a variety of cancers as they enhance the growth and proliferative potential, both important contributors to tumorigenesis. As summarized in Fig. **2C**, the majority of cancer-associated lesions that result in constitutive activation of ERK signaling have been found in upstream constituents of the ERK signaling pathway. These include overexpression of and activating mutations in receptor tyrosine kinases, sustained production of activating ligands, as well as mutations in Ras mutations and B-Raf (Dhillon Oncogene 2007) [18]. Together, these observations reflect, at least in part, the possibility that inhibition of ERK signaling pathway might have significant therapeutic activity.

PI3K-AKT-NF-κB SIGNALING

PI3K/Akt signaling is another signaling pathway that plays a role in cell growth, migration and differentiation. PI3K is a heterodimeric signaling protein composed of a catalytic subunit (p110) and a regulatory subunit (p85) that activates the downstream Akt pathway by phosphorylating specific constituents of the inner plasma membrane known as phosphatidylinositols. In response to growth factor stimulation, the p110 subunit catalyzes the phosphorylation of phosphatidylinositol-4, 5-bisphosphate (PIP2) to form phosphatidylinositol-3, 4, 5-trisphosphate (PIP3), which recruits Akt to the plasma membrane for activation of growth, proliferation and survival signaling pathways (Cantley Science 2002) [19].

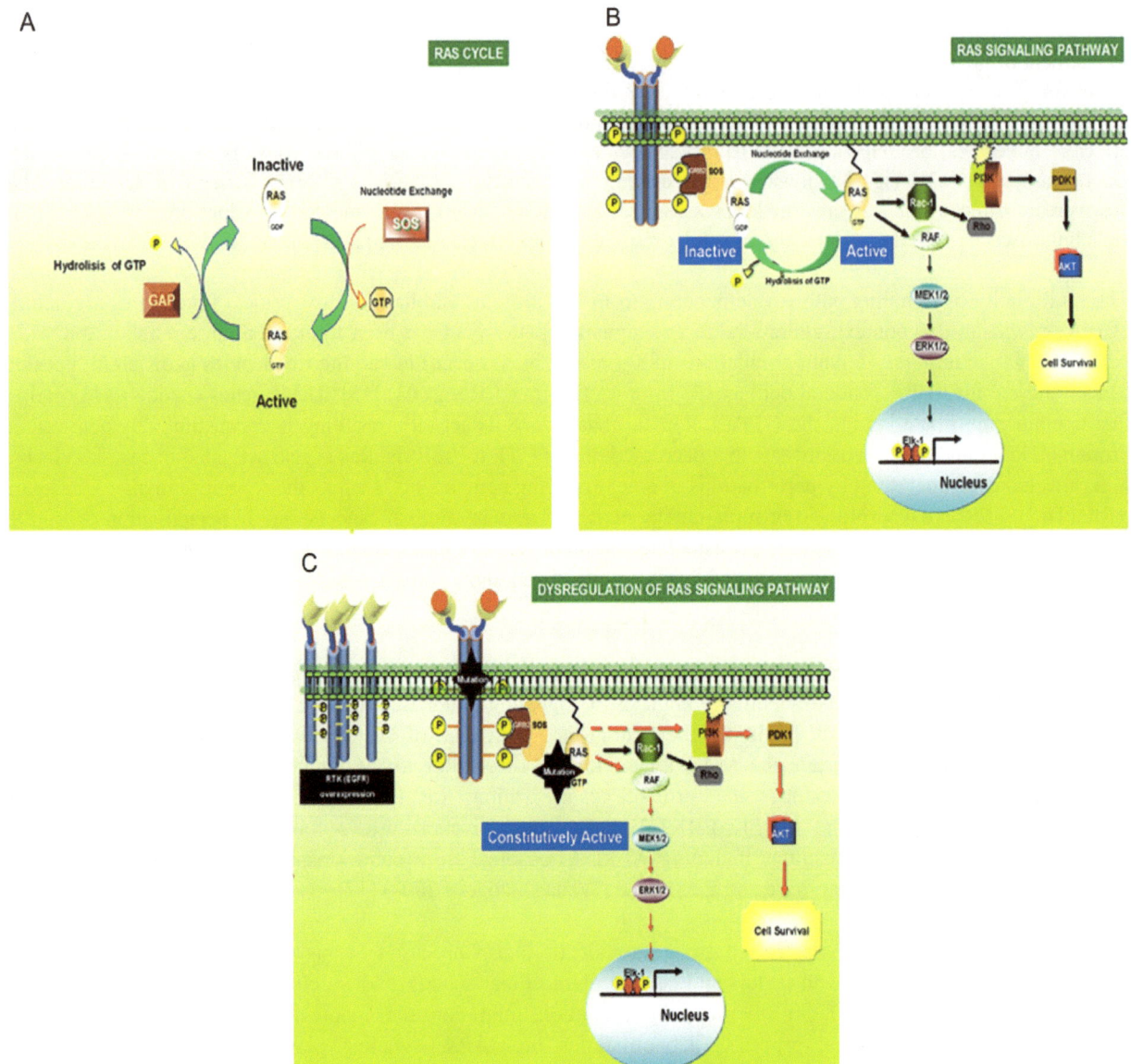

Figure 2: (A) The Ras cycle. Ras is activated by SOS that stimulates the exchange of GDP for GTP on Ras. In the GTP-bound form, Ras is in its active state; however, there exist several GAPs that are able to stimulate the GTPase activity of Ras, which convert it back to its original inactive, GDP bound. (B) The Ras signaling pathways. As discussed in the text, receptor dimerization serves as docking sites for adaptor proteins containing SH2 or PTB domains such as GRB2. GRB2 protein recruits SOS, which stimulates the exchange of GDP for GTP on Ras. Ras-GTP can activate diverse signaling pathways through their interactions with many effector molecules (eg. PI3K, Raf, and Rac-1). (C) Dysregulation of Ras signaling pathway. Expression of constitutively active mutants of Ras, or mutants of EGFR and enhanced expression of EGFR can also lead to aberrant Ras signaling. Abreviation: GAPs, GTPase-activating proteins.

Akt signaling promotes cell growth survival through a variety of mechanisms. (Burgering Nature 1995) [20]. It has been shown that Akt exerts its antiapoptotic activity in part by phosphorylating and inactivating the proapoptotic protein Bad, which blocks its complex formation with the apoptotic proteins Bcl-2 and Bcl-xL (Fig. **3A**). This prevents the release of cytochrome c from mitochondria, which in turn triggers caspase-mediated apoptosis. Akt also prevents apoptosis at the transcriptional level. Activated Akt phosphorylates and inactivates procaspase-9 and Forkhead family of transcription factors (FOXO), preventing the transcription of pro-apoptotic genes such as Fas ligand (LoPiccolo DRU 2008) [21]. In addition, Akt phosphorylates and activates the IkappaB kinase (IKK) complex leading to the transcription of antiapoptotic genes by the transcription factor NF-κB (Altomare Oncogene, 2005)

[22]. Akt also helps sustain m-TOR signaling, which plays a critical role in cell proliferation, survival, mobility and angiogenesis (LoPiccolo DRU 2008) [21], by phosphorylating and inactivating the tumor suppressor and m-TOR's negative regulator TSC2.

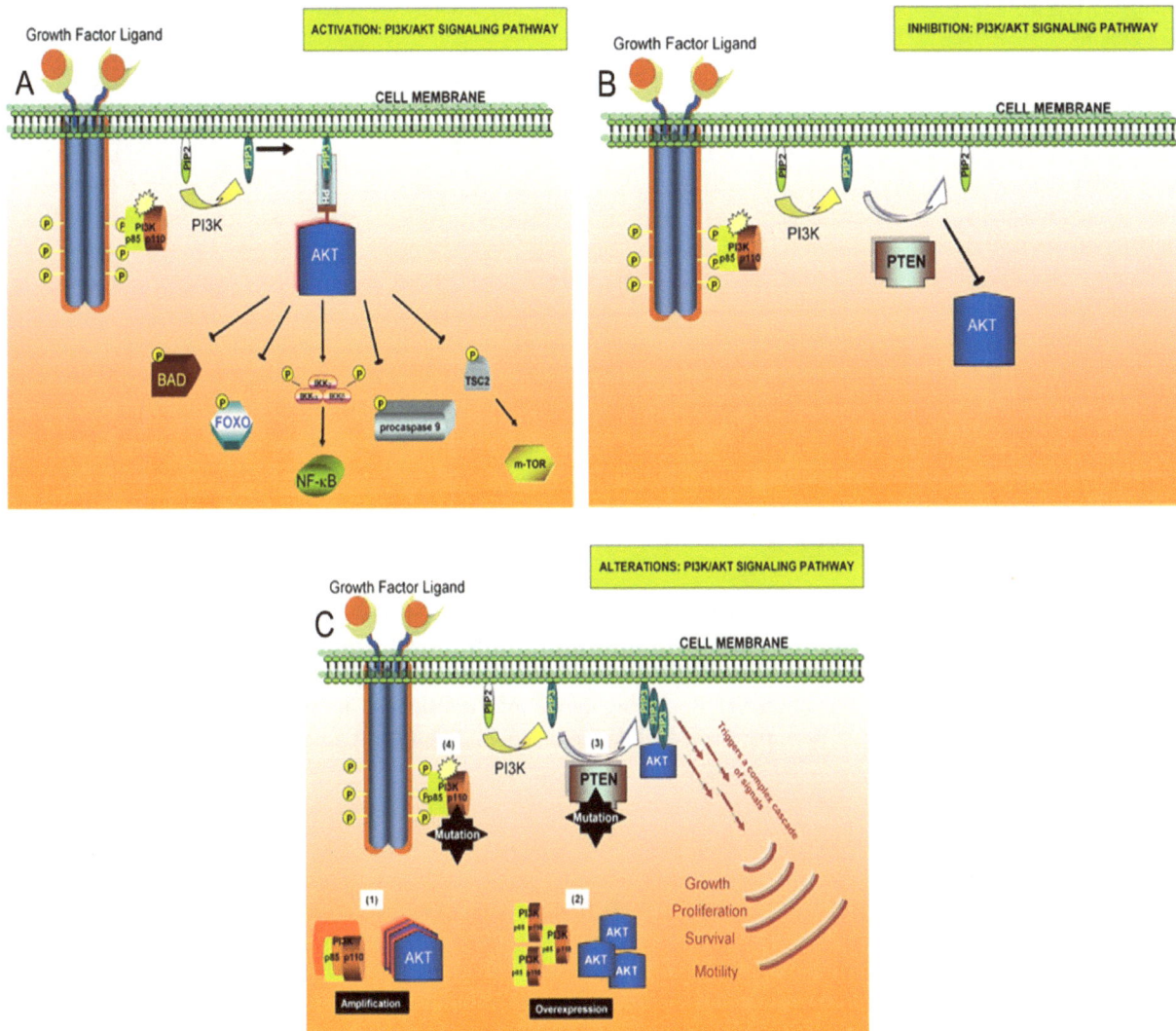

Figure 3: (A) PI3K-Akt signaling pathway. Activation of RTKs recruits PI3K, and then PI3K phosphorylates PIP2 to generate PIP3, resulting in Akt activation. Upon activation, Akt can phosphorylate and regulate multiple targets affecting a broad range of cellular activities. The specific targets phosphorylated and consequently inhibited by Akt include Bad, FOXO, procaspase-9, and TSC2, a negative regulator of m-TOR. And positively it regulates NF-κB through IKK complex. (B) Inhibition of PI3K-Akt signaling pathway. PTEN negatively regulates this signaling process through dephosphorylation of PIP3. (C) Alterations of the PI3K-Akt pathway. The mechanisms contributing to elevated Akt activity include genetic amplification of PI3K or Akt (1), and overexpresion of PI3K or Akt (2). In some instances, constitutive Akt activation may result from loss of the PTEN function resulting in elevated PIP3 levels, and consequent constitutive activation of PI3K and Akt (3), or from mutations in the catalytic or regulatory subunits of PI3K (4). Abreviations: RTK, Receptor tyrosine kinase; PI3K, phosphatidylinositol 3-kinases.

Given the role of Akt in preventing apoptosis and promoting growth, cell mobility, and cell proliferation, it is not surprising that activating alterations in this signaling pathway give rise to cancer. Fig. **3C** shows various mechanisms contributing to activation of the Akt pathway in human tumors, including perturbation of the upstream PI3K pathway. The activation of PI3K can result from gene amplifications, changes in gene regulation that lead to its overexpression or from activating mutations in its catalytic and regulatory subunits (Yuan TL. Oncogene 2008) [23]. Another frequent genetic event that occurs in human cancer is the loss or mutations in tumor suppressor genes that regulate PI3K-Akt signaling. For example, mutations in PTEN, which dephosphorylates PIP3 back to PIP2 and consequently inactivates the PI3K-Akt signaling pathway (Fig. **3B**), is a common mechanism for constitutive Akt activation in many human cancers, especially in prostate and endometrial cancers, melanoma, and glioblastoma (Sansal JCO 2004) [24]. Finally, amplification and overexpression of Akt leading to excessive activation of the Akt pathway has been linked to poorly differentiated tumors that are more invasive, grow faster, and are more resistant to treatment (Testa PNAS 2001) [25].

NF-κB Signaling Pathway

NF-κB is composed of homo-and heterodimeric complexes of Rel family proteins, comprising RelA (p65), RelB, c-Rel, p50/p105 and p52/p100. The NF-κB activation signaling pathway has been broadly classified into the classical and alternative pathways. The classical pathway involves activation of a trimeric IKK complex, composed of IKKα, IKKβ, and IKKγ (NEMO). The IKK complex phosphorylates NF-κB-bound IκB and consequently this leads to ubiquitin-dependent degradation of IκBs that allows the liberation of NF-κB dimers. The most common dimer is a p50/RelA heterodimer. In most normal cells, these p50/RelA dimers are retained in the cytoplasm as an inactive complex through the direct binding of IκB inhibitor (Fig. **4A**). Released NF-κB dimers translocate to the nucleus and bind κB sites in the promoters or enhancers of target genes, which leads to their transcription (Naugler COGD 2008) [26]. As a positive regulator of cell cycle progression, NF-κB activates genes such as cyclin D1, c-myc, and cyclooxygenase-2 (COX-2). This factor also activates the transcription of several target genes known to block the induction of apoptosis. These target genes include cellular inhibitors of apoptosis (cIAPs), caspase-8/FADD (FAS associated death domain)-like, IL-1β-converting enzyme (FLICE) inhibitory protein (c-FLIP) and members of the Bcl-2 family such as Bcl-xL (Aggarwal CC 2004) [27].

The alternative pathway does not require IκBα phosphorylation and degradation but depends on activation of IKK (Fig. **4B**). Activation of this pathway is triggered by members of the Tumor Necrosis Factor (TNF) family, which requires the activation of at least two kinases, NIK (NF-κB-inducing kinase) and IKK. The latter phosphorylates p100, resulting in its polyubiquitinylation and processing to p52. p52 translocates into the nucleus in association with RelB, where induce genes that are essential for B-cell development and lymphoid organogenesis (Senftleben Science 2001) [28].

A significant contributor to cancer related morbidity and mortality is metastasis - the spread of malignant tumor cells from the primary tumor to a secondary organ leading to colonization of this distant site. Invasion and metastatic growth are characteristics of advanced and aggressive tumors; NF-κB could well be an important player in this process since its activation leads to the activation of genes that encode several Matrix Metalloproteinases (MMP), plasminogen activator, and heparanase, all of which promote invasive growth. Chemokines represent another important class of NF-κB regulated target genes, which induce cell migration. Adhesion molecules mediate local and distant invasiveness. One example is ICAM-1, which is upregulated in some tumors with poor prognosis, Recently, NF-κB activation was found to stimulate angiogenesis, possibly by inducing expression of IL-8, VEGF, COX-2 and inducible Nitric Oxide Synthase (iNOS) (Greten CL 2004) [29] (Karin NRC 2002) [30]. Altered activation of the classical NF-κB complex and its signaling pathways plays a critical role in cancer development and progression by stimulating proliferation, metastasis and angiogenesis, as well as inhibiting apoptotic events. In addition, exacerbated activation of the alternative pathway is potentially associated with several human disorders including cancer such as B cell lymphomas and in mammary carcinogenesis (Demicco MCB 2005) [31].

JAK-STAT SIGNALING PATHWAY

JAKs enzymes are cytosolic tyrosine kinases that associate with membrane receptors and play a critical role in the transduction of signals from cell surface to the nucleus. STATs are latent cytoplasmic transcription factors that become activated by JAK on tyrosine residues. Subsequently, these active STATs translocate to the nucleus, where they induce expression of target genes (Fig. **5**). JAK-STATs regulate genes encoding apoptosis inhibitors (Bcl-xL, Mcl-1), cell cycle regulators (cyclins D1/D2, c-Myc), and inducers of angiogenesis (VEGF).

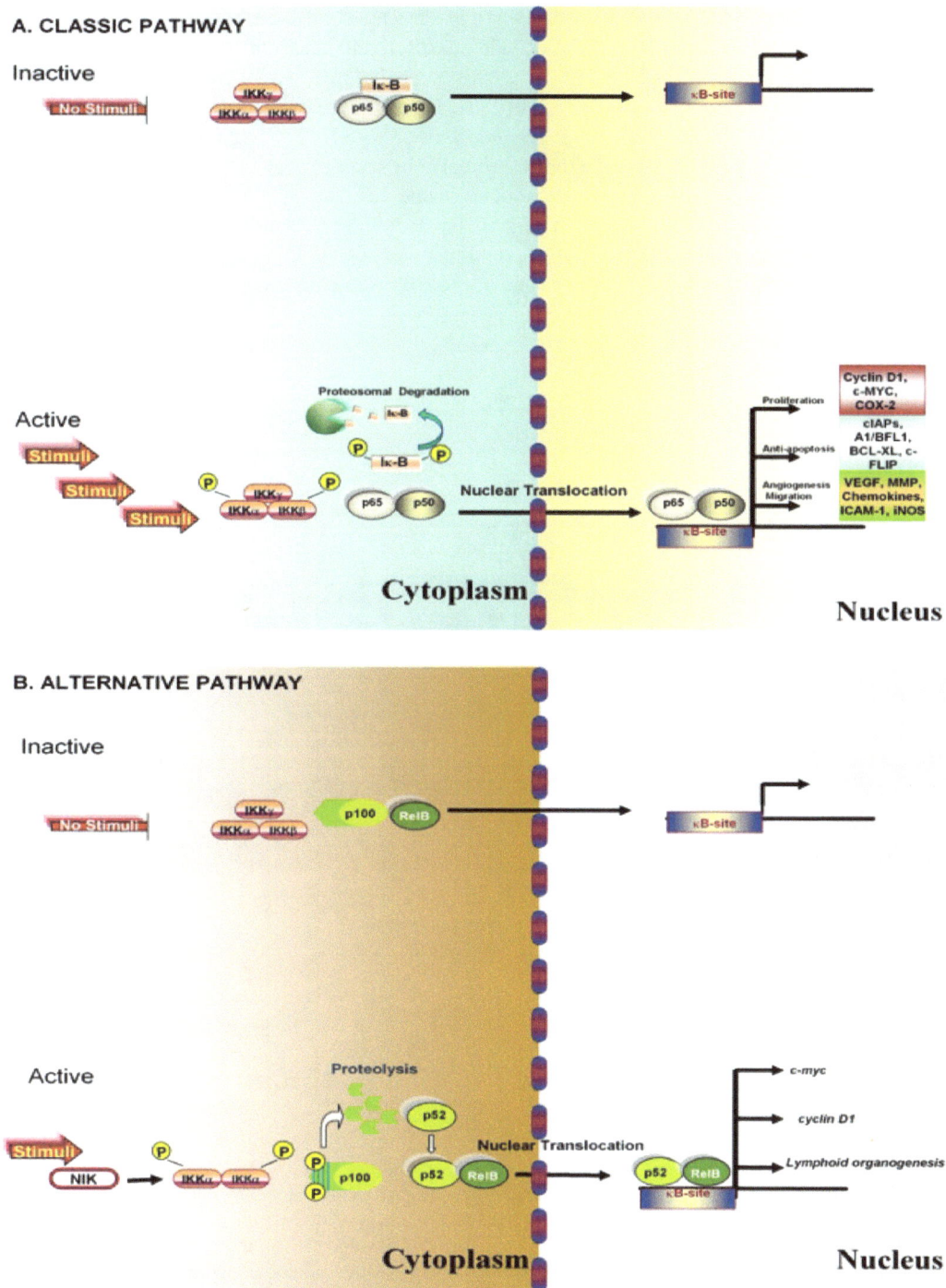

Figure 4: (A) Classical NF-κB pathway. In unstimulated cells, NF-κB dimers are inactive, since they are sequestered in the cytoplasm by interaction with inhibitory IκBs proteins. Cell stimulation activates the IKK complex (IKK-α, IKK-β, IKK-γ). Activated IKK phosphorylates IκB which is ubiquitinated and rapidly degraded by the proteosome, releasing NF-κB dimers to translocate into the nucleus and modulate gene expression involved in the proliferation, anti- apoptosis, cell angiogenesis, and migration. (B) Alternative NF-κB pathway. Receptor binding activates the NF-κB-inducing kinase NIK. NIK which phosphorylates and activates an IKKα complex, which in turn phosphorylates two serine residues adjacent to the ankyrin repeat C-terminal IκB domain of p100. This leads to partial proteolysis of p100 to generate p52 and translocation of the p52/RelB complex into nucleus. This complex activates gene expression of c-myc, cyclin D1, and genes that are essential for B-cell development and lymphoid organogenesis.

Reflecting the critical role of JAK-STAT, recent studies revealed that inappropriate activation of JAK-STAT signaling occurs with high frequency in human cancers and directly contributes to oncogenesis. In cancer cells, several JAK mutations have been identified. These encode constitutively active or hyperactive JAK proteins, which persistently activate STAT proteins. Such mutations greatly contribute to hematopoietic malignancies, especially myeloproliferative neoplasms (Lin TS Oncogene 2000) [32]. In addition, constitutive activation of the JAK-STAT pathway can be induced by mutations in negative regulators of JAK–STAT signaling such as the SOCS proteins (Fig. **5**). The SOCS proteins inhibit signaling either by direct inhibition of JAK kinase activity or by competition with STAT–SH2 domains for specific receptor phosphotyrosine residues (Croker SCDB 2008) [33]. SOCS is downregulated by methylation of the CpG island in human Hepatocellular Carcinoma (HCC), multiple myeloma and pancreatic ductal neoplasm (Yoshikawa NG 2001) [34] (Galm Blood 2003) [35] (Fukushima BJC 2003) [36]. Recent findings suggest that the inactivation of SOCS-1 was one of the targets in cancer development.

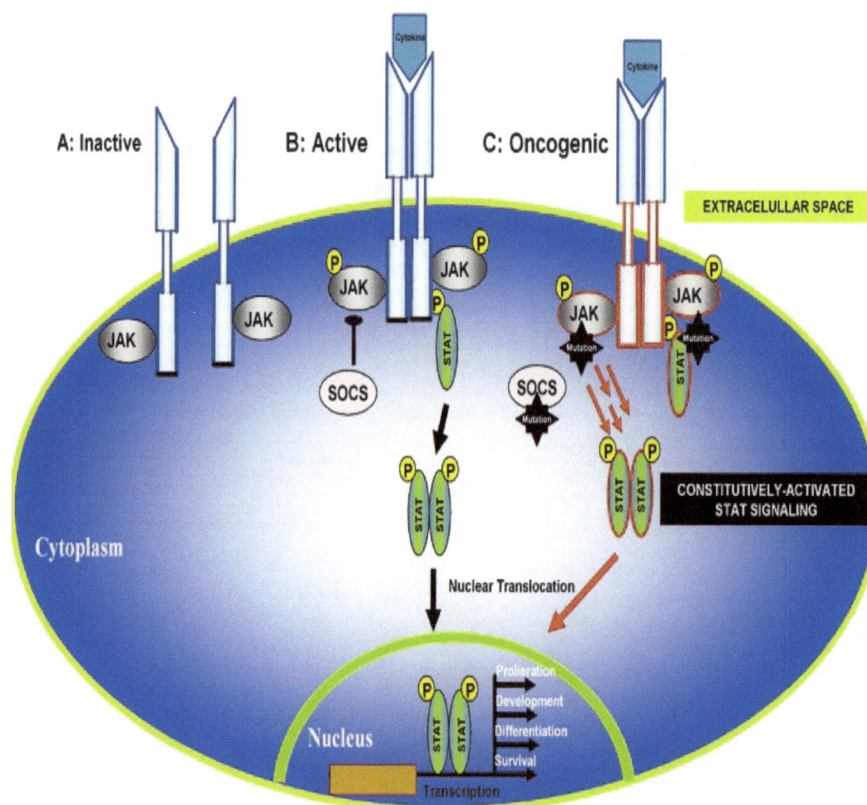

Figure 5: (A) Inactive JAK-STAT signaling pathway. (B) Activation of JAK-STAT signaling pathway. It is initiated by binding of a peptide ligand to transmembrane receptors. This leads to receptor dimerization and cross-activation of receptor-associated JAK kinases, which in turn phosphorylate tyrosine residues in the cytoplasmic tail of the receptor. These phospho-tyrosine residues lead to the recruitment of STAT proteins, which are then also tyrosine-phosphorylated by JAK. Phosphorylated STAT proteins are released from the receptor, dimerize, translocate to the nucleus, and stimulate the transcription of target genes. (C) Oncogenic activation of JAK-STAT signaling pathway. Mechanistically, mutation in JAK-STAT or mutation in SOCS, a negative regulator of the JAK/STAT, play a role in aberrant activation of JAK-STAT pathway.

FAK-SRC SIGNALING

In contrast to receptor protein tyrosine kinases, non-receptor protein tyrosine kinases are located in the cytoplasm, nucleus or anchored to the inner leaflet of the plasma membrane. The Src family kinases constitutes a family of cytosolic tyrosine kinases, including Src, Fyn and Yes which are the most ubiquitously expressed. c-Src is the prototype of a non-receptor protein tyrosine kinase which interacts with a diverse array of molecules, including growth factor receptors and cell–cell adhesion receptors, integrins and steroid hormone receptors (Ishizawar CC 2004) [37]. Src family kinases play key roles in regulating signal transduction in cellular processes. Therefore, the biological consequences of Src activation are many and can include proliferation, survival, differentiation, migration and invasion in both normal and transformed cells. The regulation of Src or other Src family kinases is through different phosphorylation and dephosphorylation events (Fig. **6A**). For enzyme activation, the tyrosine residue (Tyr530) in the C-terminal tail of the protein and the tyrosine residue (Tyr416) of the activation loop in the catalytic domain are fundamental. These two sites have opposite effects on Src activity. In fact, autophosphorylation of Tyr416 promotes the activation, while the dephosphorylation of phosphotyrosine 416 and phosphorylation of Tyr530 decreases Src kinase activity (Summy CMR 2003) [38]. This inhibitory phosphorylation is known to be catalyzed by Csk (C-terminal Src Kinase) and its relative, CHK (Csk Homologous Kinase). Dephosphorylation of phosphotyrosine 530 increases Src kinase activity. Protein Tyrosine Phosphatases (PTP) have been shown to dephosphorylate the Tyr530 of Src.

Hyper-activated Src leads to uncontrolled cell proliferation and cancer. Moreover, overexpression and/or hyperactivation of Src are correlated with tumor grade and with poor prognosis. Malignant Src activation, with constitutively high enzymatic levels, is present in many human cancers like breast, colon, pancreatic, ovarian, head, neck, lung, bladder, neuronal tumors, as well as in chronic myelogenous leukemia and multiple myeloma (Summy CMR 2003) [38] (Irby Oncogene 2000) [39].

Several mechanisms for the high levels of Src activation in human cancer have been proposed. Among them, the specific activity of Src protein kinase may be increased by direct or indirect interaction with receptor tyrosine kinases, EGFR, PDGFR, FGFR, *etc.* Other potential mechanisms for Src activation, as shown in Fig. **6A**, may relate to reductions in the levels or activity of Csk, the enzyme known to phosphorylate the negative regulatory tyrosine residue of c-Src (Tyr 530) (Masaki Hepatology 1999) [40]. Likewise, enhanced activity of phosphatases (PTP) known to dephosphorylate the regulatory Tyr 530 may cause Src activation (Bjorge CB1996) [41].

FAK, a non-receptor tyrosine kinase, can also bind and activate Src in focal complex (Irby Oncogene 2000) [39] (Schlaepfer COGD 2004) [42]. Src plays an important role in tumor cell invasion, in particular through its interaction with FAK. FAK is involved in integrin-mediated signaling that has a profound impact on cell proliferation, survival and migration through kinase-dependent signaling events affecting PI3K-Akt, Ras-MAPK, and also involves the activation of Rac and Rho GTPases (Fig. **6B**). Following integrin engagement, FAK undergoes autophosphorylation at Tyr 397 and Src becomes recruited to activated FAK *via* an interaction between the SH2 domain of Src and FAK pTyr397. Src then phosphorylates FAK at a number of tyrosine residues, creating docking sites for SH2 domain-containing signaling proteins, such as the adaptor Grb2. Both Src and FAK exhibit elevated expression in a number of different epithelial tumors, especially in invasive cancers (Mitra COCB 2000) [8].

MOLECULAR MECHANISM OF APOPTOTIC SIGNALING IN CANCER

Mammalian cells contain sophisticated molecular machinery that permits them engage in apoptosis, or programmed cell death, in response to physiological, pathogenic, or cytotoxic stimuli. Dysregulation of apoptosis is an important aspect of cancer pathogenesis and has been widely recognized as a hallmark of most types of cancer. Apoptosis can be activated through two major pathways: the extrinsic, receptor-mediated pathway, and the intrinsic, mitochondrial pathway. As apoptosis was described in detail in chapter one, this chapter will provide an overview of the key mechanisms of the intrinsic apoptotic pathway which are frequently dysregulated in human cancers.

The intrinsic pathway of apoptosis is triggered following mitochondrial damage, which leads to the release of apoptogenic factors such as cytochrome c, Apoptosis Inducing Factor (AIF) and Smac/Diablo (Fig. **7A**). Recently, much work has been done in an effort to understand the anti-apoptotic mechanisms observed in cancer. One of the most important regulators of the intrinsic pathway is the Bcl-2 family of proteins. The Bcl-2 family includes pro-apoptotic members such as Bax, Bak, Bad, and Bid, and anti-apoptotic members such as Bcl-2 and Bcl-xL. Anti-apoptotic Bcl-2 members act as repressors of apoptosis by blocking the release of cytochrome-c, whereas pro-apoptotic members act as activators by promoting the release of cytochrome-C (Ghobrial CACJC 2005) [43]. An important factor in tumorigenesis is the balance between the pro-apoptotic and anti-apoptotic members of Bcl-2 family. In a tumor cell, a mutation of the Bcl-2 gene that results in increased expression will suppress the normal function of the pro-apoptotic protein, Bax (Fig. **7B**). On the other hand, if a mutation in the Bax gene causes a downregulation of expression then the cell will also lose its ability to regulate apoptosis, again resulting in tumorigenesis (Johnstone Cell 2002) [44].

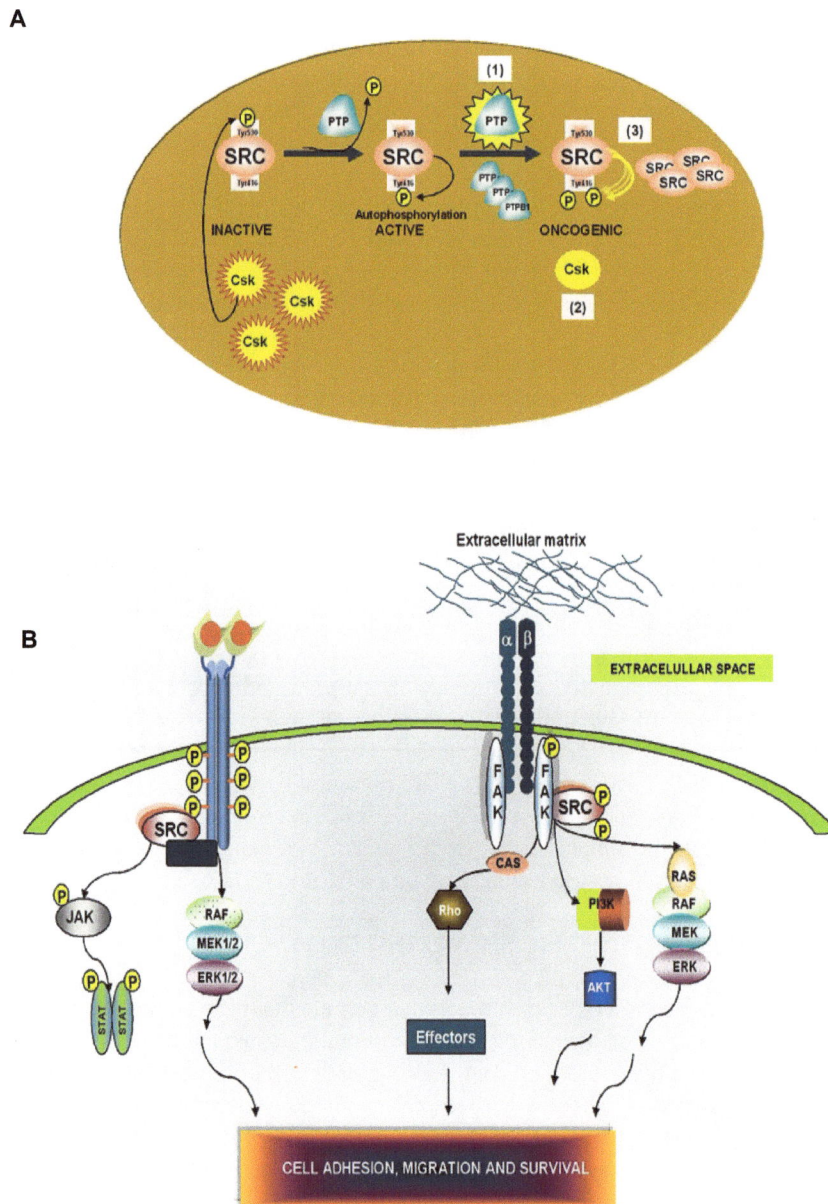

Figure 6: Regulation of Src (upper panel). Under basal conditions, the Csk tyrosine kinases phos-phorylate tyrosine-530 and inactivate Src. On the other hand, Src activation involves pTyr530 desphoshorylation by PTP, and autophosphorylation of Tyr416. Oncogenic activation of Src. The mechanisms implicated in oncogenic activation of Src include elevated expression or activity of PTP (1), reduced expression of Csk (2), or elevated Src activity (3), and in some cases protein expression. Proximal effectors in FAK/Src signaling (lower panel). Src signaling can be initiated through EGFR or integrin receptors. Integrin activation induces recruitment and stimulation of FAK and Src, which involves the activation of Rho GTPases, the PI3K and Ras GTPase. And their downstream effectors control diverse aspects of cell behavior, including growth, survival and migration. PTP, protein tyrosine phosphatase.

IAPs function as potent endogenous apoptosis inhibitors by directly binding to and effectively inhibiting three members of the caspase family of enzymes: two effector caspases (caspase-3 and -7) and one initiator caspase-9 (Schimmer CR 2004) [45]. Several lines of evidence point toward the IAP family of proteins playing a role in oncogenesis, *via* their effective suppression of apoptosis (Hunter Apoptosis 2007) [46]. High levels of IAP family of anti-apoptotic proteins, XIAP and Survivin, have been found in several cancer cells lines; in such cases, the physiological amounts of Smac/DIABLO released from the mitochondria may not be sufficient to overcome the inhibitory effect of IAPs on caspases (Mizutani IJO 2007) [47] (Lippert IJC 2007) [48]. Thus, when the IAPs are over-expressed or over-active, as is the case in many cancers, cells are no longer able to die in a physiologically programmed fashion and become increasingly resistant to standard chemo- and radiation therapies (Lopes RB IJC 2007) [49].

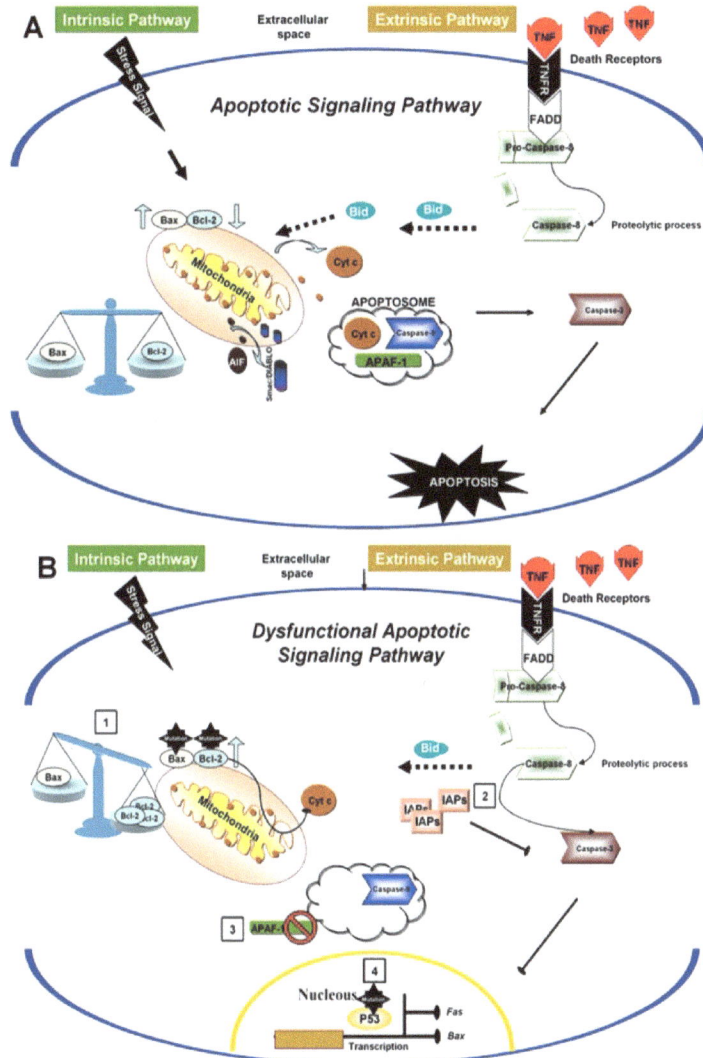

Figure 7: (A) The intrinsic pathway. Apoptotic stimuli result in the translocation of Bax from the cytosol to mitochondria and release of cytochrome c. Bcl-2 and Bcl-xL inhibit programmed cell death by preventing the release of cytochrome c, whereas pro-apoptotic Bcl-2 family members (such as Bax and Bid) promote the release of cytochrome c. Cytochrome c, released from the mitochondrial to cytoplasm, works together with the other two cytosolic protein factors, Apaf-1 and procaspase-9, to promote the assembly of a caspase-activating complex termed the apoptosome, which in return induces activation of caspase-9 and thereby activates downstream caspases such as casapase 3, leading to apoptosis. **(B)** Dysfunction in the Apoptotic Signaling Pathway. A number of alterations in apoptosis signaling occur with abnormal balance between Bcl-2 and Bax which block the pro-apoptotic signal (1). IAPs, which have been shown to directly inhibit activated caspase 3, are over-expressed or over-actived in many cancers; as a result cells are no longer able to die (2). Other alterations include the loss APAF-1 (3), and mutation in p53 protein that results in loss of transcriptional regulation of p53 target genes involved in apoptosis such as Fas and Bax, which confers advantage for tumor cells (4). Abreviation: Apaf-1, apoptotic protease activating factor-1.

Another very common cause of tumorigenesis is mutation of the p53 protein (Fig. **7B**). The product of the tumor suppressor gene p53 is a protein involved both in the extrinsic and intrinsic apoptotic pathways. P53 may function both by stimulating the function of pro-apoptotic proteins (Fas receptor, Bax and Bak) and by inactivating the function of anti-apoptotic proteins (Bcl-2) (Henry Oncogene 2002) [50].

Regardless of the mechanism, the suppression of apoptotic signaling confers an enhanced survival ability to cancer cells, which promotes their characteristic uncontrolled proliferation. Furthermore, the dysregulation of apoptotic signaling is frequently implicated in drug resistance, as many anti-neoplastic agents exert their cytotoxic effects by inducing apoptosis (Pommier Oncogene 2004) [51] (Blagosklonny CDD 2005) [52].

CONCLUSIONS

Many studies have illustrated that cell signaling is extensively involved in oncogenesis. As a result of knowledge of the molecular basis of neoplastic cell behavior, cancer can be identified as a disease of dysfunctional signaling. These observations have awoken a notable interest for the signal-transduction pathways that drive neoplastic transformation, since they may point to the design of novel therapeutic strategies that target specific molecular events and can lead to a better understanding of resistance mechanisms. Although, many signaling pathway have been linked to tumorigenesis, the targeting of few of them have shown to be promising in the treatment of cancer. In this chapter, some of the most important signaling pathways that play a major role during tumorigenesis were illustrated, and targeting them might be one of the most promising ways to conquer cancer.

REFERENCES

[1]   Martin GS. Cell signaling and cancer. Cancer Cell 2003; 4(3): 167-74.

[2]   Zandi R, Larsen AB, Andersen P, Stockhausen MT, Poulsen HS. Mechanisms for oncogenic activation of the epidermal growth factor receptor. Cell Signal 2007; 19(10): 2013-23.

[3]   Osborne C, Wilson P, Tripathy D. Oncogenes and tumor suppressor genes in breast cancer: potential diagnostic and therapeutic applications. Oncologist 2004; 9(4): 361-77.

[4]   Schlessinger J. Cell Signaling by Receptor Tyrosine Kinases. Cell 2000; 103(2): 211-25.

[5]   Joyce D, Albanese C, Steer J, Fu M, Bouzahzah B, Pestell RG. NF-κB and cell-cycle regulation: the cyclin connection. Cytokine Growth Factor Rev 2001; 12(1): 73-90.

[6]   Chow LM, Baker SJ. PTEN function in normal and neoplastic growth. Cancer Lett 2006; 2412(2):184-96.

[7]   Hayakawa F, Naoe T. SFK-STAT pathway: an alternative and important way to malignancies. Ann NY Acad Sci 2006; 1086: 213-22.

[8]   Mitra SK, Schlaepfer DD. Integrin-regulated FAK-Src signaling in normal and cancer cells. Curr Opin Cell Biol 2006; 18(5): 516-23.

[9]   Blume-Jensen P, Hunter T. Oncogenic kinase signalling. Nature 2001; 411(6835): 355-65.

[10]   Vlahovic G, Crawford J. Activation of tyrosine kinases in cancer. Oncologist 2003; 8(6): 531-8.

[11]   Bargmann CI, Weinberg RA. Oncogenic activation of the neu-encoded receptor protein by point mutation and deletion, EMBO J 1988; 7(7): 2043-52.

[12]   Segatto O, King CR, Pierce JH, di Fiore PP, Aaronson SA. Different structural alterations upregulate *in vitro* tyrosine kinase activity and transforming potency of the erbB-2 gene, Mol Cell Biol 1988; 8(12): 5570-74.

[13]   Campbell SL, Khosravi-Far R, Rossman KL, Clark GJ, Der, CJ. Increasing complexity of Ras signaling. Oncogene 998; 17(11): 1395-413.

[14]   Downward J. Targeting RAS signalling pathways in cancer therapy. Nat Rev Cancer 2003; 3(1): 11-22.

[15]   Braun BS, Shannon K. Targeting Ras in myeloid leukemias. Clin Cancer Res 2008; 15; 14(8): 2249-52.

[16]   Tsygankova OM, Prendergast GV, Puttaswamy K, *et al.* Downregulation of Rap1GAP contributes to Ras transformation. Mol Cell Biol 2007; 27(19): 6647-58.

[17]   Wada T, Penninger JM. Mitogen-activated protein kinases in apoptosis regulation. Oncogene 2004; 23(16): 2838-49.

[18]   Dhillon AS, Hagan S, Rath O, Kolch W. MAP kinase signalling pathways in cancer. Oncogene 2007; 26(22): 3279-90.

[19]   Cantley LC. The phosphoinositide 3-kinase pathway. Science 2002; 296(5573): 1655-7.

[20]   Burgering BM, Coffer PJ. Protein kinase B (c-Akt) in phosphatidylinositol-3-OH kinase signal transduction. Nature 1995; 376(6541): 599-602.

[21]   LoPiccolo J, Blumenthal GM, Bernstein WB, Dennis PA. Targeting the PI3K/Akt/mTOR pathway: effective combinations and clinical considerations. Drug Resist Updat 2008; 11(1-2): 32-50.

[22]   Altomare DA, Testa JR. Perturbations of the AKT signaling pathway in human cancer: Oncogene 2005; 24(50): 7455-64.

[23]   Yuan TL, Cantley LC. PI3K pathway alterations in cancer: variations on a theme. Oncogene 2008; 27 (41): 5497-510.

[24]   Sansal I, Sellers WR. The biology and clinical relevance of the PTEN tumor suppressor pathway. J Clin Oncol 2004; 22(14): 2954-63.

[25]   Testa JR, Bellacosa A. AKT plays a central role in tumorigenesis. Proc Natl Acad Sci USA 2001; 98(20): 10983-5.

[26]   Naugler WE, Karin M. NF-kappaB and cancer-identifying targets and mechanisms. Curr Opin Genet Dev 2008; 18(1): 19-26.

[27]   Aggarwal BB. Nuclear factor-kappaB: the enemy within Cancer. Cell 2004; 6(3): 203-8.

[28]   Senftleben U, Cao Y, Xiao G, *et al.* Activation by IKKalpha of a second, evolutionary conserved, NF-kappa B signaling pathway. Science 2001; 293(5534): 1495-9

[29]   Greten FR, Karin M. The IKK/NF-kappaB activation pathway-a target for prevention and treatment of cancer. Cancer Lett 2004; 206 (2): 193-9.

[30]   Karin M, Cao Y, Greten FR, Li ZW. NF-kappaB in cancer: from innocent bystander to major culprit. Nat Rev Cancer 2002; 2(4): 301-10.

[31]   Demicco EG, Kavanagh KT, Romieu-Mourez R, *et al.* RelB/p52 NF-κB complexes rescue an early delay in mammary gland development in transgenic mice with targeted superrepressor IκB-α expression and promote carcinogenesis of the mammary gland. Mol Cell Biol 2005; 25(22): 10136-47.

[32]   Lin TS, Mahajan S, Frank DA. STAT signaling in the pathogenesis and treatment of leukemias. Oncogene 2000; 19(21): 2496-504.

[33]   Croker BA, Kiu H, Nicholson SE. SOCS regulation of the JAK/STAT signalling pathway. Semin Cell Dev Biol 2008; 19(4): 414-22.

[34]   Yoshikawa H, Matsubara K, Qian GS, *et al.* SOCS-1, a negative regulator of the JAK/STAT pathway, is silenced by methylation in human hepatocellular carcinoma and shows growth-suppression activity. Nat Genet 2001; 28(1): 29-35

[35]   Galm O, Yoshikawa H, Esteller M, Osieka R, Herman JG. SOCS-1, a negative regulator of cytokine signaling, is frequently silenced by methylation in multiple myeloma. Blood 2003; 101(7): 2784-8.

[36]   Fukushima N, Sato N, Sahin F, Su GH, Hruban RH, Goggins M. Aberrant methylation of suppressor of cytokine signalling-1 (SOCS-1) gene in pancreatic ductal neoplasms. Br J Cancer 2003; 89(2): 338-43

[37]   Ishizawar R, Parsons SJ. c-Src and cooperating partners in human cancer. Cancer Cell 2004; 6 (3): 209-14.

[38]   Summy JM, Gallick GE. Src family kinases in tumor progression and metastasis. Cancer Metastasis Rev 2003; 22 (4): 337-58

[39]   Irby RB, Yeatman TJ. Role of Src expression and activation in human cancer. Oncogene 2000; 19(49): 5636-42.

[40]   Masaki T, Okada M, Tokuda M, *et al.* Reduced C-terminal Src kinase (Csk) activities in hepatocellular carcinoma. Hepatology 1999; 29(2): 379-84.

[41]   Bjorge JD, O'Connor TJ, Fujita DJ. Activation of human pp60c-src. Biochem Cell Biol 1996; 74(4): 477-84.

[42]   Schlaepfer DD, Mitra SK. Multiple connections link FAK to cell motility and invasion. Curr Opin Genet Dev 2004; 14(1): 92-101.

[43]   Ghobrial IM, Witzig TE, Adjei AA. Targeting apoptosis pathways in cancer therapy. CA Cancer J Clin 2005; 55(3): 178-94.

[44]   Johnstone, R. W., Ruefli, A. A., and Lowe, S. W. Apoptosis: a link between cancer genetics and chemotherapy. Cell 2002; 108(2):153-64.

[45]   Schimmer AD. Inhibitor of apoptosis proteins: translating basic knowledge into clinical practice. Cancer Res 2004; 64(20): 7183-90.

[46]   Hunter AM, LaCasse EC, Korneluk RG. The inhibitors of apoptosis (IAPs) as cancer targets Apoptosis 2007; 12(9): 1543-68.

[47]   Mizutani Y, Nakanishi H, Li YN, *et al.* Overexpression of XIAP expression in renal cell carcinoma predicts a worse prognosis. Int J Oncol 2007; 30(4): 919-25.

[48]   Lippert BM, Knauer SK, Fetz V, Mann W, Stauber RH. Dynamic survivin in head and neck cancer: molecular mechanism and therapeutic potential. Int J Cancer 2000; 121(6): 1169-74.

[49]   Lopes RB, Gangeswaran R, McNeish IA, Wang Y, Lemoine NR. Expression of the IAP protein family is dysregulated in pancreatic cancer cells and is important for resistance to chemotherapy. Int J Cancer 2007; 120(11): 2344-52.

[50]   Henry H, Thomas A, Shen Y, White E. Regulation of the mitochondrial checkpoint in p53-mediated apoptosis confers resistance to cell death. Oncogene 2002; 21(5): 748-60.

[51]   Pommier Y, Sordet O, Antony S, Hayward RL, Kohn KW. Apoptosis defects and chemotherapy resistance: Molecular interaction maps and networks. Oncogene 2004; 23(26): 2934-49.

[52]   Blagosklonny MV. Carcinogenesis, cancer therapy and chemoprevention. Cell Death Differ 2005; 12(6): 592-602.

CHAPTER 6

Metastasis

Lucrecia Márquez-Rosado[*]

Public Health Sciences Division, Fred Hutchinson Cancer Research Center, 1100 Fairview Avenue North, Seattle, WA 98109, USA

Abstract: Metastasis is a complex sequence of processes that take place when a tumor cell exits the primary tumor, and establishes a secondary tumor by traveling to a distant site *via* the circulatory system. The complex process of metastasis depends on various components for successful dissemination and tumor cell growth at a secondary site. Metastatic processes include: (1) neoplastic progression, (2) angiogenesis, (3) migration and invasion, (4) intravasation, (5) circulation and embolism, (6) extravasation, and (7) metastatic tumor establishment in the target tissue. In this chapter we will discuss the steps involved in the complex process of tumor metastasis and the molecular mechanisms that underly each one of these steps.

Keywords: Metastasis, primary tumor, tumor microenvironment, angiogenesis, invasion, epithelial mesenchymal transition, extravasation, tumor establishment, apoptosis, tumor dormancy.

1. INTRODUCTION

Metastasis is a multi-stage process in which cancer cells spread from their primary location to other organs of the body. The clinical importance of metastasis is due to the fact that most cancer mortality is linked to this process of cancer cell dissemination. Clinical evidence has indicated that patients with localized tumors have a significantly better prognosis than those with disseminated tumors (Hunter BCR 2008) [1]. The heterogeneity of cancer cells, in primary tumor and in metastases, has been an obstacle for successful treatments (Fidler NRC 2003) [2]. An improved understanding of the factors leading to tumor dissemination is of vital importance.

The metastatic process consists of a series of sequential steps all of which must be successfully completed to give rise to a metastatic tumor (Bacac ARP 2008) [3]. An initial early step in metastasis is angiogenesis, an essential phenomenon not only in tumor growth but also in the initial progression from a pre-malignant tumor to an invasive cancer (Skobe NM 1997) [4]. Another step involves the detachment or loss of cellular adhesion from the primary tumor. It requires disruption of basement membrane, which represents the first barrier to invasion by carcinoma cells, mediated by specific proteases (Weiss CMR 1983) [5]. Increased motility and invasiveness are advantageous characteristic that allow tumor cells to change position within the tissue. Following the entry of tumor cells to local lymphatic and blood vessels, their survival in the circulation is one of the most serious challenges faced by tumor cells with metastatic phenotype (Blood BBA 1990) [6]. Prior to extravasation and invasion, circulating tumor cells must be capable of resisting hemodynamic shear forces and attack by host immune cells. Finally, the development of secondary tumor at the distant site completes the metastasis process (Brooks AH 2009) [7].

The development of metastatic ability by cancer cells is a multifactorial process whose temporal events are challenging obstacles for the tumor cell. Tumor cells with metastatic capability acquire advantageous phenotypes to complete the sequence of steps outlined above. They include interaction with the local microenvironment, constitutive induction of mitogenic signals, induction of angiogenesis, migration, invasion through the basement membrane into blood vessels (intravasation), escape of cancer cells from the circulation (extravasation), and colonization to the distant organs (Bacac ARP 2008) [3] (Bernards Nature 2002) [8]. During these processes many molecules play a central role for each step, from formation of primary tumor and new blood vessels to the establishment of metastatic tumor in the secondary site. These molecules include regulators of angiogenesis, small GTPases, proteinases, adhesion molecules, Protein-Tyrosine Kinase (PTK) and chemokines. Vascular Endothelial Growth Factor (VEGF) and Fibroblast Growth Factor (FGF) are considered central molecules to the regulation of tumor angiogenesis (Cristofanilli NRDD 2002)

***Address correspondence to Lucrecia Márquez-Rosado:** Public Health Sciences Division, Fred Hutchinson Cancer Research Center, 1100 Fairview Avenue North, Seattle, WA 98109, USA. Email: lmarquez@fhcrc.org

[9]. The small GTPases, through their effects on actin remodelling, have a key role in the regulation of cell migration. The serine protease named urokinase plasminogen activator (uPA), which binds to the urokinase Plasminogen Receptor (uPAR) expressed on the cancer cells, enables tumor cells to migrate through tissue barriers (Keleg MC 2003) [10]. Matrix Metalloproteinases (MMPs) and cathepsins are defined proteinases involved in the degradation of extracellular matrix components, *e.g.* (Koblinski CCA 2000) [11]. Integrins, selectins and cadherins are adhesion molecules that determine tumor cell interaction with other cell and with the extracellular matrix (Brooks AH 2009) [7] (Jeanes Oncogene 2008) [12]. Focal Adhesion Kinase (FAK) is protein-tyrosine kinase that regulates the cycle of focal contact formation and disassembly required for efficient cell migration (Schlaepfer BBA 2004) [13]. Chemokine receptors and their corresponding chemokine ligands may potentially facilitate tumor dissemination at several key steps of metastasis (Kakinuma JLB 2006) [14].

The aim of this chapter is to detail the main steps of metastasis process including: 1) Neoplastic progression, 2) Angiogenesis, 3) Migration and Invasion, 4) Intravasation. 5) Circulation and Embolism, 6) Extravasation, and 7) Metastatic tumor establishment (Fig. **1**).

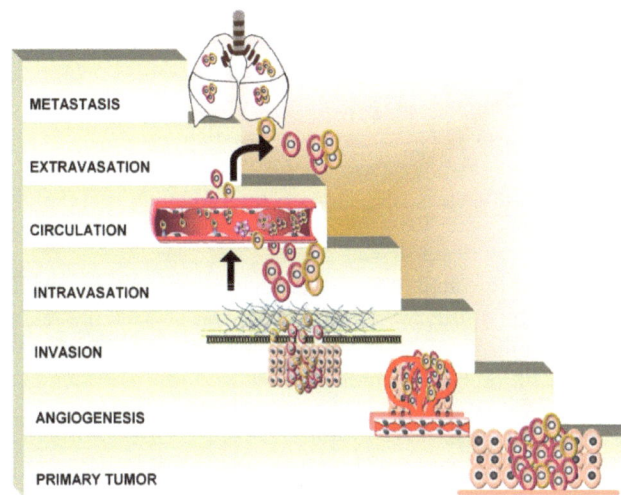

Figure 1: Steps in Tumor Metastasis.

2. NEOPLASTIC PROGRESSION

"Neoplastic progression", first described by Leslie Foulds (Foulds CR1954) [15] consists of permanent, irreversible qualitative changes in characteristics of a neoplasm. This process of neoplastic progression is gradual and can occur over periods of years where neoplastic cells acquire genetic alterations. Thus, genetic changes acquired by cells during the initial phases of neoplastic progression result in advantageous phenotypes that generate a large descendant population within the primary tumor. Other advantages involve the acquisition of constitutive mitogenic signal, resistance to growth inhibitory signaling and cell death (apoptosis) signaling, and induction of blood-vessel growth (angiogenesis) (Bernards Nature 2002) [8]. During this process, cells acquire additional mutations which enable them to metastasize, seeding new colonies at distant locations from primary tumor. Cells with such metastatic properties have the ability of progress to an advanced stage of malignancy and are genetically less stable when compared to non-metastatic cells. This genetic instability can be a key advantage that permits the evolution from a benign to the malignant tumor (Fidler NRC 2003) [2].

The process of metastasis begins early during the growth of primary tumor, which requires a source of cell heterogeneity within the population (Fig. **2**). Tumoral development can be compared with an evolutive process through which tumoral cells acquire characteristic of malignity *via* the sequential genetic and epigenetic changes (Iacobuzio ARP 2009) [16]. Cells with biological advantages, such as survival and proliferation, that allow them metastasize, are selected from a heterogeneous population. These cells become the progenitor of a successor cell population that finally will result in the predominant population of tumor (Chiang NEJM 2008) [17]. For the selection of a metastatic phenotype, tumor cells are challenged by multiple intrinsic and extrinsic barriers that limit tumor progression (Fig. **2B**, **2C**). Intrinsic barriers, which are a hallmark of primary tumors, include the genotoxic stress induced by oncogenes, the expression of growth inhibitory, apoptosis and senescence pathways, and telomere attrition (Gupta Cell 2006) [18]. Extrinsic barriers, are derived by cell-external factors, example include extracellular matrix components, basement membranes, and reactive oxygen species, attack by immune system and the limited availability of nutrients and oxygen. In this context, hypoxia is a clear example of selective pressure giving the tumor cell the advantageous property of diminished susceptibility to undergo apoptosis (Harris NRC 2002) [19].

Clinical observations of cancer patients and studies in rodent models of cancer have revealed that certain tumor types tend to mestatasize to specific organs. For example, breast cancer has the predisposition to metastasize to bones, lungs, brain, and liver. Tumors with the highest incidence of brain metastases include lung carcinoma, breast carcinoma, melanoma, and to a lesser extent, renal-cell and colorectal carcinomas (Chiang NEJM 2008) [17]. Sarcomas, renal cell carcinoma, colorectal, melanoma, and breast carcinomas have a strong preference to disseminate to the lungs. These organ preferences of metastatic spread appear to be independent of vascular anatomy, rate of blood flow and the number of tumor cells delivered to each organ (William 2008) [20]. This indicates that sites of metastasis are determined not solely by the characteristics of the neoplastic cells but also by the microenvironment of the host tissue.

Tumor Microenvironment

Cancer cell exposed to environmental stresses can acquire an aggressive phenotype. Through the activation of oncogenes and inactivation of tumor suppressor genes, cancer cells can display constitutive proliferation and survival. In addition, the surrounding normal stroma, or tumor microenvironment, not only provides essential factors for the maintenance of primary tumor but also promotes tumor formation to distant sites (Lorusso HCB 2008) [21]. Therefore, the outcome of the metastatic process depends on multiple and complex interactions of metastatic cells with host homeostatic mechanisms.

Tumor cells, directly and indirectly, alter the tumor microenvironment through the activation of many non-tumoral cells; *e.g.* blood cells, lymphatic endothelia cells, pericytes, and cells of the immune system (Coussens Nature 2002) [22]. These modifications can be observed at the transition stage from premalignant to malignant lesions. The most important ways in which tumor microenvironment promotes tumor progression is by facilitating the tumor growth, survival and angiogenesis.

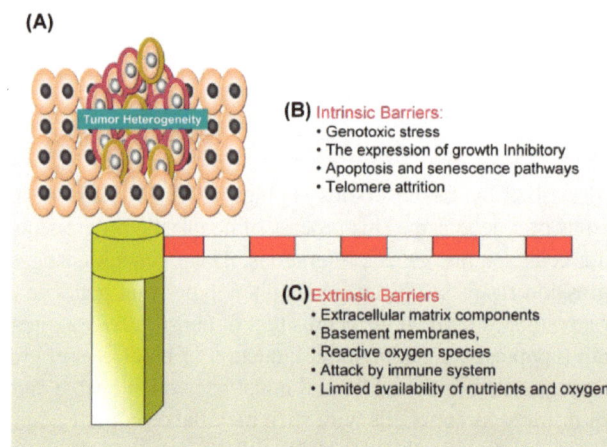

Figure 2: Neoplastic Progression. (A) Tumor heterogeneity is the presence of tumors composed of a variety of cell types with distinct morphologies and behaviors. (B) Intrinsic and extrinsic barriers that limit tumor progression.

3. ANGIOGENESIS

Although, the formation of new blood vessels is observed in many physiological processes, such as embryonic development, ovulation, and wound repair, it is also observed in many pathological conditions including arthritis, diabetes, retinopathy, and tumor growth (Hillen CMR 2007) [23]. Tumors larger than 1-2 mm^3, due to their increased metabolic demands, would be unable to obtain the oxygen and nutrients necessary to grow beyond approximately 2 mm in diameter without the formation of an intratumoral blood supply (Folkman NEJM 1971) [24]. Therefore, angiogenesis is essential to satisfy the oxygen and nutrients requirements of grown tumors. The mechanisms of neovascularization used during tumorigenesis differ from the normal physiologic process of neovascularization.

Difference Between Physiological and Tumor Angiogenesis

An example of physiological angiogenesis is embryonic vasculogenesis, in which blood vessels are created *de novo*. The first step includes proliferation and assembly of angioblasts, which create a network of primitive blood vessels, termed the primary capillary plexus. Then, the primary capillary plexus differentiates into new blood vessels that have the ability to sprout (defined as the growth of new blood vessel from pre-existing vessels) and branch (Bergers NRC 2003) [25] (Papetti APCP 2002) [26]. In contrast, in tumor cells, the first step of angiogenesis includes taking blood vessels from the surrounding stroma. After that, the sprouting angiogenesis can be initiated to induce the formation of new blood vessel from preexisting capillaries resembling normal angiogenesis (Papetti APCP 2002) [26]. Another difference between physiological and tumor angiogenesis is found in the balance between angiogenic inducers (pro-angiogenic factors) and inhibitors (anti-angiogenic factors). This balanced system in physiological angiogenesis is altered in tumors where many pro-angiogenic molecules are constitutively overexpressed, overwhelming the inhibitors, and allowing the continuous growth of new tumor blood vessels (Bergers NRC 2003) [25]. As a result, tumors develop an abnormal vascular architecture that consists of irregular blood vessels, which are dilated and convulated, resulting in abnormal blood flow. Moreover, tumor blood vessels are leaky, hemorragic and show immature vascular structures (venules, arterioles and capillaries), different from their normal counterparts (Papetti APCP 2002) [26].

Tumor Angiogenesis

Sprouting angiogenesis will provide the oxygen and nutrients that the tumor cell requires in the primary tumor stage and is required for metastasis formation and further outgrowth of metastases (Hillen CMR 2007) [23]. The process of angiogenic sprouting occurs in several well-characterized stages: (A) Growth factor release from tumor cells. (B) Extracelular matrix degradation by proteases. (C) Migration through extracellular matrix and formation of immature blood vessel. (D) Stabilisation of the immature vessels (Fig. **3**).

A. Growth Factor Release from Tumor Cells

Angiogenic sprouting is considered an active mechanism where the balance between pro-angiogenic and anti-angiogenic factors is lost in tumors. Multiple angiogenic factors are known to participate, including bFGF and members of the VEGF family (Fig. **3A**). Angiogenic growth factors, released from tumor cells, diffuse into nearby tissues and bind to receptor on the endothelial cells of pre-existing blood vessels in the vicinity of the tumor, leading to their activation (Cristofanilli.NRDD 2002) [9]. Once activated, these angiogenic growth factor receptors induce multiple signal transduction cascades, such as RAF, p38 MAPK, PI3K and FAK; these proteins play important roles in endothelial cell proliferation, migration, survival, and focal adhesion turn over, respectively (Cross TBS 2003) [27]. In addition, angiogenic growth factor receptors stimulate the production of adhesion molecules and proteolytic enzymes, including integrins, MMPs and Plasminogen activators (Brooks AH 2010) [7]. During the formation of new blood vessels, VEGF functions both as mitogen and as a potent pro-survival factor in vascular endothelial cells (Kerbel Carcinogenesis 2000) [28]. Tumor cells are a source of VEGF production, as well the tumor-associated stroma (Ferrara NM 2003) [29]. VEGF is considered one of the most potent stimulators of angiogenesis, and its production is stimulated under hypoxic conditions. Hypoxia stabilizes the transcription factor Hypoxia Inducible Factor-1 (HIF-1), which increases transcriptional activation of the VEGF gene and VEGF mRNA stability (Vaupel Oncologist 2004) [30] (Brooks AH 2009) [7]. It is therefore not surprising that hypoxic microenvironment has been associated with advanced tumor stage, metastasis, tumor recurrence and poor therapeutic response.

B. Extracellular Matrix Degradation by Proteinases

An important requirement for sprouting angiogenesis is the degradation of the basement membrane surrounding mother vessels. The membrane degradation is initiated by angiogenic factors, in particular bFGF and VEGF, which activate endothelial cells, and inducing the secretion of plasminogen activators and activation of MMPs, which are a family of zinc-binding enzymes that cleave extracellular matrix complex (Fig. **3B**) (Woodhouse Cancer1997) [31].

C. Migration Through Extracellular Matrix and Formation of Immature Blood Vessel

Once activated, angiogenic endothelial cells proliferate rapidly, migrate and invade the surrounding Extracellular Matrix (ECM) (Brooks AH 2010) [7].The migration event is facilitated by integrins and stimulated by bFGF and

VEGF growth factors (Hwang HOCNA 2004) [32] (Fig. **3C**). The migrating endothelial cells eventually differentiate to form a new and immature vessel which undergoes lumen formation (Fig. **3C**). The formation of vascular lumens is a critical step in the angiogenic process that requires co-migration of three groups of endothelial cells as a single cordlike structure. First, a group of cells shows an apoptotic process over a 12-hour period. The second group functions as a cover to the first group of cells. The adhesion of endothelial cells to each other is implied in the remodeling of the center of a solid vascular cord into a lumen. Finally, the third group of cells is required for enlargement of the luminal diameter (Meyer AR 1997) [33] (Brooks AH 2010) [7].

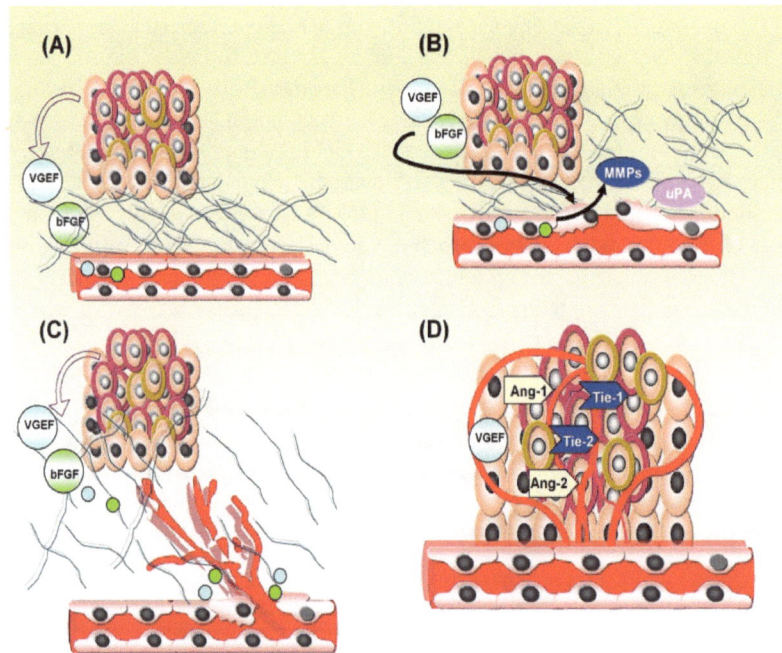

Figure 3: Angiogenesis: **(A)** Avascular Tumor. First, growth factors such as bFGF (fibroblast growth factor) and VEGF (vascular endothelial growth factor) are released from tumor cells. Then, they diffuse into nearby tissues and bind to receptors on the endothelial cells of pre-existing blood vessels in the vicinity of the tumor, leading to their activation. **(B)** Extracellular matrix degradation by proteinases. The activation of endothelial cells by bFGF and VEGF induce the secretion of plasminogen activators and activation of MMPs (Matrix metalloproteinases), in order to cleave of ECM (extracellular matrix) complex. **(C)** Migration through extracellular matrix and formation of immature blood vessel. **(D)** Stabilization of the immature vessels. The Tie receptors (Tie 1 and Tie 2) and their ligands, angiopoietin-1 and 2 (ang-1,2) play a central role in vessel formation and stabilization.

D. Stabilization of the Immature Vessels

Before blood flow begins, periendothelial cells, termed pericytes, and smooth muscle cells are attracted, and a vascular basal lamina is produced for stabilizing the newly formed vessels. Finally, the vascular system is built by the fusion of new blood-vessel sprouts (Fig. **3D**) (Bergers NRC 2003) [25]. Normally, the maturation of the vascular system includes differentiation into a macro and microvasculature, which is organized into arteries, veins, arterioles, venules and capillaries. By contrast, although the majority of tumor vasculature has a basement membrane and pericytes, it lacks further differentiation into the normal organization of perycites into the vascular wall. Moreover, there is evidence that tumor associated-perycites have abnormal morphology and produce VEGF (Jain NM 2003) [34]. While the mechanism of vascular stabilization is still in the process of being designed, it is known that abnormalities such as altered permeability and vessel diameter are associated with specific members of the VEGF family. The Tie receptors (Tie1 and Tie2) and their ligands, angiopoietin-1and 2 (ang-1, 2), also play a central role in vessel formation and stabilization. Ang1 and Tsp1 have been linked to decreased permeability and vessel diameter (Loughna MB 2001) [35]. In the absence of VEGF, Ang2 acts as an antagonist of Ang1 and destabilizes vessels, ultimately leading to vessel regression (Jain NM 2003) [34]. Thus, understanding of the mechanisms of the vascular stabilization process holds promise for the development of antiangiogenic therapy for cancer.

3. CELL MOTILITY AND INVASION

In addition to establishment of primary tumor growth and angiogenesis, tumor cells undergo changes in cell motility resulting in invasion of the basement membrane and metastasis. Cell migration is a dynamic process which is fundamental to healthy physiological events, such as tissue development and homeostasis of the immune system, but also a fundamental aspect of metastasis (Friedl CMLS 2000) [36].

Cell migration and invasion are key events in dissemination and metastatic growth of tumor cells in distant organs. Through migratory and invasive mechanisms, the cancer cell can penetrate lymphatic and blood vessels for dissemination into the circulation in order to reach the target organ (Friedl NRC 2003) [2]. Cell migration includes a series of interconnected steps such as: (A) Actin-cytoskeleton remodelling: protrusion of lamellipodia and filopodia. (B) Focal Adhesion Complexes. (C) Extracellular matrix degradation by proteinase. (D) Cell Body Contraction. (E) Cell Detachment (Fig. **4A**).

A. Actin-Cytoskeleton Remodelling: Protrusion of Lamellipodia and Filopodia

Cell protrusions, called lamellipodia and filopodia, are involved in the initial steps of cell migration and dependent on reorganization of the actin cytoskeleton. Lamellipodia are formed when the actin cytoskeleton is assembled in a particular branched pattern which appears as membrane ruffles at the leading edge. On the other hand, when actin is assembled in an unbranched pattern cells form filopodia, which are bunches of radially oriented actin filaments that sense the environment (Fig. **4B**) (Larsen NRMCBiol 2003) [37] (Carragher TCB 2004) [38].

The conservation of actin-containing structures at the leading edge of cells requires actin polymerization, depolymerization and branching. These events are controlled by families of actin-binding proteins. For example, actin polymerization is promoted by cofilins, which are small actin-binding proteins that have a key role in the direction of cell motility. Depolymerization is regulated by the actin depolymerizing factor (ADF)/cofilin family of proteins, which are essential regulators of actin filament turnover (Larsen NRMCBiol 2003) [37]. Branching is controlled by the actin-related protein 2/3 complex (ARP2/3), which is typically in an inactive state. Binding of Wiskott-Aldrich Syndrome protein (WASP) activates the ARP2/3 complex, which then organizes actin filaments into branched networks that are capable of generating protrusive force and mechanical resistance. These events are implicated both in the formation of lamellipodia and podosoma, and have an important role in the cell migration and invasion process (Goley NRMCB 2006) [39]. The small GTPases, through their affects on actin remodelling, have also a role important in the regulation of cell migration. Phosphatidylinositols activate Guanine-Nucelotide Exchange Factors (GEF) that regulate the activity of the small GTPases such as Rho, Rac and Cdc42 (Friedl NRC 2003) [2], which function in the following maner: RhoA induces focal adhesions and stress-fiber assembly, Rac stimulates lamellipodia and focal complex formation and Cdc42 promote filopodia, cell rounding and the loss actin stress fibers (Larsen NRMCBiol 2003) [37] (Ridley Cell 1992) [40].

B. Focal Adhesion Complexes

Focal adhesions are the sites of contact between the ECM and the cytoskeleton mediated through the integrin family of transmembrane proteins (Burridge ARCDB 1996) [41]. Although, the composition of a focal contact can vary widely depending on external cues and cellular responses, some of the integrin-binding proteins can be found consistently, such as talin, paxillin, vinculin and FAK (Fig. **4C**) (Mitra NRMCB 2005) [42]. Focal adhesion complexes are considered crucial determinants in the process of cell migration, serving as traction sites for migration as the cell moves forward over them. This type of migration is regulated by integrin-linked focal adhesion complexes through their association with the ECM. A consequence of linkage of these cell adhesions to the ECM, is integrin activation that regulates intracellular signaling (Berrier JCP 2007) [43]. Integrins are heterodimeric cell-surface receptors, composed of an α and β subunit, that bind ECM through the Arg-Gly-Asp (RGD) peptide sequence of proteins comprising the ECM (Woodhouse Cancer 1997) [31]. Thus, integrins can regulate the interaction between the ECM and actin cytoskeleton (Webb COCB 2003) [44]. Moreover, integrin-linked focal adhesion not only functions to support adhesion to ECM but are also implicated in the transmision of extracellular signals to intracellular signal transduction pathways (Carragher TCB 2004) [38] (Schlaepfer BBA 2004) [45]. For example, ECM binding can induce clustering of integrins which can regulate interactions between the cytoplasmic domains of integrin receptors, adaptor proteins and signaling proteins resulting in changes in the phosphorylation status of signalling proteins in cells. The integrin cytoplasmic domains are vital for its interaction with actin, talin, and FAK

(Focal Adhesion Kinase) (Friedl NRC 2003) [46]. Integrin activation can promote activation of FAK which can bind to several signaling molecules and promote cell survival and cell migration (Renshaw JCB 1999) [47]. FAK is a protein-tyrosine kinase that activates members of the Rho GTPase family such as Rho, Rac and Cdc42. As discussed above, Rho proteins are well-known for their role in the formation of stress fibers while both Rac and Cdc42 promote actin polimerization at the leading edge and, consequently, formation of filopodia and lamellipodia, respectively. Consistent with this observation, FAK and members of the Rho GTPase family have been associated with invasive tumor phenotype (Bacac ARP 2008) [3].

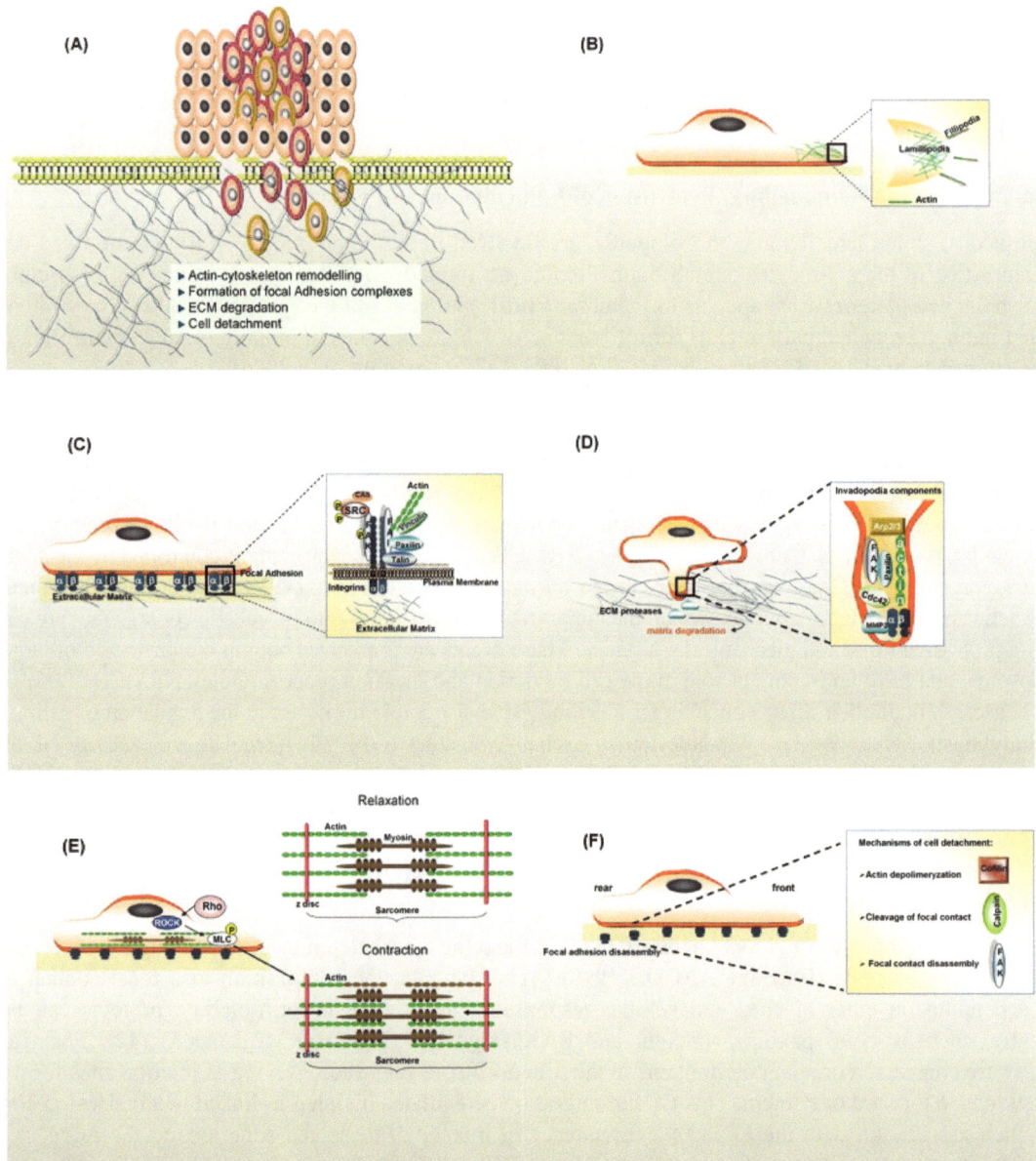

Figure 4: Migration and Invasion: (A) Cell migration results from a continuous cycle of interdependent steps. Cell migration includes a series of interconnected steps such as (B) actin-cytoskeleton remodelling: protrusion of lamellipodia and filopodia. Lamellipodia are formed when the actin filaments at the leading edge are short and highly branched. By contrast, filopodia arise when the filaments are long, unbranched, and assembled in tight, parallel bundles. (C) Focal adhesion complexes are the sites of contact between the extracellular matrix and the cytoskeleton mediated through the integrins. Within the cell, the intracellular domain of integrin binds to the cytoskeleton *via* adapter proteins such as talin, paxilin, vinculin, actin and FAK. (D) Extracellular matrix degradation by proteinases. Invadopodia are actin-rich protrusions that localize matrix-degrading activity to cell-substratum contact points. These structures are formed by proteolytic, cell signaling, adhesive, cytoskeletal proteins. (E) Cell body contraction, which is dependent on myofibrils comprised of actin and myosin myofilaments. Rho associates with ROCK (Rho-kinase), which phosphorylate myosin light

chain (MLC). The phosphorylation of MLCK stabilizes the actin filaments and promotes actin-myosin contractility. (F) Cell detachment. Mechanisms involved in the focal contact disassembly leading to cell detachment.

C. Extracellular Matrix Degradation by Proteinases

The basement membrane is the initial mechanical barrier that must be conquered in the process of tumor invasion. Degradation of the basement membrane allows neoplastic and endothelial cells to invade and migrate into surrounding tissues. In fact, altered organization or integrity of the basement membrane is considered to be a hallmark of the transition from a carcinoma *in situ* to an invasive carcinoma. Along with their function as mechanical anchor proteins, the integrins are also involved in regulating the activities of proteolytic enzymes that degrade the basement membrane (Hood NRC 2002) [48]. Localized degradation of the membrane results from the production, activation and release of several types of proteases. This proteolytic process must be tightly controlled in order to facilite cell passage while maintaining the cell traction necessary for migration to occur. An important requirement of cancer cell to migrate through a physical barrier of dense ECM and maintain a balance between remodeling and degradation of ECM, is the extension of protrusions named invadopodia. These protrusions mediate proteolysis of the ECM *via* the expression of different Matrix Metalloproteinases (MMPs) (Yamaguchi COCB 2005) [49] (Fig. **4D**). MMPs belong to a family of zinc-binding enzymes that degrade all componentes of the extracellular matrix and basement membrane. They are initially secreted as an inactive zymogen that requires proteolytic activation by extracellular proteases, and their activity is tightly regulated by specific tissue inhibitors of MMPs named TIMPs. The MMP family currently include more than 20 members that can be divided into the following 3 general classes: (1) interstitial collagenases (MMP-1) that degrade the stromal collagens types I and III; elevated expression of collagenase can result from constitutive production of the enzyme by tumor cells, neighboring stromal cells, and by interactions between tumor/stromal cell (Brinckerhoff CCR 2000) [50]; (2) stromelysins that degrade proteoglycan, laminin, fibronectin, elastin, gelatin, and collagen types III, IV, V, VII, and IX, , and (3) gelatinases that degrade denatured collagen, native collagen types IV, V, VII, IX, and X, fibronectin, and elastin (Woodhouse Cancer 1997) [31]**.**

D. Cell Body Contraction

Cell body contraction, the fourth critical step for cell migration, is dependent on actin-myosin contractility where the retraction force is generated by the sliding of myosin motors, such as myosin II, on actin filaments or actin bundles in the cell body and rear (Ananthakrishnan IJBS 2007) [51] (Kedrin JMGBN 2007) [52] (Fig. **4E**). Since actin filaments and bundles are connected to the the cell membrane and substrate, the force generated can be converted to traction forces that enable the cell to move forward. Though the roles of different molecules in regulating this complex process are still being discovered, Rho is thought to have a key role in regulation of the contraction and retraction forces required in the cell body and at the rear. Active GTP-bound Rho associates with and activates the Rho-kinase (ROCK), which can in turn phosphorylate several substrates including Myosin Light Chain (MLC). It is likely that the phosphorylation of MLCK stabilizes of actin filaments and promotes actin-myosin contractility (Olson TCB 2004) [53] (Fig. **4E**).

E. Cell Detachment

Cell detachment, considered the final stage of the cell motility process, is a critical step in metastasis. To migrate, cells must coordinately assemble and disassemble focal adhesions, with regulated adhesion formation at the cell front and release at the cell rear (Huttenlocher COCB1995) [54]. Several mechanisms are involved in the focal contact disassembly leading to cell detachment, namely: (a) actin depolymerization, in which the cofilin binds to actin filaments contributing to actin depolymerization in cells and preventing their reassembly; (b) cleavage of the focal contact, catalyzed by calpain; and (c) focal contact disassembly, which is mediated in part by FAK (Fig. **4F**). After focal contact disassembly, integrins detach from the substrate and become internalized *via* endocytic vesicles for recycling at the leading edge or deposition onto the substrate (Friedl NRC 2003) [46]. Additionally, the cell detachment process includes loss of intercellular junctional complexes, namely, tight junctions or adherens junctions. These serve as anchoring points between epithelial cells to ensure appropriate integrity, and tensile strength of epithelial sheets. Adherens junctions are constituted primarily of E-cadherin, which maintains intercellular adhesion through interaction with actin cytoskeleton *via* α-, β- and γ-catenins (Gupta Cell 2006) [18]. Like other members of the cadherin family, E-cadherins are single-pass transmembrane proteins whose extracellular regions mediate specific cell-cell interactions, are Ca^{2+}-dependent cell adhesion molecules, and display homophilic binding (binding between two identical cadherins) (Pokutta ARCDB 2007) [55]. Many studies have shown that E-cadherin is an important player in the metastatic process. It has been demonstrated that loss or reduction of E-cadherin expression is related to a highly aggressive phenotype. In addition, expression of E-cadherin and reestablishment of functional adherens can abolish the invasive phenotype of many different tumor cell lines (Bogenrieder Oncogene 2003) [56] (Jeanes Oncogene 2008) [57]. Thus, E-cadherin is considered a tumor suppressor. Mechanisms that can downregulate or cause loss of E-cadherin function in tumors include (1) transcriptional repression, (2) promoter methylation, (3) disruption of the link between E-cadherin and the cytoskeleton, (4) endocytosis of E-cadherin:β-catenin complex and (5) proteolysis of the extracellular domain of E-cadherin by MMPs (Bacac ARP 2008) [3]. The loss of E-cadherin can trigger an event termed "cadherin switch", which consists of the replacement of E-cadherin by N-cadherins, and has been observed in the most invasive tumor cells. N-cadherin can cooperate with the FGF receptor, resulting in signals that lead to the up-regulation of MMP-9 and, hence, cellular invasion (Hazan ANYAS 2004) [58].

It has long been recognized that the cell-cell adhesion molecule E-cadherin is an important determinant of tumor progression, serving as a suppressor of invasion and metastasis. Numerous studies suggest that loss of E-cadherin is required for the induction of Epithelial-Mesenchymal Transition (EMT) through loss of cell-cell adhesions (Cavallaro COID 2004) [59].

Epithelial-Mesenchymal Transition

EMT is defined as an orchestrated series of biologic events by which epithelial cells acquire mesenchymal features (Radisky DC JCS 2005) [60]. EMT is essential for embryonic development, wound healing and tissue regeneration (Kalluri JCI 2009) [61]. Nevertheless, if deregulated EMT can also be destructive, as is the case in cancer.

Epithelial cells are closely bound to one another to form continuous sheets, and they provide cell-cell junctions through E-cadherin and adhesions essential to hold them tightly together. In contrast, adhesions between mesenchymal cells are less strong compared with their epithelial counterparts. The current view is that EMT is a multi-step process in which cells obtain molecular alterations that cause disruption of cell-cell adhesions, loss of apical-baselateral polarity, cytoskeletal changes, down regulation of E-cadherin, α-catenin, β-catenin and claudins, and the gain of mesenchymal proteins including vimentin, fibronectin and N-cadherin (Thiery COCB 2003) [62] (Thiery and Sleeman NRMCB 2006 [63]). The loss of E-cadherin and converse gain of mesenchymal N-cadherin expression "cadherin switch" is thought to be a hallmark of EMT required by tumour cells to acquire invasive properties, (Cavallaro COID 2004) [59]. In addition to loss of E-cadherin, some studies also suggest that EMT is triggered by interactions with extracellular matrix molecules such as collagens, hyaluronic acid and fibronectin (Maier Cancers 2010) [64], and growth factors such as Transforming Growth Factor β (TGFβ), Hepatocyte Growth Factor (HGF), Insulin-Like Growth Factor (IGF) and Fibroblast Growth Factor (FGF). Additionally, activation of Wnt signaling and the transcription factors Snail/Slug, Twist and Six have also been implicated in EMT induction (Heuberger CSHPB 2010) [65]. Thus, a conversion from an epithelial to a more mesenchymal phenotype is a complex process involving changes in cell adhesion, cytoskeleton organization, extracellular signals and gene expression.

The activation of oncogenes, including RAS (Huber COCB 2005) [66], Her2/neu or ERBB2 and Neurotrophic Kinase Receptor 2 (NTRK2/TrkB) have also been shown to induce EMT (Smit Oncogene 2011) [67]. This differentiation is thought to allow epithelial cancer cells to escape from the primary tumor, which is followed by local invasion. EMT is thus believed to be a major mechanism by which cancer cells become migratory. Furthermore, it has also been postulated that epithelial tumor cells undergo EMT to allow their escape from the primary organ to a distant site: EMT could facilitate intravasation of tumor cells into the blood or lymph vessels, thus leading to subsequent formation of distant metastases (Radisky CSC 2008) [68]. While mechanisms that explain how EMT participates in the key steps of malignant transformation have not been fully clarified, it is well known that the acquisition of mesenchymal phenotype is typical for carcinoma cells that have gained metastatic potential. Interestingly, EMT has been described as a transient and reversible process: cells may also revert from a mesenchymal phenotype back to displaying epithelial characteristics through a process termed a Mesenchymal-Epithelial Transition (MET) during the outgrowth of tumor cells that have migrated to distant sites. While there is evidence to suggest that EMT is critical for the initial transformation from benign to invasive carcinoma, and MET critical to the latter stages of metastasis, it remains unclear at present what role MET has in metastatic dissemination. It could be important for the survival of circulating tumor cells, for seeding in distant sites or for the emergence from dormancy of tumor cells that have already established micrometastases.

4. INTRAVASATION

Once tumor cells with metastatic ability detach from the primary tumor, in order to travel to distant organs they must enter to circulation (blood vessels or lymphatic system) by a process known as intravasation. This process involves the penetration of cancer cells through the basement membrane surrounding blood or lymphatic vessel walls, which requires tumor cells to squeeze through the endothelial cell barrier (Yamaguchi COCB 2005) [49]. Although many characteristics of intravasation have not yet been defined, some metastatic cell lines have shown interesting behaviour that increases the efficiency of tumor cell dissemination to blood or lymphatic vessels. Examples include the abitily of tumor cells to properly orient themselves toward blood or lymphatic vessels, and their ability to change cell shape from a more elongated to a more rounded morphology (Wyckoff CR 2000) [69].

In many cases, migration of tumor cells from the primary site toward blood or lymphatic vessels has been characterized as an active process by following nutrient or chemokine gradients. On the other hand, there are various examples of metastases in the early stages exhibiting a relatively passive shedding process.

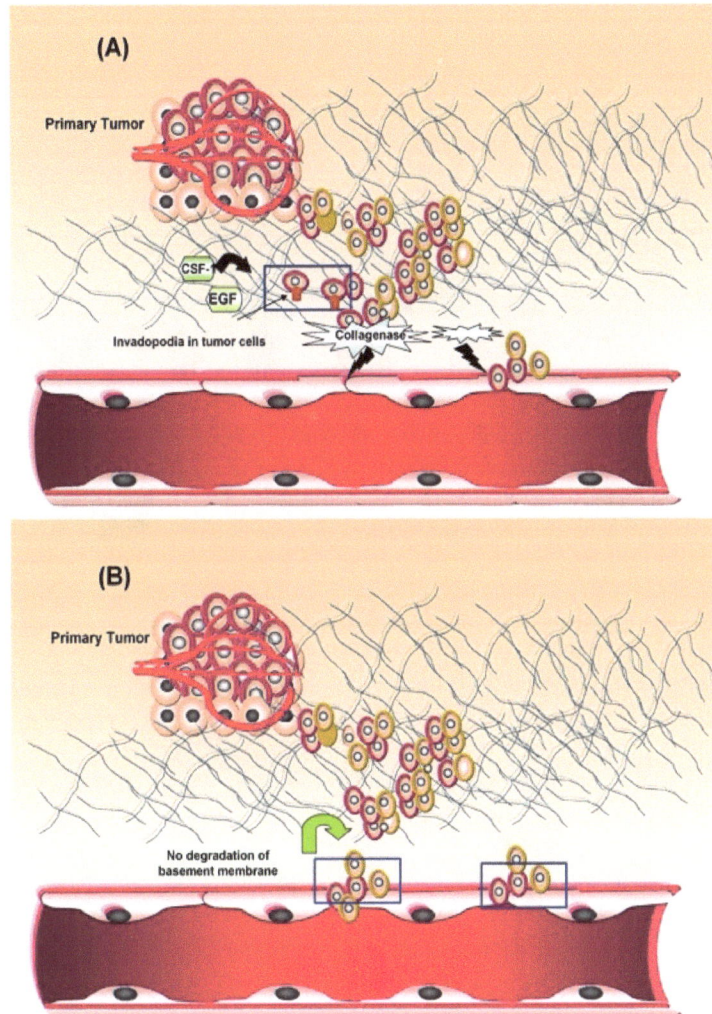

Figure 5: Intravasation. (A) Active intravasation. Tumor cells migrate in response to EGF and CSF-1 which can stimulate the formation of invadopodia. As a result, tumor cells may penetrate into a dense collagen matrix and actively digest interstitial matrix and basement membrane, mediated by IV collagenase activity, to migrate through tissue and into blood vessels. (B) Passive intravasation does not require proteolytic degradation of the basement membranes for cancer cells to enter circulation. Passive intravasation is observed in fragile blood and lymphatic vessels.

A. Active Intravasation

Active intravasation is a result of a directed migration through tissue and toward blood vessels, which requires cytoskeletal reorganization, changes in cell adhesion, degradation of ECM and basement membrane, all of which involves interactions with the surrounding tumor microenvironment (Fig. **5A**) (Gupta Cell 2006) [18]. Tumor-associated macrophages participate in ECM degradation through the podosome (actin-based adhesive structures) which in turn causes the release of chemotactic peptides that help to the migration of tumor cells (Yamaguchi COCB 2005) [49]. In animal studies, tumor cells and macrophages in primary tumors tissue with metastatic potential can migrate in response to EGF and CSF-1. As a result of this active mechanism, tumor cells may penetrate into a dense collagen matrix (Weaver CEM 2006) [70].

B. Passive Intravasation

Although passive intravasation remains poorly understood, one possible explanation includes the fragility of blood vessels, which could facilitate the shedding of tumor cells into vasculature. In addition, an altered growth of tumor cells, which can generate a mechanical stress within a limited space, could also facilitate the break down of fragile blood and lymphatic vessels (Bockhorn LO 2007) [71]. In these situations, as is observed in sarcomas, proteolytic degradation of the basement-membranes is not required for cancer cells to enter circulation (Fig. **5B**). Passive intravasation is most likely seen in tissues with thin basement membranes. For example, lung parenchyma is composed of thin-walled alveoli; each alveolus is wrapped in a fine mesh of capillaries. These vessels may require much less degradation of the basement membrane than intravasation into thick wall vessels, which could explain part of why the lungs are one of the most common sites for metastasis in the human body (Nguyen NRC 2009) [72].

6. EMBOLISMS/ CIRCULATION

Once tumor cells have penetrated the circulatory compartment, they gain access to all organs of the body. However, the metastatic spread of tumor cells from a primary tumor to distant sites in the body is considered an inefficient process: large tumor cells are frequently released into the circulation, but few develop into metastasis (Weiss ACR 1990 [73], Sahai NRC 2007) [74]. Although the reasons for the short half-life of circulating cancer cells are not completely understood, several mechanisms that threaten their survival have been proposed. Many tumor cells are morphologically rigid compared to the common property of blood cells. Thus, they may become damaged during their passage through the vasculature, which leads to tumor cells destruction (Blood BBA 1990) [6]. Other mechanisms by which circulating cancer cells are destroyed in circulation include hemodynamic shear forces caused by blood flow, and interactions with immune cells (particularly NK cells) that may lead to their destruction (Molloy COGD 2008) [75] (Palumbo Blood 2007) [76]. Although the circulatory compartment is a hostile environment for a potential metastatic cell, cancer cells can promote their survival using different mechanisms of protection. Cancer cells can physically shield one another when they travel in groups compared with single tumor cells (Fig. **6A**). While traveling through the circulatory system adhere to each other, to lymphocytes and to platelets, forming emboli that may adhere to the inner surface of capillaries (Fig. **6B, C**). This is thought to help them from immune surveillance and the shear force of blood flow (Joyce NRC 2009) [77]. Moreover, the interaction of cancer cells with the microvasculature and surrounding tissues evoke inflammatory responses that attract leukocytes and macrophages. These cells, together with endothelial cells and fibroblasts, in turn can provide a source of enzymes that could enhance both the intravasation and extravasation (pass out of the vessel) of tumor cells. The adhesion of circulating cancer cells to endothelium can involve at least some of the adhesive mechanisms required for the leukocytes recruitment, for example selectins, integrins (Fig. **6D**), and the immunoglobulin family, and their interaction with platelets and leukocytes occur mainly *via* selectins and integrins (Brooks AH 2009) [7].

As mentioned previously the blood represents an actively hostile environment for metastasizing cancer cells. Therefore, the presence of tumor cells in the circulation does not constitute metastasis, since most circulating cells die rapidly (Sahai NRC 2007) [74]. If the tumor cells survive these initial dangers, they become trapped in the microvasculature and then they can carry out the extravasation process.

7. EXTRAVASATION

Extravasation, the escape of cancer cells from circulation, is thought to be a prerequisite step during the spread of tumor cells leads to distant locations from the primary tumor. In addition to hemodynamic forces and confrontation between tumor cells and the immune system, the extravasation process is an important rate limiting-step during metastasis. Extravasation is considered to be an active process in which tumor cells have critical interactions and dynamic contacts with the microvessel endothelium. These interactions require notable cytoskeletal modifications for crossing the endothelium into the underlying matrix and stroma (Miles CEM 2008) [78]. This process also requires proteolysis and cell adhesion in wich both the endothelium and tumor cells play an active role. Extravasation can be divided into three phases. First, tumor cells interact loosely with endothelium, promoting rolling motion along the walls of blood vessels. Second, cell attachment to the vasculature endothelium, and finally, tumor cells pass through the endothelial wall, a process known as diapedesis (Fig. **7**).

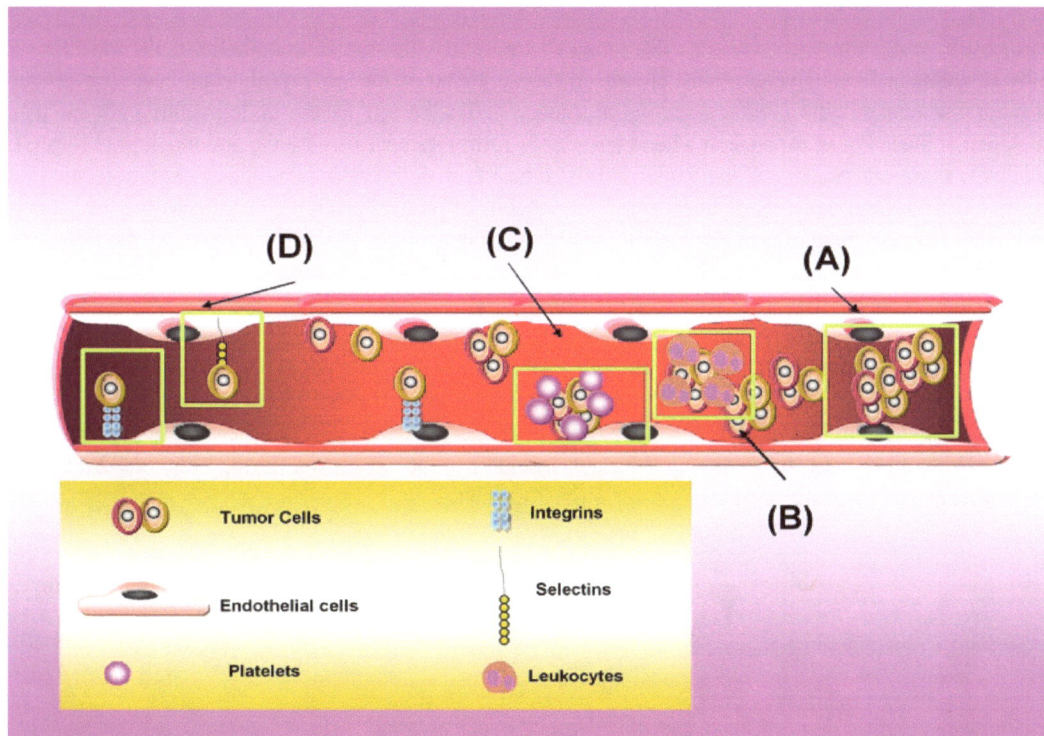

Figure 6: Embolism and Circulation. Circulating cancer cells promote their survival using different mechanisms of protection, including: (A) traveling as conglomerates, (B) adhesion to platelets, (C) adhesion to leukocytes, and (D) adhesion to vascular endothelium *via* selectins and integrins.

A. Rolling Motion of Tumor Cells

Extravasation takes place within a few hours after attachment of tumor cells to the vessel wall (it has been considered that the leukocytes are the possible cells to extravasate with tumor cells following them). Initial insight into the process of tumor cell extravasation was provided by studies with leukocytes (Miles CEM 2008) [78]. Generally, rolling of leukocytes is mediated mainly by selectins, also named as cell adhesion molecules (CAMs) (Strell CMLS 2007) [79]. CAMs belong to one of five protein families: the Immunoglobulin superfamily (IgSF CAMs), the integrins, the cadherins, the selectins and the lymphocyte homing receptors. Selectins are transmembrane molecules expressed on the surface of leukocytes and activated endothelial cells. They are grouped into three subcategories: E-selectin (in endothelial cells), L-Selectin (in leukocytes) and P-selectin (in platelets and endothelial cells) (Bertini CRC 2001) [80].

The contribution of vascular cell adhesion molecules (V-CAM) and selectins to metastasis is thought to result from specific interactions between receptors of tumor cells and ligands expressed on the endothelium (Barthel EOTT 2007) [81]. The expression of selectins on blood vessel endothelium, therefore, could initiate extravasation of tumour cells at metastatic sites (Fig. **7A**). The transient selectin-ligand binding allows cancer cells to dissociate and roll along vascular endothelia. Selectin-dependent rolling has been observed in breast, colon and prostate cancer cell lines (Tozeren IJC 1995) [82] (Dimitroff CR 2004) [83]. Furthermore, the constitutive expression of E-selectin ligands on bone vesssels has been correlated with a high potential of bone metastasis (Dimitroff CR 2005) [84]. Although carbohydrate structures, sialyl Lewis A (SLeA) and sialyl Lewis X (SLeX), are not true physiological ligands for selectins, increased adhesion of tumor cells to endothelium is mediated by binding of SLeA and SLeX on tumor cells to E-selectin (Fig. **7A**). Human colon cancer cells also express SLeA- and SLeX- glycoprotein ligands for E-selectin (Tomlinson IJO 2000) [85]. Other selectin ligands include HCELL (hematopoietic cell E-/L-selectin ligand), which functions as a high affinity E- and L-selectin ligand of colon carcimona cell lines (Burdick JBC 2006) [86] and PSGL-1 (P-selectin glycoprotein ligand-1) and ESL-1 (E-selectin-ligand-1) which are found in bone-metastatic prostate carcinoma cell lines (Dimitroff CR 2005) [84]. In conclusion, selectin-dependent rolling is a process used to recruit specific cells in the bloodstream to target tissue.

B. Adhesion to the Vasculature Endothelium

As was previously was mentioned, cancer cells establish transient adhesion to endothelial cells and this adhesion is mediated by selectins and cell glycoproteins. However, the next step of the extravasation process requires more stable adhesions with the endhothelium. Strengthening of cancer cell adhesion to the endothelium may be mediated by cytokines, which activate CAM expression when cancer cells form interactions with the endothelium (Miles CEM 2008) [78]. The *in vitro* studies demonstrated that integrin α4β1 interacts with the vascular cell adhesion molecule (V-CAM) to mediate adhesion of several cancer cell lines to the endothelium (Taichman CR1991) [87]. Moreover, animal models demonstrated that the metastatic capacity of melanoma cells is enhanced through α4β1 integrin interactions with VCAM-1 (Garofalo CR1995) [88] (Okahara CR1994) [89]. Tumor cells express intercellular adhesion molecule-1 (ICAM-1), a ligand for β2-integrins (Fig. **7B**). β2-integrins are receptors found on leukocytes but absent on tumor cells. Thus, tumor cells need to use leukocytes as linkers to connect to the endothelium and enable firm adhesion (Strell CMLS 2007) [79], (Fig. **7B**). Other molecules involved in forming strong tumor cell adhesion to the endothelium include galectin-3, a lectin upregulated in endothelial cells of cancer tissue and associated with a metastatic phenotype. CD44 is a cell-surface glycoprotein that functions as the receptor for hyaluronic acid and can interact with other ligands, such as osteopontin, collagens and MMPs. In breast cancer cells, CD44 may participate in the expression of α4β1 and αLβ2 integrins, leading to tumor-endothelial adhesion and diapedesis (Wang ECR 2005) [90].

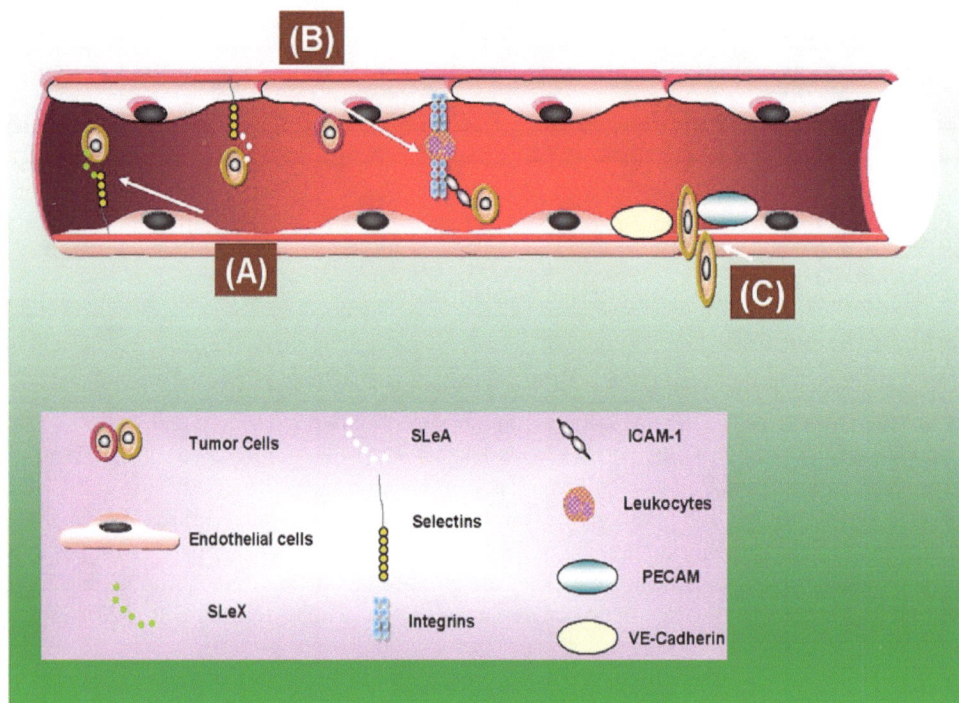

Figure 7: Extravasation. Extravasation can be divided into three sequential steps: (A) rolling motion of tumor cells. This step requires transient adhesion to endothelial cells, in which cancer cells have the ability to bind to the endothelial cell adhesion molecule E-selectin through the carbohydrate antigens, SLeA and SLeX, expressed on the surface of tumor cells. (B) Adhesion to the vasculature. In this step endothelium stable adhesions are established. (C) Diapedesis, or the passage of circulating tumor cells across the endothelium. This event is characterized by the expression of VE-cadherin (Vascular Endothelial Cadherin) and PECAM (platelet/endothelial cell adhesion molecule).

C. Diapedesis

Adhesion to the vascular endothelium is then followed by the passage of circulating tumor cells across the endothelium, which is termed diapedesis, the final step in extravasation. Diapedesis is a dynamic process that involves the constant rupture and formation of intercellular contacts. During diapedesis, tumor cells form lamellipodial and pseudopodial protrusions, which extend from the basal surface of the membrane to penetrate endothelial intercellular juctions. These protrusions are accompanied by a dramatic cell shape change (from rounded to well-spread morphology) and cytoskeletal remodeling. These events are characterized by alterations in expression of VE-cadherin (Vascular Endothelial Cadherin) and PECAM (Platelet/Endothelial Cell Adhesion Molecule) (Fig. **7C**) (Voura MRT 1998) [91]. In addition, diapedesis may require the participation of other molecules, including N-cadherin, which colocalizes with β-catenin at melanoma-endothelial junctions (Qi MBC 2005) [92]. It also has been demonstrated that metastatic cells induce changes in the vascular permeability of blood vessels in target organs through VEGF. For example, metastatic cells promote formation of the VE-cadherin/β-catenin complex, thereby disrupting endothelial cell junctions and facilitating metastatic extravasation.

During diapedesis, the endothelium is irreversibly damaged. Possible reasons for this include the induction of apoptosis by loss of cell-cell contacts (Brandt SCB 2005) [93], and the much larger size of tumor cells than leukocytes, which have difficulty squeezing between endothelial cells without damage.

8. METASTATIC TUMOR ESTABLISHMENT

Once circulating cancer cells gain access to the secondary site, their subsequent establishment requires a fertile microenvironment. Their growth is tightly regulated by the molecular interaction between cancer cells (seed) and the new environment (soil). Few extravasated cells will be competent to settle in the new site. Most undergo apoptosis within a few hours of reaching the secondary site. Others may lie dormant and only a few of these proliferate to form secondary tumors (Fig. **8**).

A. Apoptosis

Non-metastatic cells are more prone to apoptosis than those with a metastatic phenotype (Kim CL 2004) [94]. Reduction of tumor cell survival at metastatic sites can be influenced by several external factors. For example, loss of tumor cell-matrix interactions at secondary sites may lead to anoikis. In addition, high levels of nitric oxide produced by endothelial cells that surround cancer cells display cytotoxic effects. Immune surveillance identifies and eliminates cancer cells (Sahai NRC 2007) [74].

It may be indicative that survival is a key event for metastatic establishment. However, other studies have shown that not all cells that survive at secondary sites begin to proliferate due to varied replicative potential.

B. Tumor Dormancy

Tumor dormancy is a phenomenon whereby cancer cells stop growing for a period of time (Udagawa APMIS 2008) [95]. Disseminated cells may also remain dormant for prolonged periods before subsequently resuming proliferation. Although the molecular basis of dormancy is not well understood, this condition may arise due to a variety of mechanisms. These mechanisms include cell cycle arrest, immnune surveillance, and failure to obtain angiogenesis (Fig. **8**). The mechanisms leading to cell cycle arrest in tumor cells involves low expression of urokinase plasminogen activator receptor (u-PARP), which reduces ERK mitogenic signaling.

The role of immune surveillance in tumor dormancy is now well established. Some studies have indicated that the immune system recognizes cancer cells and destroys them, but other studies have shown that the immune system does not always completely eliminate tumor cells and instead maintains cancer cells in dormant condition (Koebel Nature 2007) [96]. In 1960, it was demonstrated that the absence of tumor vascularization severely restricts tumor growth (Folkman Cancer 1963) [97]. Currently, it is well established that tumor progression is dependent on recruitment of blood vessels, and failure to obtain angiogenesis may also cause tumor dormancy.

C. Proliferation and Formation of Secondary Tumors

Once tumor cells have penetrated the parenchyma of a new organ, they must create a microenvironment favorable to their survival and proliferation (Bacac ARP 2008) [3]. The organ distribution of metastasis is not a random event, and blood flow patterns alone provide only a partial explanation for preferred sites. Paget's seed and soil hypothesis proposes that sites of metastasis are determined not solely by the characteristics of the neoplastic cells (seed) but also by the microenvironment of the secondary site (soil) (Fidler NRC 2003) [2].

Several lines of evidence indicate that reciprocal cellular and molecular adaptations that occur between cancer cells and their stroma during metastatic progression influence the type of cancer cell that will evolve there. For example, prostate or breast cancer cells that metastasize to the bone are able to affect bone tissue, which is composed of diverse cell types such as osteoblasts and osteoclasts. On the one hand, prostate cancer cells may stimulate osteoblasts to form new bone, known as osteoclerotic metastasis (Reddi JBMR 2003) [98]. On the other hand, breast cancer cells may hyperactivate bone-reabsorbing osteoclasts, causing osteolytic metastasis. Consecutively, osteolytic resorption releases active factors from the bone matrix, in particular Transforming Growth Factor-beta (TGF-beta) (Guise CORR 2003) [99]. Then, increased amounts of osteolytic factors, such as parathyroid hormone-related protein, interleukin-11 and VEGF, are produced by the cancer cells to mediate the metastatic growth. These tumor cell-bone cell interactions cause a vicious cycle in which tumor cells stimulate the respective bone cells to cause bone destruction. Consequently, the bone microenvironment is enriched with growth factors that fuel tumor growth in bone (Guise JMNI 2002) [100].

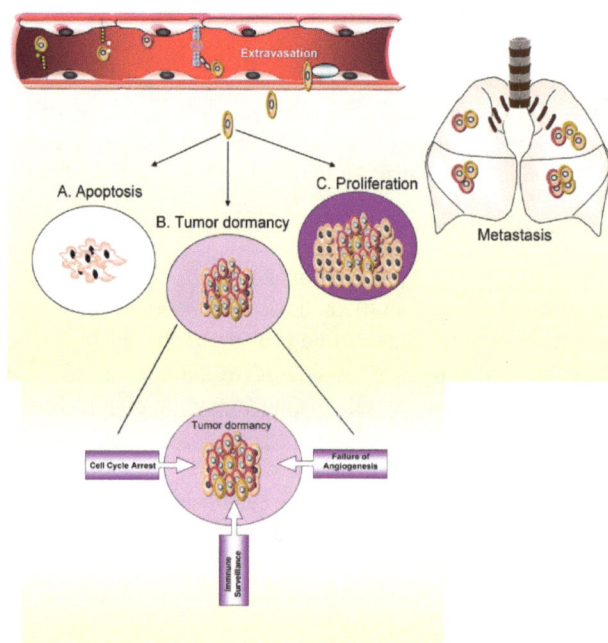

Figure 8: Metastatic Tumor Establishment. (A) The fate of post-extravasation cancer cells. (B) Mechanisms leading to tumor dormancy.

CONCLUSIONS

We have reviewed the main steps of the metastatic process which act in a concert manner and mostly rely on each other. This has suggested considering the metastasic process more as a network rather than a straight cascade (Gassmann CEM 2008) [101]. From the exhuastive effort to understand this network several clinically relevant novelties have been derived, such as anti- angiogenic agents, anti-integrin treatment (McNeel CCR 2005) [102], anti-MMPs treatment (Brown AO 1995) [103] or chemokine targeting (Ishida CS 2006) [104], among others. Although diverse therapies have been developed, in almost all situations, metastatic cancer is incurable. This may be determined by the intricacies and interrelations between the various aspects of the metastatic process, which are still only partially comprehended and may require improvement of the models used for investigation. In addition to what has been stated, the scientific community must be prepared to change paradigms in order to translate the promise (preventing neoplastic disease) into a clinical reality within a reasonable time frame. As our comprehension of the mechanisms of metastasis, the development of a variety of treatments that particullarly target metastases are needed, and such treatments must be tested in appropriate systems *in vitro* and *in vivo*. The design of clinical trial may be challenging including: identification of patients at risk by genetic profiling (overexpression of oncogenes and loss of tumor suppressor genes) and more sensitive strategies of detection of early disease and quantitation of metastases are urgently required. Prevention of metastatic outgrowth (eg, induced differentiation, stasis, or reactivation of apoptosis) is a further consideration (Eccles Lancet 2007) [105]. These investigations may lead to new methods for the treatment of cancer patients.

ACKNOWLEDGEMENTS

I would like to thank Justin Mirus and Dr Clarence A Dunn for their very helpful comments, suggestions, improvements, and corrections to this chapter.

REFERENCES

[1]   Hunter KW, Crawford NP, Alsarraj J. Mechanisms of metastasis. Breast Cancer Res 2008; 10 Suppl 1: S2.
[2]   Fidler IJ. The pathogenesis of cancer metastasis: the 'seed and soil' hypothesis revisited. Nat Rev Cancer 2003; 3: 453-8.
[3]   Bacac M, Stamenkovic I. Metastatic cancer cell. Annu Rev Pathol 2008; 3: 221-47.
[4]   Skobe M, Rockwell P, Goldstein N, Vosseler S, Fusenig NE.   Halting angiogenesis suppresses carcinoma cell invasion. Nature Med 1997; 3: 1222-7.
[5]   Weiss L, Ward PM. Cell detachment and metastasis. Cancer Metastasis Rev 1983; 2: 111-27.
[6]   Blood CH, Zetter BR. Tumor interactions with the vasculature: angiogenesis and tumor. Biochim Biophys Acta 1990; 1032: 89-118.
[7]   Brooks SA, Lomax-Browne HJ, Carter TM, Kinch CE, Hall DM. Molecular interactions in cancer cell metastasis. Acta Histochem 2010; 112: 3-25.
[8]   Bernards R, Weinberg RA. A progression puzzle. Nature 2002; 418: 823.
[9]   Cristofanilli M, Charnsangavej C, Hortobagyi GN. Angiogenesis modulation in cancer research: novel clinical approaches. Nat Rev Drug Discov 2002; 1: 415-26.
[10]   Keleg S, Büchler P, Ludwig R, Büchler MW, Friess H. Invasion and metastasis in pancreatic cancer. Mol Cancer 2003; 2: 14.
[11]   Koblinski JE, Ahram M, Sloane BF. Unraveling the role of proteases in cancer. Clin Chim Acta 2000; 291: 113-35.
[12]   Jeanes A, Gottardi CJ, Yap AS. Cadherins and cancer: how does cadherin dysfunction promote tumor progression? Oncogene 2008; 27: 6920-9.
[13]   Schlaepfer DD, Mitra SK, Ilic D. Control of motile and invasive cell phenotypes by focal adhesion kinase. Biochim Biophys Acta 2004; 1692: 77-102.
[14]   Kakinuma T, Hwang ST. Chemokines, chemokine receptors, and cancer metastasis. J Leukoc Biol 2006; 79: 639-51.
[15]   Foulds L. The experimental study of tumour progression. Cancer Res 1954; 14: 327-39.
[16]   Iacobuzio-Donahue CA. Epigenetic changes in cancer. Annu Rev Pathol 2009; 4: 229-49.
[17]   Chiang AC, Massagué J. Molecular basis of metastasis. N Engl J Med 2008; 359: 2814-23.
[18]   Gupta GP, Massagué J. Cancer metastasis: building a framework. Cell 2006; 127: 679-95.
[19]   Harris AL. Hypoxia-a key regulatory factor in tumour growth. Nat Rev Cancer 2002; 2: 38-47.
[20]   William D Figg, Judah Folkman. Angiogenesis: An Integrative Approach from Science to Medicine. Published by Springer, 2008.
[21]   Lorusso G, Rüegg C. The tumor microenvironment and its contribution to tumor evolution toward metastasis. Histochem Cell Biol 2008; 130: 1091-103.
[22]   Coussens LM, Werb Z. Infammation and cancer. Nature 2002; 420: 860-7.
[23]   Hillen F, Griffioen AW. Tumour vascularization: sprouting angiogenesis and beyond. Cancer Metastasis Rev. 2007; 26: 489-502.
[24]   Folkman J. Tumor angiogenesis: therapeutic implications. N Engl J Med 1971; 285: 1182-6.
[25]   Bergers G, Benjamin LE. Tumorigenesis and the angiogenic switch. Nat Rev Cancer 2003; 3: 401-10.
[26]   Papetti M, Herman IM. Mechanisms of normal and tumor-derived angiogenesis. Am J Physiol Cell Physiol 2002; 282: C947-70.
[27]   Cross MJ, Dixelius J, Matsumoto T, Claesson-Welsh L. VEGF-receptor signal transduction. Trends Biochem Sci 2003; 28: 488-94.
[28]   Kerbel RS. Tumor angiogenesis: past, present and the near future. Carcinogenesis 2000; 21: 505-15.
[29]   Ferrara N, Gerber HP, LeCouter J. The biology of VEGF and its receptors. Nat Med 2003; 9: 669-76.
[30]   Vaupel P. The role of hypoxia-induced factors in tumor progression. Oncologist 2004; 9 Suppl 5:10-7.
[31]   Woodhouse EC, Chuaqui RF, Liotta LA. General mechanisms of metastasis. Cancer 1997; 80: 1529-37.
[32]   Hwang R, Varner J. The role of integrins in tumor angiogenesis. Hematol Oncol Clin North Am 2004; 18: 991-1006.
[33]   Meyer GT, Matthias LJ, Noack L, Vadas MA, Gamble JR. Lumen formation during angiogenesis *in vitro* involves phagocytic activity, formation and secretion of vacuoles, cell death, and capillary tube remodeling by different populations of endothelial cells. Anat Rec 1997; 249: 327-40.
[34]   Jain RK. Molecular regulation of vessel maturation. Nat Med 2003; 9: 685-93.
[35]   Loughna, S. Sato, T.N. Angiopoietin and Tie signaling pathways in vascular development. Matrix Biol 2001; 20: 319-325.
[36]   Friedl P, Bröcker EB. The biology of cell locomotion within three-dimensional extracellular matrix. Cell Mol Life Sci 2000; 57: 41-64.

[37]   Larsen M, Tremblay ML, Yamada KM. Phosphatases in cell-matrix adhesion and migration. Nat Rev Mol Cell Biol 2003; 4: 700-11.

[38]   Carragher NO, Frame MC. Focal adhesion and actin dynamics: a place where kinases and proteases meet to promote invasion. Trends Cell Biol 2004; 14: 241-9.

[39]   Goley ED, Welch MD. The ARP2/3 complex: an actin nucleator comes of age. Nat Rev Mol Cell Biol 2006; 7: 713-26.

[40]   Ridley AJ, Paterson HF, Johnston CL, Diekmann D, Hall A. The small GTP-binding protein rac regulates growth factor-induced membrane ruffling. Cell 1992; 70: 401-10.

[41]   Burridge K, Chrzanowska-Wodnicka M. Focal adhesions, contractility, and signaling. Annu Rev Cell Dev Biol 1996; 12: 463-518.

[42]   Mitra SK, Hanson DA, Schlaepfer DD. Focal adhesion kinase: in command and control of cell motility. Nat Rev Mol Cell Biol 2005; 6: 56-68.

[43]   Berrier AL, Yamada KM. Cell-matrix adhesion. J Cell Physiol 2007; 213(3): 565-73.

[44]   Webb DJ, Brown CM, Horwitz AF. Illuminating adhesion complexes in migrating cells: moving toward a bright future. Curr Opin Cell Biol 2003; 15: 614-20.

[45]   Schlaepfer DD, Mitra SK, Ilic D. Control of motile and invasive cell phenotypes by focal adhesion kinase. Biochim Biophys Acta 2004; 1692: 77-102.

[46]   Friedl P, Wolf K. Tumour-cell invasion and migration: diversity and escape mechanisms Nat Rev Cancer 2003; 3: 362-74.

[47]   Renshaw MW, Price LS, Schwartz MA. Focal adhesion kinase mediates the integrin signaling requirementfor growth factor activation of MAP kinase. J Cell Biol 1999; 147: 611-8.

[48]   Hood JD, Cheresh DA. Role of integrins in cell invasion and migration. Nat Rev Cancer 2002; 2: 91-100.

[49]   Yamaguchi H, Wyckoff J, Condeelis J. Cell migration intumors. Curr Opin Cell Biol 2005; 17: 559-64.

[50]   Brinckerhoff CE, Rutter JL, Benbow U. Interstitial collagenases as markers of tumor progression. Clin Cancer Res 2000; 6: 4823-30.

[51]   Ananthakrishnan R, Ehrlicher A. The forces behind cell movement. Int J Biol Sci 2007; 3: 303-17.

[52]   Kedrin D, van Rheenen J, Hernandez L, Condeelis J, Segall JE. Cell motility and cytoskeletal regulation in invasion and metastasis. J Mammary Gland Biol. Neoplasia 2007; 12: 143-52.

[53]   Olson MF. Contraction reaction: mechanical regulation of Rho GTPase. Trends Cell Biol 2004; 14: 111-4.

[54]   Huttenlocher, A., Sandborg, R. R. and Horwitz, A. F. Adhesion in cell migration. Curr Opin Cell Biol 1995; 7: 697-706.

[55]   Pokutta S, Weis WI. Structure and mechanism of cadherins and catenins in cell-cell contacts. Annu Rev Cell Dev Biol 2007; 23: 237-61.

[56]   Bogenrieder T, Herlyn M. Axis of evil: molecular mechanisms of cancer metastasis. Oncogene 2003; 22: 6524-36.

[57]   Jeanes A, Gottardi CJ, Yap AS. Cadherins and cancer: how does cadherin dysfunction promote tumor progression? Oncogene 2008; 27: 6920-9.

[58]   Hazan RB, Qiao R, Keren R, Badano I, Suyama K. Cadherin switch in tumor progression. Ann N Y Acad Sci 2004; 1014: 155-63.

[59]   Cavallaro U. N-cadherin as an invasion promoter: a novel target for antitumor therapy? Curr Opin Investig Drugs 2004; 5: 1274-8.

[60]   Radisky DC. Epithelial-mesenchymal transition. J Cell Sci 2005; 118: 4325-6.

[61]   Kalluri R, Weinberg RA. The basics of epithelial-mesenchymal transition. J Clin Invest 2009; 119: 1420-8.

[62]   Thiery JP. Epithelial-mesenchymal transitions in development and pathologies. Curr Opin Cell Biol 2003; 15: 740-6.

[63]   Thiery JP, Sleeman JP. Complex networks orchestrate epithelial-mesenchymal transitions. Nat Rev Mol Cell Biol. 2006; 7: 131-42.

[64]   Maier HJ, Wirth T, Beug H. Epithelial-Mesenchymal Transition in Pancreatic Carcinoma. Cancers 2010; 2: 2058-83.

[65]   Heuberger J, Birchmeier W. Interplay of cadherin-mediated cell adhesion and canonical Wnt signaling. Cold Spring Harb Perspect Biol 2010; 2: a002915.

[66]   Huber MA, Kraut N, Beug H. Molecular requirements for epithelial-mesenchymal transition during tumor progression. Curr Opin Cell Biol 2005; 17: 548-58.

[67]   Smit MA, Peeper DS. Zeb1 is required for TrkB-induced epithelial-mesenchymal transition, anoikis resistance and metastasis. Oncogene. 2011; [Epub ahead of print].

[68]   Radisky DC, LaBarge MA. Epithelial-mesenchymal transition and the stem cell phenotype. Cell Stem Cell 2008; 2: 511-2.

[69]   Wyckoff JB, Jones JG, Condeelis JS, Segall JE. A critical step in metastasis: *in vivo* analysis of intravasation at the primary tumor. Cancer Res 2000; 60: 2504-11.

[70]   Weaver AM. Invadopodia: specialized cell structures for cancer invasion. Clin Exp Metastasis 2006; 23(2): 97-105.

[71]   Bockhorn M, Jain RK, Munn LL.Active versus passive mechanisms in metastasis: do cancer cells crawl into vessels, or are they pushed?. Lancet Oncol 2007; 8: 444-8.

[72]   Nguyen DX, Bos PD, Massagué J. Metastasis: from dissemination to organ-specific colonization. Nat Rev Cancer 2009; 9: 274-84.

[73]   Weiss L. Metastatic inefficiency. Adv Cancer Res 1990; 54: 159-211.

[74]   Sahai E. Illuminating the metastatic process. Nat Rev Cancer 2007; 7: 737-49.

[75]   Molloy T, van'tVeer LJ. Recent advances in metastasis research. Curr Opin Genetics and Development 2008; 18: 35-41.

[76]   Palumbo JS, Talmage KE, Massari JV, *et al.* Tumor cell-associated tissue factor and circulating hemostatic factors cooperate to increase metastatic potential through natural killer cell-dependent and -independent mechanisms. Blood 2007; 110: 133-141.

[77]   Joyce JA, Pollard JW. Microenvironmental regulation of metastasis. Nat Rev Cancer 2009; 9: 239-52.

[78]   Miles FL, Pruitt FL, van Golen KL, Cooper CR. Stepping out of the flow: capillary extravasation in cancer metastasis. Clin Exp Metastasis 2008; 25: 305-24.

[79] Strell C, Lang K, Niggemann B, Zaenker KS, Entschladen F. Surface molecules regulating rolling and adhesion to endothelium of neutrophil granulocytes and MDA-MB-468 breast carcinoma cells and their interaction. Cell Mol Life Sci 2007; 64: 3306-31.

[80] Bertini I, Sigel A, Sigel H. Hanbook on Metalloproteins. New York, 2001.

[81] Barthel SR, Gavino JD, Descheny L, *et al.* Targeting selectins and selectin ligands in inflammation and cancer. Expert Opin Ther Targets 2007; 11: 1473-91.

[82] Tozeren A, Kleinman HK, Grant DS. E-selectin mediated dynamic interactions of breast- and colon-cancer cells with endothelial-cell monolayers. Int J Cancer 1995; 60: 426-31.

[83] Dimitroff CJ, Lechpammer M, Long-Woodward D, *et al.* Rolling of human bone-metastatic prostate tumor cells on human bone marrow endothelium under shear flow is mediated by E-selectin. Cancer Res 2004; 64: 5261-9.

[84] Dimitroff CJ, Descheny L, Trujillo N, *et al.* Identification of leukocyte E-selectin ligands, P-selectin glycoprotein ligand-1 and E-selectin ligand-1, on human metastatic prostate tumor cells. Cancer Res 2005; 65 (13):5750-60.

[85] Tomlinson J, Wang JL, Barsky SH *et al.* Human colon cancer cells express multiple glycoprotein ligands for E-selectin. Int J Oncol 2000; 16:347-53.

[86] Burdick MM, Chu JT, Godar S, *et al.* HCELL is the major E and L-selectin ligand expressed on LS174T colon carcinoma cells. J Biol Chem 2006; 281:13899-905.

[87] Taichman DB, Cybulsky MI, Djaffar I, *et al.* Tumor cell surface alpha 4 beta 1 integrin mediates adhesion to vascular endothelium: demonstration of an interaction with the N-terminal domains of INCAM-110/VCAM-1. Cell Regul 1991; 2:347-55.

[88] Garofalo A, Chirivi RG, Foglieni C, *et al.* Involvement of the very late antigen 4 integrin on melanoma in interleukin 1-augmented experimental metastases. Cancer Res 1995; 5: 414-9.

[89] Okahara H, Yagita H, Miyake K, *et al.* Involvement of very late activation antigen 4 (VLA-4) and vascular cell adhesion molecule 1 (VCAM-1) in tumor necrosis factor alpha enhancement of experimental metastasis. Cancer Res 1994; 54: 3233-6.

[90] Wang HS, Hung Y, Su CH, *et al.* CD44 cross-linking induces integrin-mediated adhesion and transendothelial migration in breast cancer cell line by up-regulation of LFA-1 (alpha L beta2) and VLA-4 (alpha4beta1). Exp Cell Res 2005; 304: 116-26.

[91] Voura EB, Sandig M, Siu CH. Cell-cell interactions during transendothelial migration of tumor cells. Microsc Res Tech 1998; 43: 265-75.

[92] Qi J, Chen N, Wang J, *et al.* Transendothelial migration of melanoma cells involves N-cadherin-mediated adhesion and activation of the beta-catenin signaling pathway. Mol Biol Cell 2005; 16: 4386-97.

[93] Brandt B, Heyder C, Gloria-Maercker E, *et al.* 3D-extravasation model - selection of highly motile and metastatic cancer cells. Semin Cancer Biol 2005; 15: 387-95.

[94] Kim JW, Wong CW, Goldsmith JD, *et al.* Rapid apoptosis in the pulmonary vasculature distinguishes non-metastatic from metastatic melanoma cells. Cancer Lett 2004; 213: 203-12.

[95] Udagawa T. Tumor dormancy of primary and secondary cancers. APMIS. 2008; 116: 615-28.

[96] Koebel CM, VermiW, Swann JB, *et al.* Adaptive immunity maintains occult cancer in an equilibrium state. Nature 2007; 450: 903-7.

[97] Folkman J, Long DM Jr, Becker FF. Growth and metastasis of tumor in organ culture. Cancer 1963; 16: 453-67.

[98] Reddi AH, Roodman D, Freeman C, *et al.* Mechanisms of tumor metastasis to the bone: challenges and opportunities. J Bone Miner Res 2003; 18:190-4.

[99] Guise TA, Chirgwin JM. Transforming growth factor-beta in osteolytic breast cancer bone metastases. Clin Orthop Relat Res 2003; 415 Suppl: S32-8.

[100] Guise TA. The vicious cycle of bone metastases. J Musculoskelet Neuronal Interact 2002; 2: 570-2.

[101] Gassmann P, Haier J. The tumor cell-host organ interface in the early onset of metastatic organ colonisation. Clin Exp Metastasis 2008; 25: 171-81.

[102] McNeel DG, Eickhoff J, Lee FT, *et al.* Phase I trial of a monoclonal antibody specific for alphavbeta3 integrin (MEDI-522) in patients with advanced malignancies, including an assessment of effect on tumor perfusion. Clin Cancer Res 2005; 11: 7851-60.

[103] Brown PD, Giavazzi R. Matrix metalloproteinase inhibition: a review of anti-tumour activity. Ann Oncol 1995; 6: 967-74

[104] Ishida T, Ueda R. CCR4 as a novel molecular target for immunotherapy of cancer. Cancer Sci 2006; 97:1139-46.

[105] Eccles SA, Welch DR. Metastasis: recent discoveries and novel treatment strategies. Lancet 2007; 369: 1742-57.

CHAPTER 7

Cancer Immunology and Novel Strategies for Immunotherapy

Alberto Monroy-García[1,2,*], María de Lourdes Mora-García[2] and Jorge Hernández-Montes[2]

[1]*Oncology Research Unit, Oncology Hospital, National Medical Centre, IMSS, México City, México and* [2]*Laboratory of Immunobiology, Cellular Differentiation and Cancer Research Unit, FES-Zaragoza, National University of México, México City, México*

Abstract: It is known that the immune system through innate and adaptive immune responses plays an important role to detect and eliminate primary chemically induced or spontaneous tumors. However, according to clinical data and experimental studies using *de novo* immune-competent mouse models of cancer development, the immune system can also participate as cancer-promoter. In this regard, deficient anti-tumor cell-mediated immunity, in combination with enhanced pro-tumor humoral and/or innate immunity (inflammation), are significant factors influencing malignant outcome. This review describes current knowledge of the interaction between tumors and the immune system, cellular and molecular events that favor tumor immune tolerance and current approaches to control tumor growth trough immunotherapy as well as novel strategies to block immunosuppressive elements.

Keywords: Inflamation and cancer, cancer immunoediting, immune tolerance, immunological escape, immunosuppression, suppressive molecules, T regulatory cells, dysfunctional dendritic cells, cancer immunotherapy, tumor antigens, adoptive T cell immunotherapy, novel tumor immunotherapy, combinatorial therapy.

INTRODUCTION

The main function of the immune system is to discriminate between ranges of stimuli, allowing some to provoke immune responses, which lead to immunity, and preventing others which lead to ineffective immune response against proper or specific antigens (tolerance). To this end, the immune system includes an early immune response mediated by the innate immune system (*i.e.*, phagocytes, NK cells, NKT cells, cytokines, and complement proteins) and later by the adaptive immune system (*i.e.*, B cells and T cells). In this context the major challenge for the immune system is to recognize and eliminate cells undergoing carcinogenesis. On the other hand, tumor microenvironment is complex; it is composed by immune cells, tumor cells, stromal cells and the extracellular matrix. Several mechanisms are maintained during the neoplastic process, such as proliferation, survival and migration of tumor cells. However, the interplay between innate and adaptive immunity may contribute to cancer development through dysregulated interactions that can result in excessive activation of the immune system and chronic inflammation, culminating in tissue damage and malignant conversion, as well as, the establishment of tolerating conditions in favor of tumor escape. A better understanding of this immunosuppressive network in the course of tumour development and progression should lead towards refine novel immune-boosting strategies to achieve successful tumor immunotherapy.

IMMUNE RESPONSE, INFLAMMATION AND CANCER

The immune system is composed of a large variety of cells and mediators that interact in a complex and dynamic network to ensure protection against all foreign pathogens possibly encountered during life-time, while simultaneously maintaining self-tolerance. The immune system can be divided into two subsets, the innate immune system, also referred to as the first line of immune defense against infection, and the adaptive immune system. Innate immune cells, *e.g.*, granulocytes (neutrophils, basophils, and eosinophils), Dendritic Cells (DCs), macrophages,

Address correspondence to Alberto Monroy-García: Oncology Research Unit, Oncology Hospital, National Medical Centre, IMSS and Laboratory of Immunobiology, Cellular Differentiation and Cancer Research Unit, FES-Zaragoza, National University of México, México City, México; E-mail: albertomon@yahoo.com

Natural Killer Cells (NK cells) and mast cells, express germline encoded pattern-recognition Toll-Like Receptors (TLRs) with which they recognize conserved molecular patterns, *e.g.*, Lipopolysaccharide (LPS), Lipoteichoic Acid (LTA), mannans, unmethylated CpG DNA motifs and glycans, found on microbes but not in self-tissue (Murphy GS 2007) [1]. Activation of TLRs triggers a cascade of intracellular events, including activation of NF-kB signaling pathways, resulting in increased production of proinflammatory mediators, increased nitric oxide synthesis and increased antigen presentation, thus, further enhancing recruitment and activation of additional leukocytes (Akira NRI 2004) [2]. When tissue homeostasis is perturbed, sentinel macrophages and mast cells immediately release soluble mediators, such as cytokines, chemokines, matrix remodelling proteases and reactive oxygen species (ROS), and bioactive mediators such as histamine, that induce mobilization and infiltration of additional leukocytes into damaged tissue (a process that is known as inflammation). Macrophages and mast cells can also activate vascular and fibroblast responses in order to orchestrate the elimination of invading organisms and initiate local tissue repair. DCs, on the other hand, take up foreign antigens and migrate to lymphoid organs where they present their antigens to adaptive immune cells. They are, therefore, key players in the interface between innate and adaptive immunity. NK cells also participate in cellular crosstalk between innate and adaptive immune cells through their ability to interact bidirectionally with DCs; certain NK-cell subsets eliminate immature DCs, whereas others promote DC maturation, which can then also reciprocally regulate activation of NK cells (Murphy GS 2007) [1]. In addition, activation of the complement system, represented by a complex network of more than 30 serum proteins and cell surface receptors, is a central event during innate immune defense after pathogenic tissue attack (Sahu IR 2001) [3]. Activation of the complement system by pathogens and immune complexes results in lysis of foreign cells and bacteria, opsonization and uptake of complement-coated antigens by phagocytosis, recruitment of innate immune cells *via* engagement of complement receptors and clearance of immune complexes (Walport NEJ 2001) [4, 5]. These different pathways of innate immune cell activation not only form the first line of immune defense against invading pathogens, but are also involved in activation and modulation of more specific adaptive immune responses (Carroll NI 2004) [6].

In contrast to innate immune cells that express germline encoded receptors, adaptive immune cells, *e.g.*, B and T lymphocytes, express highly diverse, somatically generated, antigen-specific receptors. T Cell Receptors (TCRs) and B Cell Receptors (BCRs) are generated by random rearrangement of the T cell receptor and Immunoglobulin (Ig) gene segments, respectively, allowing generation of extremely diverse T and B lymphocyte repertoires that provide organisms with a flexible and broader repertoire of responses to pathogens as compared to the innate immune system (Goldrath Nature 1999) [7] (Tonegawa Nature 1983) [8]. Mature B lymphocytes can undergo additional processes upon initial activation resulting in modifications in their capacity to recognize antigens, *i.e.*, somatic hypermutation of Ig genes, Ig affinity maturation and Ig class switching (isotype switching) (Mc Heyzer COI 2003) [9]. The two major T lymphocyte subsets, *e.g.*, CD4+ T cells (helper T cells) and CD8+ T cells (cytotoxic T cells), are activated upon interaction of their TCRs with nonself antigens presented by Major Histocompatibility Complex (MHC) class II and I, respectively, in combination with simultaneous interactions with costimulatory molecules (Murphy GS 2007) [1]. Fully activated T lymphocytes subsequently exert various effector functions such as cytokine production, B cell help (CD4+ T cells) and cytotoxic killing of cells expressing the antigen of specificity (CD8+ T cells). On the other hand, B lymphocytes recognize soluble antigens, require additional signals derived from helper T cells for full activation and subsequently exert their effector function by secreting antibodies with the same antigen specificity as the BCR (Mc Heyzer COI 2003) [9]. As individual B and T lymphocytes are antigenically committed to a specific unique antigen, clonal expansion of antigen-specific lymphocytes is required upon antigen recognition to obtain a sufficient number of antigen-specific T and/or B lymphocytes to counteract infection (Mc Heyzer COI 2003) [9] (Sprent ARI 2002) [10]. Therefore, the kinetics of primary adaptive immune responses are slower than innate immune responses; however, during a primary adaptive immune response, a subset of lymphocytes differentiates into long-lived memory cells resulting in heightened states of immune reactivity to subsequent exposure with the same antigen (Sprent ARI 2002) [10].

On the other hand, in the particular case of cancer, current dogma suggests that the adaptive immune system protects organisms from nascent tumors, a process referred to as immune surveillance (Dunn I 2004) [11] (Pardoll NB 2002) [12]. Immune surveillance protects individuals against certain pathogen-associated cancers, either by protecting against chronic pathogen infections or by preventing viral re-activation (Boshoff NRC 2002) [13]. The importance of immune surveillance in protecting against viral-induced malignancy is underscored by the increased incidence of HPV16-related cervical and squamous carcinomas, Herpesvirus 8-associated Kaposi's sarcoma and Epstein-Barr virus-related non-Hodgkin's lymphoma in immunocompromised patients (Euvrard NEJM 2003) [14] (Penn TP

1999) [15], as well as in nonviral-associated malignancies such as melanoma and lung carcinoma, appears to be increased (Euvrard NEJM 2003) [14]. On the other hand, several epidemiological studies have shown that patients with autoimmune disease, in particular, rheumatoid arthritis, SLE, celiac disease and inflammation-induced pulmonary fibrosis, are predisposed to certain types of nonhematogenous malignancies, *e.g.*, lung carcinoma, nonmelanoma skin cancer and cervical atypia (Alaedini AIM 2005) [16] (Artinian COPM 2004) [17], suggesting that an altered balance between innate and adaptive immunity might contribute to cancer development.

Based on the observed importance of the adaptive immune system in initiating and/or maintaining the innate immune response during pathogenesis of various autoimmune diseases (Ji I 2002) [18] (Korganow I 1999) [19], it would be anticipated that adaptive immunity may also play a promoting role in inflammation-associated cancer development. The earliest reports revealing a potential tumor-enhancing effect of adaptive immunity demonstrated that passive transfer of tumor-specific antibodies could enhance *in vivo* outgrowth of transplanted tumor cells or chemically induced tumors (Agassy IL 1988) [20]. In addition, absence of B lymphocytes was reported to protect against transplanted and chemically induced tumors (Brodt CII 1982) [21] (Monach T 1993) [22]. Recently, availability of *de novo* carcinogenesis mouse models has allowed more accurate analysis of a possible tumor-enhancing role of the adaptive immune system. For example, active immunization of mice carrying a mutant *ras* oncogene resulted in the activation of humoral immune responses and enhanced papilloma formation upon chemical promotion (Schreiber SCB 2000) [23] (Siegel JEM 2000) [24]. In addition, some studies have reported that antitumor humoral immune responses potentiate *in vivo* growth and invasion of injected murine and human tumor cell lines *via* recruitment and activation of granulocytes and macrophages (Barbera N 1999) [25]. An interesting study to functionally assess whether the adaptive immune system exerts a regulatory role during *de novo* carcinogenesis, was showed by de Visser et al 2005, who intercrossed K14-HPV16 mice with Recombination-Activating Gene-1 homozygous null (RAG-1-/-) mice deficient for mature B and T lymphocytes and found that genetic deletion of adaptive immune cells resulted in failure to initiate and/or sustain leukocyte infiltration during premalignancy (de Visser CC 2005) [26]. In this model, chronic inflammation, tissue remodeling, angiogenesis and epithelial hyperproliferation were significantly reduced, culminating in attenuated premalignant progression to carcinoma (de Visser CC 2005) [26]. Genetic elimination of CD4+ and/or CD8+ T lymphocytes did not affect chronic inflammation or alter characteristics of premalignant progression in these K14-HPV16 mice. However, when B lymphocytes or serum isolated from K14-HPV16 mice were adoptively transferred into K14-HPV16/RAG-1-/- mice, it was found that chronic inflammation in neoplastic skin as well as hallmarks of premalignant progression were restored, suggesting that B lymphocytes play a crucial role in the onset of chronic inflammation associated with premalignant progression, thus potentiating neoplastic cascades downstream of oncogene expression (de Visser CC 2005) [26]. Taken together, these data hypothesize that the activation of adaptive immune response in early neoplastic tissues, can result in both protection against viral-induced malignancies or tumour-promoting due to potentiated development of chronic inflammation-associated malignancy. In this place, innate immune cells, such as mast cells, granulocytes and macrophages, promote tumour development by the release of potent pro-survival soluble molecules that modulate gene-expression programmes in initiated neoplastic cells, culminating in altered cell-cycle progression and increased survival. In addition, inflammatory cells positively influence tissue remodelling and development of the angiogenic vasculature by production of pro-angiogenic mediators and extracellular proteases (Fig. **1**) (de Visser CC 2005) [26].

FROM IMMUNOSURVEILLANCE TO IMMUNOESCAPE IN CANCER

The concept that the immune system protects the host against cancer was first posited by Ehrlich in 1909 and modified in the 1950s by Burnet and Thomas, who proposed that it was instrumental in eliminating precancerous or cancerous cells, through a "surveillance" function (Burnet BMB 1964) [27] (Thomas CHAHS 1959) [28]. However, the concept fell out of favor when studies in the 1980s indicated that tumors failed to develop more rapidly in nude mice (which lack T cells and B cells, but not NK cells) than in wild-type mice. It was resurrected in the 1990s, when a body of evidence emerged indicating that immunodeficient mice were at greater risk for spontaneous tumor development (Dunn NI 2002) [29]. These studies led to further refinement of the theory, now referred to as "cancer immunoediting", encompassing three phases: elimination, equilibrium, and escape (Fig. **1**).

Elimination

During the elimination phase, nascent tumor cells are destroyed by elements of the innate and adaptive immune systems. Molecules involved in antigen processing and presentation and mediators of cytotoxic pathways are also critical for controlling tumor growth. Evidence for the existence of this phase comes from animal experiments examining spontaneous or carcinogen induced tumors in mice that lack specific immune effector cells, molecules, or pathways that are important for suppressing tumor growth. For example, RAG2-deficient mice, which lack T cells, B cells, and NK cells, spontaneously develop adenomas of the intestine and lung (Street JEM 2004) [30]. Similarly, mice lacking key cytokines such as IFN-γ (Shankaran Nature 2001) [31] have a higher incidence of tumor development with age than wild-type mice. Although these studies provide very strong support for immune surveillance, point out that models in which tumors develop spontaneously and then undergo autochthonous regression, provide definitive evidence of immunoediting (Swann JCI 2007) [32]. In humans, it has been observed that immunosuppressed patients have a higher incidence of tumors, especially those of viral etiology (Penn ARM 1988) [33]. In contrast, individuals whose tumors are infiltrated with T cells have a more favorable prognosis (Camus CR 2009) [34].

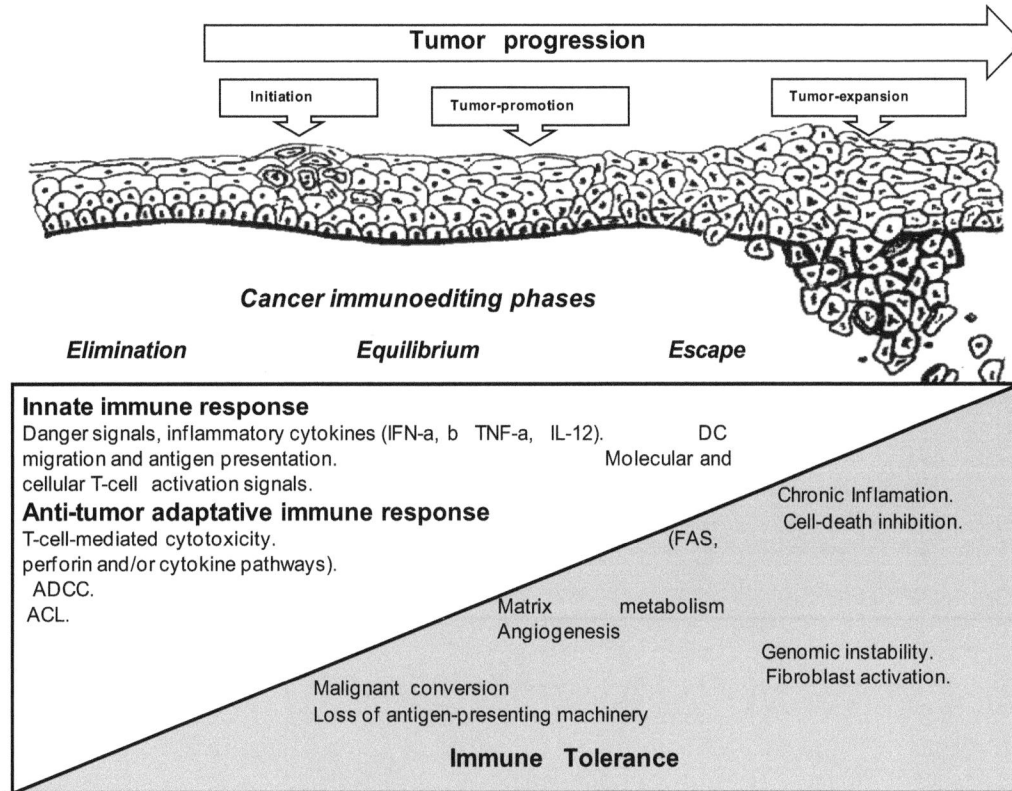

Figure 1: Tumor progression and immunoediting phases. Cancer immunoediting encompassing three phases: elimination, equilibrium, and escape. During elimination phase, innate and adaptive immune responses are active. Antigens that are present in normal or pre-neoplastic tissues are transported to lymphoid organs by dendritic cells (DCs) that activate adaptive immune responses resulting in antitumor effect (Open triangle). B and T activated cells elicit effector mechanisms such as: T-cell-mediated cytotoxicity (FAS, perforin and/or cytokine pathways); antibody-dependent cell-mediated cytotoxicity (ADCC) and antibody-induced complement-mediated lysis (ACL). On the other hand, during equilibrium phase, activation of B cells and humoral immune responses can result in chronic activation of innate immune cells that can initiate and promote tumor development. Activated innate immune cells, such as mast cells, granulocytes and macrophages, promote tumor development by the release of potent pro-survival soluble molecules that modulate gene-expression programmes in initiated neoplastic cells, culminating in altered cell-cycle progression and increased survival (shaded triangle). Through tumor progression, inflammatory cells positively influence tissue remodelling and development of the angiogenic vasculature by production of pro-angiogenic mediators and extracellular proteases. Finally during the escape phase, the immune tolerance is dominant with the concomitant tumor expansion.

Equilibrium

The second phase of immunoediting is the equilibrium phase, in which tumor cells persist but are "equilibrated" by the immune system. Indirect evidence of this phase comes from studies in which spontaneous or carcinogen-derived tumors have been transplanted into immunodeficient and wild-type mice. Although these tumors are eliminated in wild-type mice, they grow progressively in syngeneic immunodeficient animals (Shankaran Nature 2001) [31] (Crowe JEM 2002) [35]. These data suggest that tumors normally undergo sculpting by the immune system. More direct evidence of the equilibrium phase comes from experiments showing that if wild-type mice that are tumor free after low-dose methylcholanthrene administration are depleted of CD4+ and CD8+ T cells, they rapidly develop sarcomas that have unusual growth characteristics when transplanted into naive recipients (Ostrand COGD 2008) [36].

Escape

The final phase of immunoediting is termed escape, in which tumors actively disable immune recognition by co-opting immune cells for growth, angiogenesis, and invasion. Escape constitutes several complex events and processes, including loss of antigen-presenting machinery, tumor antigens, and sensitivity to immune effector molecules; expression of inhibitory molecules that induce T cell apoptosis or anergy; and induction of Tregs (Swann JCI 2007) [32] (Blank CII 2007) [37] (Dong NM 2002) [38]. In this regard, production of indoleamine 2,3-dioxygenase (IDO) and the induction of Myeloid-Derived Suppressor Cells (MDSCs) and T regulatory cells (Treg) in the tumoral environment, constitute three of the most important mechanisms of tumor escape.

IDO enzyme catalyzes the ratelimiting step of tryptophan degradation along the kyneurenine pathway, in tumor-induced tolerance (Munn JCI 2007) [39]. IDO is produced by several cells, including tumor cells and antigen presenting cells (APCs, that include both conventional and plasmacytoid DCs), and its function is dependent on activation signals imparted to the APCs (Chen JI 2008) [40] (Orabona Blood 2006) [41]. IDO-mediated immune suppression is due to the production of tryptophan metabolites and local reduction of tryptophan levels, which cause T cell apoptosis and suppress T cell proliferation (Terness JEM 2002) [42]. The stress-responsive kinase General Control Nonderepressible 2 (GCN2), activated by amino acid deficiency, was recently shown to participate in IDO-mediated T cell anergy (Chen JI 2008) [43]. In addition, IDO expression in APCs has been associated with the induction of immunosuppressive Tregs (Mello JI 2005) [44]. DC subsets expressing IDO have been described in tumor-draining lymph nodes, and IDO expression has been linked to poor clinical outcome (Lee CCR 2005) [45].

On the other hand, tumors can also induce the differentiation of circulating myeloid cells into suppressor cells, termed collectively myeloid-derived suppressor cells (Gabrilovich NRI 2009) [46] or MDSCs, which impact on immune surveillance mechanisms. MDSCs, are a complex mix of CD11b+ and Gr-1+ mononuclear cells that mediate the suppression of T cells in cancer and other pathological conditions (Sica JCI 2007)[47]. MDSCs apparently require activation by T cells, after which they inhibit CD4+ and CD8+ T cells in an MHC-independent manner (Sica JCI 2007)[47]. They express the inducible forms of NOS2 and arginase (ARG1), enzymes involved in the metabolism of arginine. NOS2 and ARG1 are expressed in MDSCs by in an IL-13- and IFN-γ-dependent manner and function synergistically to induce T cell dysfunction or apoptosis through the production of reactive nitrogen and oxygen species (Gallina JCI 2006) [48]. In addition MDSCs can also induce the development of Tregs (Huang CR 2006) [49]. Tumor-Associated Macrophages (TAMs), another type of myeloid suppressor cell, are recruited to tumors and promote tumor growth by enhancing inflammation and angiogenesis (Colombo CR 2005) [50]. The expression of angiopoietin receptor TIE2 in monocytes for tumor vessel formation, constitute an evidence of their role in promoting angiogenesis (De Palma CC 2008) [51]. On the other hand, induction of B7-H1 on myeloid DCs by factors within the tumor microenvironment is a novel mechanism for immune evasion by a tumor (Colombo CR 2005) [50]. Tumor environmental B7-H1+ myeloid DCs, profoundly affect the functional capacity of DCs to activate T-cell toward specific immunity, by triggering myeloid DC B7-H1 expression (Colombo CR 2005) [50]. B7.1 and B7.2 (also known as CD80 and CD86, respectively) are B7 family members with co-stimulatory functions for T-cell activation. B7-H1 is a recently identified B7 family member. There is approximately 25% homology between B7.1, B7.2 and B7-H1 (Choi JI 2003) [52]. A significant fraction of tumor-associated T cells are Treg cells (Barnett AEMB 2008) [53], which express PD-1, the ligand for B7-H1 (Chen NRI 2004) [54]. Tumor-associated T cells can then, through reverse signaling through B7-H1, suppress IL-12 production by myeloid DCs, and therefore reduce their immunogenicity (Curiel NM 2003) [55]. The expression of B7-H1 on human cancers such as ovarian cancer, lung cancer, melanoma, glioblastoma and squamous-cell carcinoma also contributes to immune evasion by inducing apoptosis of effector T cells, so facilitating tumor growth (Dong NM 2002) [56]. PD-1 is one of the ligands for B7-H1. PD-1 blockade by genetic manipulation (producing *PD-1-/-* cells) or antibody treatment efficiently inhibits mouse B16 melanoma and CT26 colon cancer dissemination and metastasis accompanied with increased effector T-cell number and enhanced function (Iwai II 2002) [57]. Similar to B7-H1, B7-H4 (also known as B7X or B7S1) negatively regulates T cell responses *in vitro* by inhibiting T cell proliferation, cell-cycle progression and cytokine production (Prasad I 2003) [58]. B7-H4 is commonly detectable in the human cancer, for example, human ovarian cancers express high levels of B7-H4 protein (Kryczek JEM 2006) [59], and low levels of soluble B7-H4 protein were found in the sera from patients with ovarian cancer (Simon GO 2007) [60]. In addition to tumor cells, tumor-infiltrating macrophages and endothelial cells of small blood vessels in the cancer microenvironment are also found to constitutively express B7-H4 (Kryczek CR 2007) [61]. Another type of DCs involved intumor environment is the plasmacytoid DC, a subset of dendritic cells with a microscopic appearance similar to plasmablasts with phenotype HLA- DR+CD11c- (Wei CR 2005) [62]. Plasmacitoid DCs are the main producers of type I IFN. Functional plasmacytoid DCs are found in the local tumor environment of patients with ovarian cancer (Wei CR 2005) [62], melanoma (Salio EJI 2003) [63] and head and neck squamous-cell carcinoma (Hartman CR 2003) [64]. For example, tumor cells produce the chemokine ligand CXCL12 (also known as stromal-cell-derived factor 1) and plasmacytoid DCs express CXCR4, the receptor for CXCL12 (Hartman CR 2003) [64]. Tumor-derived CXCL12 mediates trafficking of plasmacytoid DCs into the tumor and protects tumor plasmacytoid DCs from apoptosis (Wei CR 2005) [62]. Interestingly, plasmacytoid DCs within the tumor microenvironment show reduced expression of toll-like receptor 9 (TLR9) which is the most specific TLR pathway for inducing IFN-α (Hartman CR 2003) [64]. Likewise plamacytoid DCs induce significant IL-10 production by T cells that suppresses myeloid-DC-induced TAA (Tumor Associated Antigen)-specific T-cell effector functions (Wei CR 2005) [62]. These results suggest that plasmacytoid DCs can be phenotypically and functionally modulated in the tumor microenvironment.

Finally, Treg cells have an important role in impeding tumor immune surveillance (Curiel JCI 2007) [65]. They were initially described by Gershon *et al.* in the early 1970s and were called suppressive T cells (Gershon I 1970) [66]. Five years later, Sehon and colleagues suggested that these Treg cells negatively regulated tumor immunity and contributed to tumor growth in mice. After another five years, North and colleagues published a series of experiments providing evidence that CD4+CD25+ T cells from tumor bearing mice inhibited tumor rejection, indicating the existence of tumor-suppressor T cells (Berendt JEM 1980) [67]. These pioneering studies established the field of Treg cells in tumor immunology. Unfortunately, despite the importance of these studies there was extensive skepticism in the immunological field about the existence of these cells, and suppressive T cells left the centre stage of immunology for decades. However, in 1995, Sakaguchi and colleagues showed that the interleukin-2 (IL-2) receptor α-chain, CD25, could serve as a phenotypic marker for CD4+ suppressor T cells or CD4+ Treg cells (Sakaguchi JI 1995) [68]. More recent studies have shown that the transcription factor forkhead box P3 (FOXP3) is not only a key intracellular marker but is also a crucial developmental and functional factor for CD4+CD25+ Treg cells (Hori Science 2003) [69]. Thereafter, the notion of Treg cells was revived and the field of Treg cells has evolved rapidly. Indeed, over the past few years, several phenotypically distinct regulatory T-cell populations have been suggested (Sakaguchi JI 1995) [68] (Zou NI 2003) [69]. CD4+ Treg cells typically express CD25 (the α-chain of the IL-2 receptor), cytotoxic T lymphocyte-associated antigen 4 (CTLA-4), glucocorticoid-induced TNF receptor-related protein (GITR), and the transcription factor forkhead box P3 (FOXP3). They are generated in the thymus and the periphery (Liston COI 2007) [71] (Liu NI 2008) [72] and exert their suppressive activity on multiple immune cells (T cells, NK cells, NKT cells, B cells, and APCs), through both contact-dependent and contact-independent mechanisms. (Zou W 2006) [70] (Liston COI 2007) [71] (Liu NI 2008) [72]. Treg accumulation has been documented in various tumors, in tumor-draining lymph nodes, and in the peripheral circulation of individuals with cancer, and tumor antigen-specific Tregs have also been described (Ke FB 2008) [73] (van der Burg PNAS 2007) [74] . An inverse correlation between the number of Tregs in the tumor and clinical outcome has also been noted (Liu NI 2008) [72].

CANCER IMMUNOTHERAPY

Immunotherapy aims to enhance immune responses that will effectively kill all tumor cells while leaving healthy tissue intact. The potential benefits include the stimulation of cytotoxic and helper T cells, natural killer cells, dendritic cells, and antibodies that can kill disseminated tumors, in addition to the development of immunological memory to guard against cancer recurrence. After decades of intensive investigation, considerable progress has been made in many areas, and the development of improved methods for tumor antigen identification, molecular and genetic manipulation of the immune system, and fundamental new insights into immunobiology have paved the way for further advances that are now reaching the clinic.

In order to attain effective, reliable and consistent clinical efficacy, improving the tumor-associated immune response can be achieved by either boosting components of the immune system that produce an effective immune response or by inhibiting components that suppress the immune response. In this regard, conventional immunotherapy supplements the immune system and provides essential immune elements, including tumor-associated antigen, antigen-presenting cells, effector T cells and cytokines and/or chemokines with the aim of boosting TAA-specific immunity. Meanwhile, novel immunotherapeutic strategies target the immunosuppressive network of tumors, including Treg cells, suppressive molecules and dysfunctional APCs, with the aim of recovering TAA-specific immunity.

Boosting Immune Elements

Adoptive T cell immunotherapy. Adoptive cell therapy is an alternative way to isolate and expand antigen specific T cells for potent tumor immunity for the treatment of cancer. The challenges faced by immunologists using adoptive T cell therapy relate not only to generating large numbers of cells for transfusion, but also to developing cells that have specificity for tumor antigens; retain proliferative, homing, and effector function; and can engraft long-term. The ability to transfer central memory T cells with stem cell-like self-renewing qualities and that rapidly acquire effector function remains a challenge (Sallusto ARI 2004) [75]. Active immunization of characterized Ags has been explored for many years and success remains limited. Although infused T cells infiltrate tumors and exhibit tumor control in some patients, tumor antigen evasion still remains a major problem. Thus, targeted antigen selection is important for treatment. The solution is to select over-expressed oncogenes indispensable for the tumor phenotype. This is illustrated by the dramatic regression of some tumors that is seen following the adoptive transfer and clonal expansion of tumor-infiltrating lymphocytes recognizing melanoma-associated antigens and administration of IL-2 (Dudley JCO 2008) [76]. Nevertheless, a problem has previously existed in terms of the failure of the adoptively transferred cells to engraft and persist, although lymphodepletion seems to have overcome this issue to some extent (Rosenberg NRC 2008) [77]. For example, nonmyeloablative lymphodepletion prior to adoptive T cell transfer allows the transferred T cells to undergo homeostasis-driven proliferation in response to increased synthesis and accessibility to the endogenous growth factors (Rosenberg NEJM 2008) [78]. On the other hand, it is difficult to generate large numbers of high avidity tumor-reactive CD8+ T cells in individual patients in time and maintain their survival *in vivo*. The solution is gene therapy, by engineering T cells with high avidity through insertion of cloned TCRs of known specificity and affinity. T cell avidity can be further improved by mutating low affinity TCRs prior to insertion into host T cells (Tsuji Blood 2005) [79] (Roszkowski CR 2005) [80]. This allows autologous T cells to be directly equipped with the desired specificity without requiring a prior antigen presentation step—a strategy that can overcome self-tolerance to tumor antigens (Stanislawski NI 2001) [81]. The primary drawback here is the scarcity of cloned T-cell receptors with characteristics that would be suitable for universal use. In the meantime, to improve the survival of transferred T cells *in vivo*, pro-survival molecules/signals or receptor genes are engineered into T cells that inherently survive better *in vivo*. A novel strategy to improve T cell recognition of poorly processed/presented tumor antigens or MHC class I loss tumors, is to create chimeric receptors that take advantage of Ab-recognition structures, which have higher affinities than TCRs and do not require MHC (Alajez Blood 2005) [82]. Chimeric TCR structures can be further modified with costimulatory and/or signal transducing molecules to improve signaling and promote survival. In some cases, they have been engineered to be completely artificial, for example Morgan *et al.* used retroviral vector-mediated *ex vivo* delivery to genetically reprogram autologous T cells with melanoma antigen-specific T-cell receptor, and achieved sustained regression of locally advanced and metastatic melanoma in 2 of 17 patients, both of whom have remained disease free for more than a year after treatment (Heemskerk HGT 2008) [83]. Finally an important obstacle is how to maintain effective T cell response in the hostile micro- and macro-environment created by a progressive tumor, molecular disruption of T cell regulatory checkpoints would help transferred T cells resist the tumor inhibitory microenvironment. For example, CTLA-4 blockade is a potential strategy to be combined with adoptive cell transfer for effective host responses against tumor.

Tumor antigen identification and therapeutic exploitation. Tumor antigens can elicit immune lead to tumor elimination. In most cases in cancer, tumor cells transform and mutate frequently, resulting in immune equilibrium and finally escape immune surveillance. A rational way of fighting cancer is to identify tumor antigens and utilize them in vaccines to boost anti-tumor immunity. Many approaches have been used to discover tumor antigens, including: 1. Direct immune approach, starting with T-cells or antibodies that recognize tumors and identifying the antigens by cDNA cloning techniques (Kreiter JI 2008) [84] (Nicholaou ICB 2006) [85]; 2. reverse immune approaches, starting with candidate antigens that are over-expressed by tumors and determining whether T-cells can recognize these antigens (Nussbaum COI 2003) [86]. Numerous human tumor antigens have been discovered using the above approaches, covering shared tumor-specific antigens (MAGE, NY-ESO-1, etc), antigens resulting from mutations (MUM-1, CDK4, *etc.*), differentiation antigens (MART-1, gp100), overexpressed antigens (p53, HER2/neu), and viral antigens (EBV, HPV16) (Nabeta MAI 2000) [87] (Kawakami CS 2004) [88]. Characterization of antigen fragments derived from these tumor antigens, denominated T cytotoxic cell determinants (DTc), has allowed the design of immunization strategies based on the use of subunit vaccines (Melief NRC 2008) [89] (Cavallo ERV 2009) [90]. Thus, by combining DTc with peptides recognized by T helper cells, different adjuvants or vectors, CTL responses against many antigens have been induced (Cavallo ERV 2009) [90]. Because of the potential of CTL to kill cells expressing tumour antigens, immunotherapy based on the activation of this lymphocyte population has been suggested as a strategy for cancer treatment (Cavallo ERV 2009) [90]. Several approaches of subunit vaccines using DTc have been considered for the induction of anti-tumour CTL. Some of these approaches have relied on the use of immunodominant DTc belonging to the main tumour antigen expressed by malignant cells, whereas in other cases full antigens encoding all the DTc contained in a protein have been used as antigens (Kessler IR 2008) [91]. To avoid the effect of appearance of tumour antigen loss variants, it would be desirable to combine different DTc as well as DTc belonging to different tumour antigens, inducing thus CTL responses against a wide target repertoire. One of the most common strategies has been the inclusion of several DTc in minigene constructs encoding these antigenic sequences. A number of reports have shown that by immunizing with these constructs CTL responses can be induced (van Baren JCO 2005) [92] (Mc Conkey NM 2003) [93], but it has also been reported that a high heterogeneity exists between responses induced against the different DTc (Depla JV 2008) [94]. However, immunization with chimerical vector containing immunodominant epitopes (multiepitopes), using antigenic peptides, whole proteins, or virus-like particles (recombinant viruses/bacteria/DNA encoding tumor DTc) has led to the induction of better and long lasting immune responses (Durántez SJI 2008) [95] . In this regard, we recently have shown that using a plant derived chimeric virus like particles, containing the HPV 16 L1 sequence and a string of T-cell epitopes from HPV 16 E6 and E7 (Monroy MM 2007) [96] fused to the C-terminus, were able to induce a significant antibody and cytotoxic T-lymphocytes response in mice (Paz de la Rosa VJ 2009) [97]. Intraperitoneal administration in mice was able to elicit both neutralizing antibodies against the viral particle and cytotoxic T-lymphocytes activity against the epitopes as well as tumor reduction (Paz de la Rosa VJ 2009) [97]. Then employing virus vectors as adjuvants and as carrier of multiepitopes, can be important to achieve mass reduction and immunostimulation, as well as tools for genetic re-programming of antigen presentation and effector function in the immune system.

DC-based immunotherapy. Dendritic cells are the natural immune adjuvant to help tumor antigen presentation. Multiple signals can mature DC, such as microbial products, tissue damage, and innate/adaptive immune components (O´Neill Blood 2004) [98]. DC can be induced into mature status either as tolerogenic (by β-catenin, NO, IL-10) or immunogenic (by type I IFN, IL-12). Great attention has to be paid on the selection of DC as immune adjuvants for vaccination, because different types of DCs have distinct functions, such as pDC, mDC (langerhans DC, interstitial DC) (O´Neill Blood 2004) [98]. As a perfect example, skin DC can be CD14+, DC-SIGN+ (IntDC), or CD1a+, Langerin+ (LC-DC) . LC-DC are more efficient in CD8+ T cell priming and proliferation than IntDC, thus, LC-DC are better for cross priming/presentation (Lanzavecchia COI 2001) [99]. However, IntDC prime follicular CD4+ T cells more efficiently to induce B cell antibody responses (O´Neill Blood 2004) [98] (Lanzavecchia COI 2001) [99]. To design tumor vaccines, peptides (tumor associated Ags) or killed allogenic cancer cells were pulsed onto DCs. DCs have directly induced immunity in many clinical trials, but only limited success has been achieved in terms of inducing partial or complete remissions in cancer patients (Stagg IR 2007) [100]. The main problem is the lack of functional mature DCs and abundance of suppressive DCs, that significantly reduce the TAA-specific T-cell priming in draining lymph nodes, as well as the TAA-specific effector immunity in the tumour microenvironment. In addition, the absence of "danger signals", including inflammatory cytokines, molecular and cellular T-cell activation signals in the tumour microenvironment, has been considered the main cause of poor tumour immunity (Matzinger Science 2002) [101]. In many cases DCs used in the treatment of patients with cancer are differentiated *in vitro* from blood monocytes and activated *in vitro* by cytokines and PGE2, which render them resistant to *in vivo* licensing by costimulatory molecules such as CD40. These DCs fail to induce cytokines such as IL-12 that skew the immune response to a Th1 response, and they might even induce Treg cells *in vivo* (Fuchs SI 1996) [102]. By contrast, exposure to pathogen components (TLR agonists) resulted in fully activated DCs that promoted Th cell responses. Therefore, preferential activation of DCs with natural activators such as TLR agonists (particularly when physically linked with antigens to facilitate endosomal processing) might be a preferable way to generate therapeutically useful DCs. DC function might be further improved by inhibiting negative regulatory pathways in the cells or by inducing the cells to express costimulatory molecules and antiapoptotic proteins to enhance viability. Improving the delivery of antigens to DCs is also required. Although several vehicles have been used for this purpose (viral vectors and apoptotic or necrotic tumor lysates), there is no consensus on the optimal approach, but transfection of human DCs with mRNA encoding tumor antigens is effective at inducing tumor-specific immunity *in vitro* and *in vivo* (Gilboa IR 2004) [103]. Recent studies indicate that immature mouse DCs (unlike macrophages) express few proteases, with reduced capacity for lysosomal degradation (Delamarre Science 2005) [104]. *In vivo*, mouse DCs degrade internalized antigens slowly and retain them for long periods. Evidently this translates into more favorable antigen presentation to both T cells and B cells. Therefore, modification of antigens to resist lysosomal proteolysis might render them more immunogenic when acquired by immature DCs (Delamarre JEM 2006) [105]. Other issues in the design of DC-based immunotherapies include the type(s) of antigen to be administered, the number of DCs to use per vaccination, the frequency of vaccinations, the mode and site of injection, the utility of targeting DCs *in situ* with TLR agonists in place of the whole-cell approach, and the incorporation of danger signals as a strategy to boost tumor immunity (Matzinger Science 2002) [101] (Fuchs SI 1996) [102].

Antibody therapies. Antibodies provide the opportunity to target a very specific population of cells by virtue of the expression of a single type of protein on the cell surface. However, such antibodies are of limited use for the targeting of a large number of tumor antigens that are expressed only within the cell (Li CII 2004) [106]. Perhaps so many tumor-associated antigens provide poor targets for immune mediated tumor eradication because of the destruction of tumor cells that express highly antigenic proteins early in the course of tumor evolution, in a process described as "tumor editing" (Chan CII 2006) [107]. Furthermore, the stimulated T cells that can target such antigens may be clonally deleted or exhausted or become anergic, in a process known as "immune editing" (Dunn IR 2005)[108]. The antigens present on the remaining tumor cells, which are able to escape immune surveillance, are unlikely to induce effective CD8+ T-cell responses and are much more likely to induce CD4+ and B-cell immune responses. However, where antibodies can be used to target a malignant cell population, and where the tumor burden is low enough to prevent subsequent patient toxicity as a result of tumor lysis syndrome, antibody therapy can be exquisitely specific and effective. Among the most effective monoclonal antibody therapies has been Rituximab, which targets anti-CD20 on the surface of B cells, effectively removing the malignant cells in B-cell leukemia and CD20+ non-Hodgkins lymphoma (Mc Laughlin JCO 1998) [109]. Rituximab has shown very promising results in the treatment of B-cell lymphomas, 90% of which express the CD20 antigen. In a seminal phase II multi-institutional clinical trial of 166 patients with relapsed low-grade follicular lymphoma, the chimeric anti-CD20 antibody IDEC-C2B8 led to a 48% response rate, similar to single-agent cytotoxic chemotherapy (Cohen H 2003) [110]. Rituximab showed enhanced efficacy when used in combination with chemotherapy in four clinical trials (Coiffier CRB 2006) [111]. Among the drawbacks of this treatment has been the expansion of escape mutants which do not express CD20, and again this treatment cannot be used on bulky disease owing to the toxicity associated with tumor lysis syndrome. However, anti-CD20 therapy, when used as an adjuvant after conventional therapy, has been highly effective at eliminating the malignant clone at diffuse sites. Other monoclonal antibody products have been successful in the clinic, albeit as adjunct therapies, and have been approved by the US Food and Drug Administration, including Herceptin (trastuzumab, anti-HER2/neu) for metastatic breast cancer, and Avastin (bevacizumab, anti-vascular endothelial growth factor) and Erbitux (cetuximab, anti-epidermal growth factor receptor) for metastatic colorectal cancer (Adams NB 2005) [112]. Although the antibody continues to convey some specificity for the target, toxicity against normal tissues remains a problem, for this reason is necessary to identify a surface-expressed tumor antigen whose normal tissue expression is limited to non-essential cell types. In this regard, vaccination strategies are advantageous in educating the body to select target epitopes on its own, where it can determine an antigen's expression to be abnormal.

Cytokines in cancer immunotherapy. The development of anti-cancer cytokines is an active area for investigators in the field of cancer immunotherapy. Both immune or non-immune cells can be the focus of biological rationals for cytokine therapy, including: 1) T cells: to enhance the development, proliferation and/or function of either endogenous or adoptively transferred effector T cells; 2) NK cells: to enhance NK activity and improve ADCC; 3) tumor cells: to upregulate Ag and MHC expression, or induce an anti-proliferative effect; 4) DC/APC: to generate and mature DC/APC *in vitro*, and to increase DC/APC number and function *in vivo*. Although over 20 cytokines have been developed for the treatment of cancer, only IL-2, IFN-α and TNF-α have been approved in the US and/or Europe for immunologic anticancer therapy. Multiple issues for clinical development of cytokines have been highlighted over decades of studies, such as their context-dependent biological effects, secondary effects, and differences in response between individuals (Li JTM 2009) [113]. IL-2 was one of the first cytokines to be applied to cancer therapy (Lotze I 1986) [114]. IL-2 induces T cell activation and proliferation and stimulates NK cell cytotoxicity; however, IL-2 also causes vascular leak syndrome, which can lead to significant side effects. IL-2 regimens have been tested in several types of cancers, with a 15% response rate only in human metastatic renal cell carcinoma and melanoma (Lotze I 1986) [114]. Adoptive cell transfer of tumor infiltrating lymphocytes to lymphodepleted patients with melanoma in combination with high dose IL-2 has been shown to achieve clinical responses in the range of 50% (Rosenberg PM 1994) [115]. However, minimal activity of IL-2 in the treatment of other cancers has been observed. Mechanistic studies involving T cells activation, Treg cells and B7 costimulatory family members are under investigation to address how IL-2 works or fails in therapy (Maker ASO 2005) [116] (Powell JI 2007) [117] . IL-2, IL-15 and IL-21 all belong to the common gamma chain receptor family. Targeting NK, NKT and memory CD8+ T cells, IL-15 exerts its functions preferentially through trans-presentation. Murine models demonstrated that IL-15 enhances *in vivo* anti-tumor activity of adoptively transferred T cells, which is further enhanced in combination with an anti-IL-2 antibody (Klebanoff PNAS 2004) [118]. IL-21 may be a promising candidate for cancer immunotherapy as it has pleiotropic roles in immune cells, yet does not support Treg function (Hinrichs Blood 2008) [119]. A combination of IL-15 and IL-21 may be a choice for future therapeutic regimens, as suggested by some mouse studies (Kowalczyk CII 2007) [120]. In the particular case of IL-12, local administration is recommended due to its excessive systemic toxicity (Sotiriadou CI 2005) [121]. Future applications of new cytokines include *in vitro* expansion of antigen-specific T cells and the support for adoptively transferred cells; local application as a vaccine adjuvant; and antibodies to neutralize selected cytokines to enhance immune responses.

Blocking Suppressive Elements

Regulatory T cells (Treg). Recent evidence has demonstrated that regulatory-T-cell-mediated immunosuppression is one of the crucial tumour immune-evasion mechanisms and the main obstacle of successful tumour immunotherapy (Shevach NRI 2002) [122] (Zou NRC 2005) [123]. However, utilizing CD4+ CD25+ T cell depletion experiments, tumor immunity has been closely examined in regard to Treg cells (Sakaguchi JI 1995) [68]. Induction of anti-tumor immunity by CD4+ CD25+ T regulatory depletion was first proved in mouse models (Shimizu JI 1999) [124]. Anti-IL-2 treatment reduced CD25+ Treg cells and mice developed autoimmune disease. IL-2 is crucial for self-tolerance maintenance (Malek NRI 2004) [125]. Foxp3 is a master transcription factor in Treg cells, and Foxp3+ Treg have constitutive expression of CTLA-4 (Hori S 2003) [126]. CTLA-4 blockade abrogates Treg suppression (Hodi PNAS 2008) [127]. Further effective tumor immunity was provoked in Treg restricted-CTLA-4-/- mice (Tang EJI 2004) [128]. Through microarray analysis, folate receptor 4 (FR4) was discovered to have high expression on activated Treg cells. Functional analysis indicated that FR4 differentiate activated Teff into Treg, and its blockade leads to Treg depletion *in vivo*, in turn improving tumor rejection (Yamaguchi Immunity 2007) [129]. GITR is another molecule preferentially expressed by Treg, DTA-1, an antibody for GITR, can abrogate Treg suppression while not depleting Treg, can reverse Teff/Treg ratio and increase CD4 T cell infiltration into tumors, and can synergize with CTLA-4 blockade to enhance anti-tumor immunity (Shimizu NI 2002) [130]. On the other hand, depletion of CD25+ T cells *in vivo* is another strategy to deplete Treg. Given that treatment with CD25-specific antibody efficiently depletes Treg cells, improves tumour immunity and results in mouse tumour regression, it is predicted that depletion of Treg cells would be beneficial for cancer patients. Denileukin diftitox (Ontak) is a ligand-toxin fusion protein that consists of full-length IL-2 fused to the enzymatically active and translocating domains of diphtheria toxin (Duvic FO 2008) [131]. This drug has been approved by the Food and Drug Administration in the United States for treatment of CD25+ cutaneous T-cell leukaemia and lymphoma. This fusion protein is internalized into CD25+ T cells by endocytosis. The ADP-ribosyltransferase activity of diphtheria toxin is cleaved in the endosome and is translocated into the cytosol, where it inhibits protein synthesis, leading to apoptosis (Duvic FO 2008) [131]. It has been reported that a single dose of denileukin diftitox reduced the prevalence and absolute numbers of peripheral Treg cells and increased effector T-cell activation in patients with lung, ovarian or breast cancer (Ruter FB 2009) [132].

Targeting suppressive molecules. T cell response requires two signals: the first signal is the recognition and binding of the T Cell Receptor (TCR) to antigen bound within the Major Histocompatibility Complex (MHC) presented by APCs; the second is the binding of costimulatory ligands, expressed on APC, to receptors on the T cells (Melero NRC 2007) [133]. The discovery of multiple costimulatory molecules that influence the course of T cell activation has increased our appreciation of the complexity of the T cell response. CD28 and cytotoxic T lymphocyte antigen 4

(CTLA-4) are the critical costimulatory receptors that determine the early outcome of stimulation through TCR. CTLA-4 plays a critical role in the down-regulation of T cell responses (Melero NRC 2007) [133]. Its inhibition may restrict T cell activation during both the initiation and progression of the antitumor response. Thus, blockade of CTLA-4 inhibitory signals during T cell-APC interactions can result in enhanced tumor immunity (Korman AI 2006) [134]. Some of the more promising strategies involve the coadministration of agonistic antibodies specific for the costimulatory molecules that are expressed on activated T cells (Melero NRC 2007) [133]. Antagonistic antibodies specific for the coinhibitory receptors CTLA-4 and Programmed Death 1 (PD1) (Korman AI 2006) [134] are also being evaluated. In mouse models, CTLA-4-specific antibody, in combination with cancer vaccines (*e.g.*, a GM-CSF-transduced tumor cell vaccine), functions in a cell intrinsic manner on both effector T cells and Tregs to increase the rejection of poorly immunogenic tumors. The net effect is greater infiltration of tumor-reactive T cells in the tumor and a change in the balance of effector T cells and Tregs (in favor of the effector T cells) at this site (Quezada JCI 2006) [135]. CTLA-4 blockade might also release DCs from B7-mediated engagement, with either effector T cells or Tregs, which causes the induction of IDO and immune suppression due to tryptophan depletion and the production of proapoptotic factors (Fallrino TI 2006) [136]. In humans, CTLA-4 blockade increased tumor immunity in a number of previously vaccinated cancer patients (Hodi NCPO 2008) [137] and was associated with objective tumor regression in some melanoma patients who received peptide/adjuvant vaccines (Phan ASO 2008) [138], although it was accompanied by serious side effects in some cases (hypophysitis and enterocolitis). An ongoing phase III clinical trial will resolve whether CTLA-4-specific antibodies as a single agent or administered in combination with peptide vaccine are efficacious in treating metastatic melanoma. T cells become functionally impaired in chronic viral infections and in the tumor setting and express high levels of PD1, an inhibitory molecule induced after T cell activation (Blackburn PNAS 2008) [139]. PD1 interacts with B7-H1 (also known as PDL1) and B7-DC (also known as PDL2) (Iwai II 2005) [140]. It has been appointed a marker of disease progression in HIV infection, as it correlates positively with plasma viral load and inversely with CD4+ T cell numbers (Day N 2006) [141]. Blockade with antibodies specific for B7-H1 augmented HIV-specific CD4+ and CD8+ T cell function *in vitro* (Trautman NM 2006) [142]. Similar analyses of T cells in the tumor setting are being undertaken. B7-H1 has been shown to be expressed by mouse melanoma cells, and their *in vivo* growth was inhibited by administering B7-H1-specific antibody (Iwai II 2005) [140]. PD1 blockade is currently being evaluated in humans, and it remains to be seen whether blockade of other functionally related coinhibitory molecules, such as B7-H3, B7-H4 (also known as B7x), B and T lymphocyte attenuator (BTLA), and the recently described V-set and Ig domain-containing 4 (VSIG4) will achieve antitumor effects in humans (Vogt JCI 2006) [143].

Suppressing dysfunctional DCs. Tumor microenvironment lacks functionally mature myeloid Dendritic Cells (DCs) capable of inducing tumor-specific T-cell immunity, whereas it is abundant in immunosuppressive Antigen-Presenting Cell (APC) subsets, including partially differentiated myeloid DCs, B7-H1+ DCs, indoleamine-2,3-deoxygenase (IDO)+ DCs, Plasmacytoid DCs (PDCs) and myeloid suppressor cells (MSCs). These suppressive APC subsets induce arrest of the T-cell cycle, suppressive T cells and T-cell apoptosis. This APC-subset imbalance favours the formation of immune tolerance. As mentioned above, tumour immunotherapies including DC vaccines often target late-stage tumours with the aim of boosting TAA immunity. Fully activated DCs are less sensitive to suppression and able to rescue suboptimal activated T cells (Tyagi ERA 2009) [144] (O'Neill MB 2007) [145]. However, it remains to be defined whether fully activated DCs alone would subvert the suppressive capacity of Treg cells and of regulatory (or dysfunctional) APCs in tumor-bearing patients (O'Neill MB 2007) [145]. For instance, in patients with ovarian cancer, repetitive stimulation with fully matured myeloid DCs is not able to recover T-cell dysfunction mediated by tumor-associated plasmacytoid DCs (Wei CR 2005) [146]. Tolerizing conditions will have already been established in these patients and will remain present after surgery. Adoptively transferred DCs will face identical tolerizing situations as the 'original' DCs did in the tumour microenvironment and could partially explain the poor clinical efficiency of DC vaccinations (Kryczek CR 2007) [147]. Furthermore, fully activated DCs would possibly expand and activate CD4+CD25+ Treg cells (Kryczek CR 2007) [147]. Thus, tackling these tolerizing conditions might improve the efficacy of DC vaccines. For example, administration of AMD3100 or other CXCR4-CXCL12 signalling antagonists could block the trafficking of plasmacytoid DCs into tumors, interrupt the interaction between tumors and plasmacytoid DCs, and in turn disable tumor plasmacytoid-DC-mediated immunosuppression and vascularization. CXCL12-CXCR4 antagonists would further suppress CXCL12-CXCR4-mediated tumor neoangiogenesis (Kryczek CR 2007) [147] and metastasis (Müller Nature 2001) [148]. In addition, activated plasmacytoid DCs in the tumor microenvironment remain as a chief source of type I IFN, potentially bridging innate and adaptive immunity. IFNα derived from plasmacytoid DCs might induce maturation of myeloid DCs and activate

NK cells in the tumor microenvironment, and also provide important T-cell survival signals (Le Bon CGFR 2008) [149]. IFN is also a potent inhibitor of tumor angiogenesis (Persano C 2009) [150]. On the other hand, the immunosuppressive activity of IDO-expressing APCs or tumor cells can be inhibited by the IDO inhibitor 1-methyltryptophan (Lob Blood 2008) [151] (Ou JCRCO 2008) [152]. The immunosuppressive activity of arginase-expressing myeloid suppressor cells might be inhibited by an arginase inhibitor, *N*-hydroxy-nor-L-arginine (Nor-NOHA). The injection of Nor-NOHA and Nor-NOHA plus L-arginine in tumor-bearing mice significantly inhibits tumor growth in a dose-dependent manner (Bak MI 2008) [153]. As most of human epithelial tumors and APCs express B7-H1 and B7-H4 (Files JI 2007) [154], these molecules represent additional attractive new targets for cancer immunotherapy. As *in vitro* and *in vivo* experiments in mice demonstrate that blocking B7-H1 and B7-H4 pathways improves TAA-specific T-cell immunity, it would be therapeutically meaningful to develop the related signal pathway blocking molecules for human clinical trials (Wei CR 2008) [155] (Ozao CR 2009) [156].

CONCLUDING REMARKS

Several clinical and experimental studies have found that tumors actively develop different mechanisms to escape tumor immunity and defeat conventional tumor immunotherapy strategies. This panorama is now more complicated, due to the tumor-promoting properties of innate immune cells. For this reason, researchers are now investigating the efficacy of novel anticancer strategies that are based on an understanding of the mechanism at each step of immunological tumor evasion in order to either bolster antitumour adaptive immunity or neutralize cancer-promoting properties of innate immune cells.

In spite of clinical trials performed to date show hopeful immunologic results, appears not be sufficient to passively supplement the essential immune elements, such as immunogenic peptides, T cells, cytokines and Dendritic Cells. This limited succes may also be due to tumour tolerization as result of imbalances in the tumour microenvironment, including alterations in antigen-presenting-cell subsets, co-stimulatory and co-inhibitory molecule alterations, antigen/MHC loss, altered ratios of effector T cells and regulatory T cells among others. A better understanding of this immunosuppressive network in the course of tumor development and progression should lead towards refine novel immune-boosting strategies. In this context, is necessary to consider combinatorial tumor therapies that include: subversion of tolerizing conditions; supplementation of immune elements including new adyuvants, and suppression of tumor angiogenesis and growth (Fig. **2**).

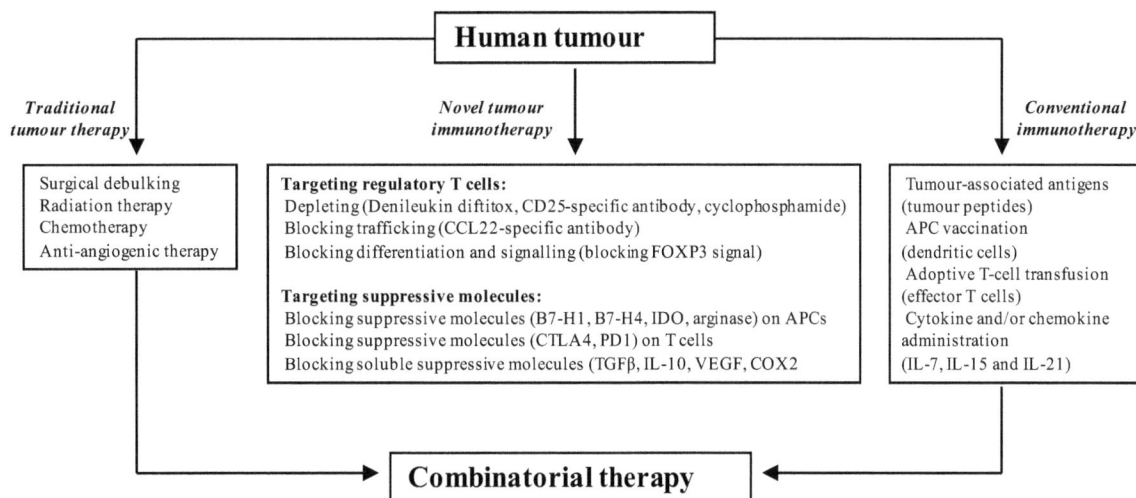

Figure 2: Combinatorial tumor immunotherapy. After clinical and/or pathological diagnosis, patients with cancer might be subjected to traditional tumour therapy, including surgical debulking, radiation therapy, chemotherapy and antitumour angiogenic therapy. Depending on their clinical situation, patients could receive a combination of these strategies. Traditional tumor therapy targets the tumor itself and remains the 'gold standard' therapy. Conventional immunotherapy supplements the immune system and provides essential immune elements, including tumor-associated antigen (TAA), antigen-presenting cells (APCs), effector T cells and cytokines and/or chemokines with the aim of boosting TAA-specific immunity. Early clinical trials with conventional tumor immunotherapy have been encouraging, but improvements in clinical efficacy are needed. Novel immunotherapeutic strategies target the immunosuppressive network of tumors, including regulatory T cells, suppressive molecules and dysfunctional

APCs, with the aim of recovering TAA-specific immunity. To attain effective, reliable and consistent clinical efficacy, it might be essential to combine traditional tumour therapy, conventional immunotherapy and novel tumor immunotherapy. COX2, cyclooxygenase 2; CTLA-4, cytotoxic T-lymphocyte-associated antigen 4; FOXP3, forkhead box P3; IDO, indoleamine 2,3-dioxygenase; IL, interleukin; PD1, programmed cell death 1; TGFβ, transforming growth factor-β; VEGF, vascular endothelial growth factor. Data from reference [70].

ACKNOWLEDGEMENTS

CONACyT (grants 47615-Q and 106591) and IMSS (grant FIS/IMSS/PROT/060, 762 and 876) support to AMG; and CONACyT (grant 82827) support to MLMG, are gratefully acknowledged.

REFERENCES

[1]   Murphy K, Tranvers P, Walport M. Immunobiology. 7th ed. USA: Garland Science 2008

[2]   Akira S, Takeda K. Toll-like receptor signalling. Nat Rev Immunol 2004; 4: 499-511.

[3]   Sahu A, Lambris JD. Structure and biology of complement protein C3, a connecting link between innate and acquired immunity. Immunol Rev 2001; 180: 35-48.

[4]   Walport MJ. Complement. First of two parts. N Engl J Med 2001; 344: 1058-66.

[5]   Walport MJ. Complement. Second of two parts. N Engl J Med 2001; 344: 1140-4.

[6]   Carroll MC. The complement system in regulation of adaptive immunity. Nat Immunol 2004; 5: 981-6.

[7]   Goldrath AW, Bevan MJ. Selecting and maintaining a diverse T-cell repertoire. Nature 1999; 402:255-62.

[8]   Tonegawa S. Somatic generation of antibody diversity. Nature 1983; 302: 575-81.

[9]   McHeyzer-Williams MG. B cells as effectors. Curr Opin Immunol 2003; 15: 354-61.

[10]   Sprent J, Surh CD. T cell memory. Annu Rev Immunol 2002; 20: 551-79.

[11]   Dunn GP, Old LJ, Schreiber RD. The immunobiology of cancer immunosurveillance and immunoediting. Immunity 2004; 21: 137-48.

[12]   Pardoll DM. Tumor reactive T cells get a boost. Nat Biotechnol 2002; 20: 1207-8.

[13]   Boshoff C, Weiss R. AIDS-related malignancies. Nat Rev Cancer 2002; 2: 373-82.

[14]   Euvrard S, Kanitakis J, Claudy A. Skin cancers after organ transplantation. N Engl J Med 2003; 348: 1681-91.

[15]   Penn I. Posttransplant malignancies. Transplant Proc 1999; 31: 1260-2.

[16]   Alaedini A, Green PH. Narrative review: celiac disease: understanding a complex autoimmune disorder. Ann Intern Med 2005; 142: 289-98.

[17]   Artinian V, Kvale PA. Cancer and interstitial lung disease. Curr Opin Pulm Med 2004; 10:425-34.

[18]   Ji H, Ohmura K, Mahmood U, *et al.* Arthritis critically dependent on innate immune system players. Immunity 2002; 16: 157-68.

[19]   Korganow AS, Ji H, Mangialaio S, *et al.* From systemic T cell self-reactivity to organ-specific autoimmune disease *via* immunoglobulins. Immunity 1999; 10: 451-61.

[20]   Agassy-Cahalon L, Yaakubowicz M, Witz IP, *et al.* The immune system during the precancer period: naturally-occurring tumor reactive monoclonal antibodies and urethane carcinogenesis. Immunol Lett 1988; 18: 181-9.

[21]   Brodt P, Gordon J. Natural resistance mechanisms may play a role in protection against chemical carcinogenesis. Cancer Immunol Immunother 1982; 13: 125-7.

[22]   Monach PA, Schreiber H, Rowley DA. CD4+ and B lymphocytes in transplantation immunity. II. Augmented rejection of tumor allografts by mice lacking B cells. Transplantation 1993; 55: 1356-61.

[23]   Schreiber H, Wu TH, Nachman J, *et al.* Immunological enhancement of primary tumor development and its prevention. Semin Cancer Biol 2000; 10: 351-7.

[24]   Siegel CT, Schreiber K, Meredith SC, *et al.* Enhanced growth of primary tumors in cancer-prone mice after immunization against the mutant region of an inherited oncoprotein. J Exp Med 2000; 191: 1945-56.

[25]   Barbera-Guillem E, May KF Jr, Nyhus JK, *et al.* Promotion of tumor invasion by cooperation of granulocytes and macrophages activated by anti-tumor antibodies. Neoplasia 1999; 1: 453-60.

[26]   de Visser KE, Korets LV, Coussens LM. De novo carcinogenesis promoted by chronic inflammation is B lymphocyte dependent. Cancer Cell 2005; 7: 411-23.

[27]   Burnet M. Immunological factors in the process of carcinogenesis. Br Med Bull 1964; 20: 154-8.

[28]   Thomas L. In: Lawrence HS, Ed. Reactions to homologous tissue antigens in relation to hypersensitivity. New York, Hoeber-Harper 1959; 529-32.

[29]   Dunn GP, Bruce AT, Ikeda H, *et al.* Cancer immunoediting: from immunosurveillance to tumor escape. Nat Immunol 2002; 3: 991-8.

[30]   Street SE, Hayakawa Y, Zhan Y, *et al.* Innate immune surveillance of spontaneous B cell lymphomas by natural killer cells and gammadelta T cells. J Exp Med 2004; 199: 879-84.

[31]   Shankaran V, Ikeda H, Bruce AT, *et al.* IFNγ and lymphocytes prevent primary tumour development and shape tumour immunogenicity. Nature 2001; 410: 1107-11.

[32]   Swann JB, Smyth MJ. Immune surveillance of tumors. J Clin Invest 2007; 117: 1137-46.

[33]   Penn I. Tumors of the immunocompromised patient. Annu Rev Med 1988; 39:63-73.

[34]   Camus M, Tosolini M, Mlecnik B, *et al.* Coordination of intratumoral immune reaction and human colorectal cancer recurrence. Cancer Res 2009; 69: 2685-93

[35]   Crowe NY, Smyth MJ, Godfrey DI. A critical role for natural killer T cells in immunosurveillance of methylcholanthrene-induced sarcomas. J Exp Med 2002; 196: 119-27.

[36]   Ostrand-Rosenberg S. Immune surveillance: a balance between protumor and antitumor immunity. Curr Opin Genet Dev 2008; 18:11-8.

[37]   Blank C, Mackensen A. Contribution of the PD-L1/PD-1 pathway to T-cell exhaustion: an update on implications for chronic infections and tumor evasion. Cancer Immunol Immunother 2007; 56: 739-45.

[38]   Dong H, Strome SE, Salomao DR, *et al.* Tumor-associated B7-H1 promotes T-cell apoptosis: a potential mechanism of immune evasion. Nat Med 2002; 8: 793-800.

[39]   Munn DH, Mellor AL. Indoleamine 2,3-dioxygenase and tumor-induced tolerance. J Clin Invest 2007; 117: 1147-54.

[40]   Chen W, Liang X, Peterson AJ, *et al.* The indoleamine 2,3-dioxygenase pathway is essential for human plasmacytoid dendritic cell-induced adaptive T regulatory cell generation. J Immunol 2008; 181: 5396-404.

[41]   Orabona C, Puccetti P, Vacca C, *et al.* Toward the identification of a tolerogenic signature in IDO-competent dendritic cells. Blood 2006; 107: 2846-54.

[42]   Terness P, Bauer TM, Röse L, *et al.* Inhibition of allogeneic T cell proliferation by indoleamine 2,3-dioxygenase-expressing dendritic cells: mediation of suppression by tryptophan metabolites. J Exp Med 2002; 196: 447-57.

[43]   Chen W, Liang X, Peterson AJ, *et al.* The indoleamine 2,3-dioxygenase pathway is essential for human plasmacytoid dendritic cell-induced adaptive T regulatory cell generation. J Immunol 2008; 181: 5396-404.

[44]   Mellor AL, Baban B, Chandler PR, *et al.* Cutting edge: CpG oligonucleotides induce splenic CD19+ dendritic cells to acquire potent indoleamine 2,3-dioxygenase dependent T cell regulatory functions *via* IFN type 1 signaling. J Immunol 2005; 175: 5601-5.

[45]   Lee JH, Torisu-Itakara H, Cochran AJ, *et al.* Quantitative analysis of melanoma-induced cytokine-mediated immunosuppression in melanoma sentinel nodes. Clin Cancer Res 2005; 11: 107-12.

[46]   Gabrilovich DI, Nagaraj S. Myeloid-derived suppressor cells as regulators of the immune system. Nat Rev Immunol 2009; 9: 162-74.

[47]   Sica A, Bronte V. Altered macrophage differentiation and immune dysfunction in tumor development. J Clin Invest 2007; 117:1155-66.

[48]   Gallina G, Dolcetti L, Serafini P, *et al.* Tumors induce a subset of inflammatory monocytes with immunosuppressive activity on CD8+ T cells. J Clin Invest 2006; 116: 2777-90.

[49]   Huang B, Pan PY, Li Q, *et al.* Gr-1+CD115+ immature myeloid suppressor cells mediate the development of tumor-induced T regulatory cells and T-cell anergy in tumor-bearing host. Cancer Res 2006; 66: 1123-31.

[50]   Colombo MP, Mantovani A. Targeting myelomonocytic cells to revert inflammation-dependent cancer promotion. Cancer Res 2005; 65: 9113-16.

[51]   De Palma M, Mazzieri R, Politi LS, *et al.* Tumor-targeted interferon-alpha delivery by Tie2-expressing monocytes inhibits tumor growth and metastasis. Cancer Cell 2008; 14: 299-311.

[52]   Choi IH, Zhu G, Sica GL, *et al.* Genomic organization and expression analysis of B7-H4, an immune inhibitory molecule of the B7 family. J Immunol 2003; 171: 465-54.

[53]   Barnett BG, Rüter J, Kryczek I, *et al.* Regulatory T cells: a new frontier in cancer immunotherapy. Adv Exp Med Biol 2008; 622: 255-60.

[54]   Chen L. Co-inhibitory molecules of the B7-CD28 family in the control of T-cell immunity. Nature Rev Immunol 2004; 4: 336-47.

[55]   Curiel TJ, Wei S, Dong H, *et al.* Blockade of B7-H1 improves myeloid dendritic cell-mediated antitumor immunity. Nature Med 2003; 9: 562-67.

[56]   Dong H, Strome SE, Salomao DR, *et al.* Tumor-associated B7-H1 promotes T-cell apoptosis: a potential mechanism of immune evasion. Nature Med 2002; 8: 793-800.

[57]   Iwai Y, Ishida M, Tanaka Y, *et al.* Involvement of PD-L1 on tumor cells in the escape from host immune system and tumor immunotherapy by PD-L1 blockade. Proc Natl Acad Sci USA 2002; 99: 12293-97.

[58]   Prasad DV, Richards S, Mai XM. *et al.* B7S1, a novel B7 family member that negatively regulates T cell activation. Immunity 2003; 18: 863-73.

[59]   Kryczek I, Zou L, Rodriguez P, *et al.* B7-H4 expression identifies a novel suppressive macrophage population in human ovarian carcinoma. J Exp Med 2006; 203: 871-81.

[60]   Simon I, Katsaros D, Rigault de la Longrais I, *et al.* B7-H4 is over-expressed in early-stage ovarian cancer and is independent of CA125 expression. Gynecol Oncol 2007; 106: 334-41.

[61]   Kryczek I, Wei S, Zhu G, *et al.* Relationship between B7-H4, Regulatory T cells, and patient outcome in human ovarian carcinoma. Cancer Res 2007; 67: 8900-5.

[62]   Wei S, Kryczek I, Zou L, *et al.* Plasmacytoid dendritic cells induce CD8+ regulatory T cells in human ovarian carcinoma. Cancer Res 2005; 65: 5020-6.

[63]   Salio M, Cella M, Vermi W, *et al.* Plasmacytoid dendritic cells prime IFN-gamma- secreting melanoma-specific CD8 lymphocytes and are found in primary melanoma lesions. Eur J Immunol 2003; 33: 1052-62.

[64]   Hartmann E, Wollenberg B, Rothenfusser S, *et al.* Identification and functional analysis of tumor-infiltrating plasmacytoid dendritic cells in head and neck cancer. Cancer Res 2003; 63: 6478-87.

[65]   Curiel TJ. Tregs and rethinking cancer immunotherapy. J Clin Invest 2007; 117:1167-74.

[66]   Gershon RK, Kondo K. Cell interactions in the induction of tolerance: the role of thymic lymphocytes. Immunology 1970; 18: 723-37.

[67]   Berendt MJ, North RJ. T-cell-mediated suppression of anti-tumour immunity. An explanation for progressive growth of an immunogenic tumour. J Exp Med 1980; 151: 69-80.

[68]   Sakaguchi S, Sakaguchi N, Asano M, *et al.* Immunologic self-tolerance maintained by activated T cells expressing IL-2 receptor alpha-chains (CD25). Breakdown of a single mechanism of selftolerance causes various autoimmune diseases. J Immune 1995; 155: 1151-64.

[69]   Hori S, Nomura T, Sakaguchi S. Control of regulatory T cell development by the transcription factor Foxp3. Science 2003; 299: 1057-61.

[70]   Zou W. Regulatory T cells, tumor immunity and immunotherapy. Nature Immunol 2006; 6: 295-307.

[71]   Liston A, Rudensky AY. Thymic development and peripheral homeostasis of regulatory T cells. Curr Opin Immunol 2007; 19: 176-85.

[72]   Liu Y, Zhang P, Li J, *et al.* A critical function for TGF-beta signaling in the development of natural CD4+CD25+Foxp3+ regulatory T cells. Nat Immunol 2008; 9: 632-40.

[73]   Ke X, Wang J, Li L, *et al.* Roles of CD4+CD25 (high) FOXP3+ Tregs in lymphomas and tumors are complex. Front Biosci 2008; 13: 3986-4001.

[74]   van der Burg SH, Piersma SJ, de Jong A, *et al.* Association of cervical cancer with the presence of CD4+ regulatory T cells specific for human papillomavirus antigens. Proc Natl Acad Sci USA 2007; 104: 12087-92.

[75]   Sallusto F, Geginat J, Lanzavecchia A. Central memory and effector memory T cell subsets: function, generation, and maintenance. Annu Rev Immunol 2004; 22: 745-63.

[76]   Dudley ME, Yang JC, Sherry R, *et al.* Adoptive cell therapy for patients with metastatic melanoma: evaluation of intensive myeloablative chemoradiation preparative regimens. J Clin Oncol 2008; 26: 5233-9.

[77]   Rosenberg SA, Restifo NP, Yang JC, *et al.* Adoptive cell transfer: a clinical path to effective cancer immunotherapy. Nat Rev Cancer 2008; 8: 299-308.

[78]   Rosenberg SA, Dudley ME, Restifo NP. Cancer immunotherapy. N Engl J Med 2008; 359: 1072.

[79]   Tsuji T, Yasukawa M, Matsuzaki J, *et al.* Generation of tumor-specific, HLA class I-restricted human Th1 and Tc1 cells by cell engineering with tumor peptide-specific T-cell receptor genes. Blood 2005; 106: 470-6.

[80]   Roszkowski JJ, Lyons GE, Kast WM, *et al.* Simultaneous generation of CD8+ and CD4+ melanoma-reactive T cells by retroviral-mediated transfer of a single T-cell receptor. Cancer Res 2005; 65: 1570-6.

[81]   Stanislawski T, Voss RH, Lotz C, *et al.* Circumventing tolerance to a human MDM2-derived tumor antigen by TCR gene transfer. Nat Immunol 2001; 2: 962-70.

[82]   Alajez NM, Schmielau J, Alter MD, *et al.* Therapeutic potential of a tumor-specific, MHC-unrestricted T-cell receptor expressed on effector cells of the innate and the adaptive immune system through bone marrow transduction and immune reconstitution. Blood 2005; 105: 4583-9.

[83]   Heemskerk B, Liu K, Dudley ME, *et al.* Adoptive cell therapy for patients with melanoma, using tumor-infiltrating lymphocytes genetically engineered to secrete interleukin-2. Hum Gene Ther 2008; 19: 496-510.

[84]   Kreiter S, Selmi A, Diken M, *et al.* Increased antigen presentation efficiency by coupling antigens to MHC class I trafficking signals. J Immunol 2008; 180: 309-18.

[85]   Nicholaou T, Ebert L, Davis ID, *et al.* Directions in the immune targeting of cancer: lessons learned from the cancer-testis Ag NY-ESO-1. Immunol Cell Biol 2006; 84: 303-17.

[86]   Nussbaum AK, Kuttler CH, Tenzer S, *et al.* Using the word wide web for predicting CTL epitopes. Curr Opin Immunol 2003; 15: 69-74.

[87]   Nabeta Y, Kawaguchi Y, Sato Y, *et al.* Identification strategy and cataloguing of antigenic cancer epitopes. Mod Asp Immunobiol 2000; 1: 17-9.

[88]   Kawakami Y, Fujita T, Matsuzaki Y, *et al.* Identification of human tumor antigens and its implications for diagnosis and treatment of cancer. Cancer Sci 2004; 95: 784-91.

[89]   Melief CJ, van der Burg SH. Immunotherapy of established (pre)malignant disease by synthetic long peptide vaccines. Nat Rev Cancer 2008; 8:351-60.

[90]   Cavallo F, Forni G. Recent advances in cancer immunotherapy with an emphasis on vaccines. Expert Rev Vaccines 2009; 8: 25-8.

[91]   Kessler JH, Melief CJ. Identification of T-cell epitopes for cancer immunotherapy. Leukemia 2007; 21: 1859-74.

[92]   van Baren N, Bonnet MC, Dréno B, *et al.* Tumoral and immunologic response after vaccination of melanoma patients with an ALVAC virus encoding MAGE antigens recognized by T cells. J Clin Oncol 2005; 23:9008-21.

[93]   McConkey SJ, Reece WH, Moorthy VS, *et al.* Enhanced T-cell immunogenicity of plasmid DNA vaccines boosted by recombinant modified vaccinia virus Ankara in humans. Nat Med 2003; 9: 729-35.

[94]   Depla E, Van der Aa A, Livingston BD, *et al.* Rational design of a multiepitope vaccine encoding T-lymphocyte epitopes for treatment of chronic hepatitis B virus infections. J Virol 2008; 82: 435-50.

[95]   Durántez M, López-Vázquez AB, de Cerio ALD, *et al.* Induction of multiepitopic and long-lasting immune responses against tumor antigens by immunization with peptides, DNA and recombinant adenoviruses expressing minigenes. Scandinavian J of Immunol 2009; 69: 80-89.

[96]   Monroy GA, Hernández MJ, Mora GML. In: Mas OJ, Ed. Advances in Cancer Research at UNAM (Universidad Nacional Autónoma de México). México, Manual Moderno, UNAM y PUIS. 2007; pp. 1-32.

[97]   Paz RG, Monroy GA, Mora GML, *et al.* An HPV 16 L1-based chimeric human papilloma virus-like particles containing a string of epitopes produced in plants is able to elicit humoral and cytotoxic T-cell activity in mice. Virol J 2009; 6: 2.

[98]   O'Neill DW, Adams S, Bhardwaj N. Manipulating dendritic cell biology for the active immunotherapy of cancer. Blood 2004; 104: 2235-46.

[99]   Lanzavecchia A, Sallusto F. The instructive role of dendritic cells on T cell responses: lineages, plasticity and kinetics. Curr Opin Immunol 2001; 13: 291-8.

[100]   Stagg J, Johnstone RW, Smyth MJ. From cancer immunosurveillance to cancer immunotherapy. Immunol Rev 2007; 220: 82-101.

[101]   Matzinger P. The danger model: a renewed sense of self. Science 2002; 296: 301-5.

[102]   Fuchs EJ, Matzinger P. Is cancer dangerous to the immune system? Semin Immunol 1996; 8:271-80.

[103]   Gilboa E, Vieweg J. Cancer immunotherapy with mRNA-transfected dendritic cells. Immunol Rev 2004; 199: 251-63.

[104]   Delamarre L, Pack M, Chang H, *et al.* Differential lysosomal proteolysis in antigen-presenting cells determines antigen fate. Science *2005*; 307: 1630-34.

[105]   Delamarre L, Couture R, Mellman I, *et al.* Enhancing immunogenicity by limiting susceptibility to lysosomal proteolysis. J Exp Med 2006; 203: 2049-55.

[106]   Li G, Miles A, Line A *et al.* Identification of tumour antigens by serological analysis of cDNA expression cloning. Cancer Immunol Immunother 2004; 53: 139-43.

[107]   Chan L, Hardwick NR, Guinn BA, *et al.* An immune edited tumour versus a tumour edited immune system: prospects for immune therapy of acute myeloid leukaemia. Cancer Immunol Immunother 2006; 55: 1017-24.

[108]   Dunn GP, Ikeda H, Bruce AT, *et al.* Interferon-gamma and cancer immunoediting. Immunol Res 2005; 32: 231-45.

[109]   McLaughlin P, Grillo-Lopez AJ, Link BK, *et al.* Rituximab chimeric anti-CD20 monoclonal antibody therapy for relapsed indolent lymphoma: half of patients respond to a four-dose treatment program. J Clin Oncol 1998; 16: 2825-33.

[110]   Cohen Y, Solal-Celigny P, Pollack A. Rituximab therapy for follicular lymphoma: a comprehensive review of its efficacy as primary treatment, treatment for relapsed disease, re-treatment and maintenance. Haematologica 2003; 88: 811-23.

[111]   Coiffier B. Monoclonal antibody as therapy for malignant lymphomas. C R Biol 2006; 329:241-54.

[112]   Adams GP, Weiner, LM. Monoclonal antibody therapy of cancer. Nat Biotechnol 2005; 23: 1147-57.

[113]   Le Y, Liu S, Margolin K. Summary of the primer on tumor immunology and the biological therapy of cancer. J Translat Med 2009; 7: 11.

[114]   Lotze MT, Rosenberg SA. Results of clinical trials with the administration of interleukin 2 and adoptive immunotherapy with activated cells in patients with cancer. Immunobiol 1986; 172: 420-37.

[115] Rosenberg SA. The gene therapy of cancer. Prev Med 1994; 23: 624-6.

[116] Maker AV, Phan GQ, Attia P, *et al.* Tumor regression and autoimmunity in patients treated with cytotoxic T lymphocyte-associated antigen 4 blockade and interleukin 2: a phase I/II study. Ann Surg Oncol 2005; 12: 1005-16.

[117] Powell DJ Jr, de Vries CR, Allen T, *et al.* Inability to mediate prolonged reduction of regulatory T Cells after transfer of autologous CD25-depleted PBMC and interleukin-2 after lymphodepleting chemotherapy. J Immunother 2007; 30: 438-47.

[118] Klebanoff CA, Finkelstein SE, Surman DR, *et al.* L-15 enhances the *in vivo* antitumor activity of tumor-reactive CD8+ T cells. Proc Natl Acad Sci USA 2004; 1017: 1969-74.

[119] Hinrichs CS, Spolski R, Paulos CM, *et al.* IL-2 and IL-21 confer opposing differentiation programs to CD8+ T cells for adoptive immunotherapy. Blood 2008; 111: 5326-33.

[120] Kowalczyk A, Wierzbicki A, Gil M, *et al.* Induction of protective immune responses against NXS2 neuroblastoma challenge in mice by immunotherapy with GD2 mimotope vaccine and IL-15 and IL-21 gene delivery. Cancer Immunol Immunother 2007; 56:1443-58.

[121] Sotiriadou NN, Perez SA, Gritzapis AD, *et al.* Beneficial effect of short-term exposure of human NK cells to IL15/IL12 and IL15/IL18 on cell apoptosis and function. Cell Immunol 2005; 234: 67-75.

[122] Shevach EM. CD4+ CD25+ suppressor T cells: more questions than answers. Nature Rev Immunol 2002; 2: 389-400.

[123] Zou W. Immunosuppressive networks in the tumour environment and their therapeutic relevance. Nature Rev Cancer 2005; 5: 263-274.

[124] Shimizu J, Yamazaki S, Sakaguchi S. Induction of tumour immunity by removing CD25+CD4+ T cells: a common basis between tumour immunity and autoimmunity. J Immunol 1999; 163: 5211-8.

[125] Malek TR, Bayer AL. Tolerance, not immunity, crucially depends on IL-2. Nature Rev Immunol 2004; 4: 665-74.

[126] Hori S, Nomura T, Sakaguchi S. Control of regulatory T cell development by the transcription factor Foxp3. Science 2003; 299: 1057-61.

[127] Hodi FS, Butler M, Oble DA, *et al.* Immunologic and clinical effects of antibody blockade of cytotoxic T lymphocyte-associated antigen 4 in previously vaccinated cancer patients. Proc Natl Acad Sci USA 2008; 105: 3005-10.

[128] Tang Q, Boden EK, Henriksen KJ, *et al.* Distinct roles of CTLA-4 and TGF-b in CD4+CD25+ regulatory T cell function. Eur J Immunol 2004; 34: 2996-3005.

[129] Yamaguchi T, Hirota K, Nagahama K, *et al.* Control of immune responses by antigen-specific regulatory T cells expressing the folate receptor. Immunity 2007; 27: 145-59.

[130] Shimizu J, Yamazaki S, Takahashi T, *et al.* Stimulation of CD25+CD4+ regulatory T cells through GITR breaks immunological self-tolerance. Nature Immunol 2002; 3: 135-42.

[131] Duvic M, Talpur R. Optimizing denileukin diftitox (Ontak) therapy. Future Oncol 2008; 4: 457-69.

[132] Ruter J, Barnett BG, Kryczek I, *et al.* Altering regulatory T cell function in cancer immunotherapy: a novel means to boost the efficacy of cancer vaccines. Front Biosci 2009; 14: 1761-70.

[133] Melero I, Hervas-Stubbs S, Glennie M, *et al.* Immunostimulatory monoclonal antibodies for cancer therapy. Nat Rev Cancer 2007; 7: 95-106.

[134] Korman AJ, Peggs KS, Allison JP. Checkpoint blockade in cancer immunotherapy. Adv Immunol 2006; 90: 297-339.

[135] Quezada SA, Peggs K.S., Curran, M.A., and Allison, J.P. CTLA-4 blockade and GM-CSF combination immunotherapy alters the intratumor balance of effector and regulatory T cells. J Clin Invest 2006; 116:1935-45. doi: 10.1172/JCI27745.

[136] Fallarino F, Grohmann U, You S, *et al.* Tryptophan catabolism generates autoimmune-preventive regulatory T cells. Transpl Immunol 2006; 17: 58-60.

[137] Hodi FS, Oble DA, Drappatz J, *et al.* CTLA-4 blockade with ipilimumab induces significant clinical benefit in a female with melanoma metastases to the CNS. Nat Clin Pract Oncol 2008; 5: 557-61.

[138] Phan GQ, Weber JS, Sondak VK. CTLA-4 blockade with monoclonal antibodies in patients with metastatic cancer: surgical issues. Ann Surg Oncol 2008; 15: 3014-21.

[139] Blackburn SD, Shin H, Freeman GJ, *et al.* Wherry EJ.Selective expansion of a subset of exhausted CD8 T cells by alphaPD-L1 blockade. Proc Natl Acad Sci USA 2008; 105: 15016-21.

[140] Iwai Y, Terawaki S, Honjo T. PD-1 blockade inhibits hematogenous spread of poorly immunogenic tumor cells by enhanced recruitment of effector T cells. Int Immunol 2005; 17: 133-44.

[141] Day CL, Kaufmann DE, Kiepiela P, *et al.* PD-1 expression on HIV-specific T cells is associated with T-cell exhaustion and disease progression. Nature 2006; 443: 350-4.

[142] Trautmann L, Janbazian L, Chomont N, *et al.* Upregulation of PD-1 expression on HIV-specific CD8+ T cells leads to reversible immune dysfunction. Nat Med 2006; 12: 1198-202.

[143] Vogt L, Schmitz N, Kurrer MO, *et al.* VSIG4, a B7 family-related protein, is a negative regulator of T cell activation. J Clin Invest 2006; 116: 2817-26.

[144] Tyagi RK, Mangal S, Garg N, *et al.* RNA-based immunotherapy of cancer: role and therapeutic implications of dendritic cells. Expert Rev Anticancer Ther 2009; 9: 97-114.

[145] O'Neill DW, Bhardwaj N. Exploiting dendritic cells for active immunotherapy of cancer and chronic infections. Mol Biotechnol 2007; 36: 131-41.

[146] Wei S, Kryczek I, Zou L, *et al.* Plasmacytoid dendritic cells induce CD8+ regulatory T cells in human ovarian carcinoma. Cancer Res 2005; 65: 5020-6.

[147] Kryczek I, Wei S, Zhu G, *et al.* Relationship between B7-H4, regulatory T cells, and patient outcome in human ovarian carcinoma. Cancer Res 2007; 67: 8900-5.

[148] Müller A, Homey B, Soto H, *et al.* Involvement of chemokine receptors in breast cancer metastasis. Nature 2001; 410: 50-6.

[149] Le Bon A, Tough DF. Type I interferon as a stimulus for cross-priming. Cytokine Growth Factor Rev 2008; 19: 33-40.

[150] Persano L, Moserle L, Esposito G, *et al.* Interferon-{alpha} counteracts the angiogenic switch and reduces tumor cell proliferation in a spontaneous model of prostatic cancer. Carcinogenesis 2009.

[151] Lob S, Konigsrainer A, Schafer R, *et al.* Levo- but not dextro-1-methyl tryptophan abrogates the IDO activity of human dendritic cells. Blood 2008; 111: 2152-4.

[152] Ou X, Cai S, Liu P, *et al.* Enhancement of dendritic cell-tumor fusion vaccine potency by indoleamine-pyrrole 2,3-dioxygenase inhibitor, 1-MT. J Cancer Res Clin Oncol 2008; 134: 525-33.

[153] Bak SP, Alonso A, Turk MJ, *et al.* Murine ovarian cancer vascular leukocytes require arginase-1 activity for T cell suppression. Mol Immunol 2008; 46: 258-68.

[154] Flies DB, Chen L. The new B7s: playing a pivotal role in tumor immunity. J Immunother 2007; 30: 251-60.

[155] Wei S, Shreiner AB, Takeshita N, *et al.* Tumor-induced immune suppression of *in vivo* effector T-cell priming is mediated by the B7-H1/PD-1 axis and transforming growth factor beta. Cancer Res 2008; 68: 5432-8.

[156] Ozao-Choy J, Ma G, Kao J, *et al.* The novel role of tyrosine kinase inhibitor in the reversal of immune suppression and modulation of tumor microenvironment for immune-based cancer therapies. Cancer Res 2009; 69: 2514-22.

CHAPTER 8

In Vitro and *In Vivo* Models for Cancer Research

Julio I. Pérez Carreón* and Jorge M. Zajgla

Instituto Nacional de Medicina Genómica México (INMEGEN), Periférico Sur No. 4809, Col. Arenal Tepepan, Delegación Tlalpan. México, D.F. C.P. 14610

Abstract: Nowadays cancer kills thousands of humans around the world, so its research presents an important challenge to decrease cancer mortality. Strategies for cancer research have made great advancement in the last century, providing major insight into the complexity of tumor development. Numerous experimental protocols for many years have been performed to mimic features of cancer cells in humans; for example, to generate tumors in living organisms and study cancer in cultured cells. This chapter describes several of theses biological models: 1) chemical carcinogenesis protocols 2) genetically modified animals (transgenic and knockout mice), 3) cancer cell lines culture, 4) gene manipulation in cultured cells such as DNA transfection and RNA interference for gene knockdown and 5) the concept of cancer stem cells. The significance of *in vivo* and *in vitro* models for cancer research lies in the possibility of providing improved understanding of cancer biology and cancer treatment.

Keywords: Carcinogenesis, cell culture, transgenic mice, DNA damage, cancer stem cells, knockout mice, chemical carcinogen, cytochrome p450, metabolic activation, DNA adducts, dysplasia, solid tumors, DNA transfection, gene silencing, RNA interference.

INTRODUCTION

Interest for cancer research is sustained by the need to understand causes, mechanisms and genesis of malignant tumors and to develop methods for diagnosis, prevention and treatment of cancer patients. Although the main goal of cancer research is to reduce mortality of patients with different types of cancer, researchers have developed models that mainly are not of human origin. These experimental models use a wide variety of biological systems to mimic features of cancer cells. Experiments in cancer research are usually designed to identify chemical carcinogens, test preventive or therapeutic effect of drugs, understand cancer biology and look for biomarkers that could be used for diagnosis or as targets for therapeutic strategies. *In vivo* models are designed to study cancer in living organisms such as drosophila [1], zebrafish [2], chicken [3], monkey [4], dog [5], being the most frequently used rodents such as hamsters, rats and mice. *In vitro* models to investigate molecular aspects of cancer research are usually performed under controlled conditions impossible in the intact organism; examples include a variety of cell lines that can be cultured under different conditions. Researchers select a particular model depending on the goals and scope of the investigation and it is frequent to do comparative analyses of findings in both experimental models and human samples of cancer. Usually, models for cancer research included treatment with etiological factors associated to human cancer, such as experiments with chemical carcinogens, virus infection, genetic alteration and modification of biomolecules. Although environmental risk factors for cancer may differ between countries [6, 7], it is generally accepted that major contributors to cancer are; 1) smoking, to date 28 chemical carcinogens have been identified in tobacco being the major group N-nitrosamines [8], 2) occupational exposition to chemical carcinogens, 3) dietary imbalances such as low intake of fruits and vegetables and excessive lipids and calories 4) specific chronic infections leading to inflammation and 5) hormonal factors primarily influenced by life style.

Tumor formation in humans is a complex process that usually proceeds over many decades explaining why advanced age of patients is a frequent factor related to the incidence of cancer. Tumorigenesis in most types of tissues arise from a sequence of cellular events in which cancer is the end step, thus, the clinical oncologist often faces the final evolutive stage of multi-step tumor formation. Both *in vivo* and *in vitro* models offer to scientists a wide variety of experimental possibilities to help understand the origin of cancer, detect cancer etiological agents, characterization of

---

*Address correspondence to Julio Isael Pérez Carreón: Instituto Nacional de Medicina Genómica México (INMEGEN), Periférico Sur No. 4809, Col. Arenal Tepepan, Delegación Tlalpan. México, D.F. C.P. 14610; E-mail; jiperez@inmegen.gob.mx

tumor-biomarkers, and elucidate molecular regulation of cancer cells such as metabolic reactions and cellular signaling pathways, and the opportunity of evaluation therapeutic strategies for cancer treatment. This chapter describes the most important *in vivo* animal models used for cancer research, from classical chemical-carcinogenesis to the genetically modified animals such as transgenic and knockout mouse models, furthermore it underlines the advantages of *in vitro* models for the study of molecular regulation in cancer cells as well the concept of cancer stem cells an their application in cancer research.

IN VIVO MODELS FOR CANCER RESEARCH

The first evidence that cancer could be induced experimentally in laboratory animals was shown at the beginning of the twentieth century by Katsusaburo Yamagiwa [9]. He and his assistant, Koichi Ichikawa induced squamous cell carcinoma in rabbits-ears by painting them with crude coal tar during 250 days. Yamagiwa concluded that chronic irritation of skin could cause cancer, further investigations found diverse chemical carcinogens on coal tar extracts, mainly polycyclic aromatic hydrocarbons (PHA) responsible of skin cancer such as the widely studied benzo[a]pyrene [10].   Several chemical carcinogens such as PHA, nitrosamines in cigarette smoke, the mycotoxin aflatoxin B1, vinyl chloride and other chemicals have been recognized as cancer-causing agents in humans. Parallel to the beginning of chemical carcinogenesis as a field of study, tumor virology research was introduced by Peyton Rous, he induced sarcoma in healthy chickens using filtered cell-free sarcoma extracts [11]. This result led to discovery of the first tumor virus the Rous Sarcome Virus (RSV) and also stimulated the discovery of virus that induce tumors in humans, such as the Epstein-Barr Virus (EBV), Hepatitis B and C Virus (HBV and HCV) and Human Papillomavirus (HPV). The use of animal models in the 20th century led the discovery of cancer-etiological agents, such as chemical carcinogens and tumor viruses; moreover, they contributed to the recognition of DNA as the cellular-target for carcinogenic agents.

Chemical Carcinogenesis

A chemical carcinogen is defined as a substance that induces or increases cancer in animals or humans. Chemicals may be classified according to their origin, structure, metabolic activation and/or mechanism of action on cells. Substances that depend on metabolic activation to be carcinogenic may be defined as indirect, while substances that act themselves as carcinogens are defined as direct.   Most chemical carcinogens with genotoxic activity are not themselves active but instead require bioactivation to form electrophilic molecules that could bind covalently to DNA forming adducts [12]. Metabolic activation is executed mainly by a group of proteins that conform the cytochrome P450 (Cyp450) family, these enzymes uses oxygen and NADPH as electron source to activate through hydroxylation a wide number of endo- and exo-biotic molecules. Cyp450 enzymes are involved in phase I of xenobiotic detoxification and recent research have shown the importance of variations (single nucleotide polymorphisms) in genes of this group that confers the susceptibility or resistance to carcinogens, drugs and endogenous chemicals [13]. A genotoxic carcinogen is often named cancer-initiating agent because of its capability to induce cellular mutations, therefore a cell with irreversible DNA damage is termed initiated cell and it is believed to be the origin of a malignant tumor (Fig. **1**). Cell mutations can happen in the genome by inadequate removal of DNA adducts (deficient DNA repair) or by increased DNA replicative rate, since each round of cell cycle creates the possibility of genome alterations.

Other important groups of chemicals that induce tumor with a non-genotoxic mechanism are tumor-promoting carcinogens; they induce tumor development without directly interacting with DNA. Promoter substances share the ability to induce clonal expansion of initiated cells that yield large population of altered cells seen in precancerous lesions. Non-genotoxic mechanisms of carcinogenesis are more heterogeneous than the genotoxic mechanism; in general tumor-promoting carcinogens induce cellular proliferation in specific organs [14]. These substances can induce cellular proliferation by a diversity of mechanisms; 1) chronic cell injury and tissue regeneration, 2) growth factor receptors activation, 3) signal transduction pathways perturbation, 4) cell survival promotion by increased secretion of trophic hormones, 5) cellular stress induction by overproduction of reactive oxygen species, 6) immunosuppression, and 7) metabolic activation of carcinogens by Cyp450 enzymes.

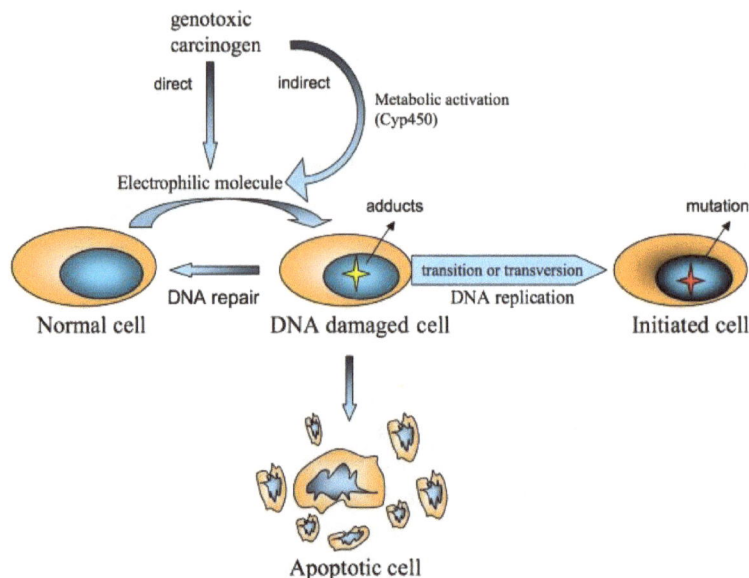

Figure 1: Mechanism of action of genotoxic carcinogens. Chemical carcinogens may directly or indirectly (metabolic activation) be converted to electrophilic molecules that interact with DNA. Depending of the cell injury level (formation of DNA-adducts), different ways of cellular response may occur; with low damage level, cells can be reverted to a normal by DNA repair, with excessive damage, cells can undergo programmed cell death, however, under cellular replicative pressure, damaged DNA allows cell mutation, thus initiated cells carry permanent and heritable DNA changes that may predispose to cancer development.

Initiating and promoting carcinogens act cooperatively to induce tumors; however, the order of exposition of these substances to experimental animals is a relevant factor that influences success for cancer induction. A single exposition to a carcinogen would be not enough for cancer induction in animals, but when genetic damage by an initiating carcinogen is followed by cellular proliferation induced by promoting agents, a large population of genetically altered cells will be formed (Fig. **2**). The cluster of mutated cells induced experimentally in animals form a lesion that seems to be comparable to the preneoplastic lesions found in human patients, such as papillomas, nodules and polyps. Some carcinogenic agents named complete carcinogens individually induce tumors after repeated applications; they include both initiating and promoting activities, but the strength of carcinogenicity will depend of balance between genotoxic potential and cell proliferation inducing activities. Furthermore, there are many chemicals termed co-carcinogens that are not themselves carcinogens but can enhance carcinogenic potential of initiating or promoting agents. These substances can stimulate metabolic activation of carcinogens through increase Cyp450 activities, or block activities of the enzymes responsible for carcinogen detoxification such as phase II detoxification enzymes. Other chemicals that can interfere with carcinogens are cancer chemopreventive substances, these are able to inhibit, delay or reverse carcinogenesis though a wide of cellular mechanism. Among chemopreventive substances are some micronutrients of food that can modulate carcinogen metabolism and their genotoxic or tumor-promoting effects. Some chemopreventive substances contain antioxidant properties; therefore they can improve cellular response to oxidative stress induced during carcinogenesis [15].

Because several types of human cancer are likely associated with chemical carcinogens from synthetic or natural origin the identification of new carcinogens continues as an important field for life sciences. Animal models in association with epidemiological observations, have allowed identification of hundreds of potential chemical carcinogens to humans. During the past 6 decades, animal cancer tests mainly in mice and rats have been done to identify hazardous chemicals to human. The Carcinogenic Potency Database (CPDB) http://potency.berkeley.edu/ is an important database that systematically unifies and analyzes published reports of chronic long-term chemical expositions on animal. This database includes results of carcinogenicity for more than 1485 natural and synthetic chemicals of which 751 (52 %) were reported with positive carcinogenic effect [16, 17]. Other important organization, the International Agency for Research on Cancer (IARC) http://www.iarc.fr/en/, is dedicated to the identification of causes of cancer through evaluation of epidemiological and experimental data. This organism has published monographs containing a complete list of agents, mixtures and exposures, that have been evaluated and classified to provide a source of information which reflect cancer risk to humans [18].

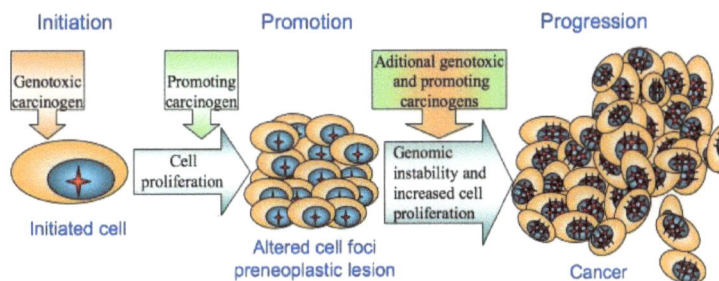

Figure 2: Mechanism of chemical carcinogenesis. The three stages of carcinogenesis; initiation, promotion and progression. The genotoxic carcinogen produces initiated cells with a mutant genotype, during promotion these cells can be stimulated to proliferate by tumor promoting carcinogens to form clusters of initiated cells, the formed lesion is predisposed to progress into a cancer, but, additional exposition to genotoxic and tumor promoting substances accelerates progression stage by increasing genomic instability and cell proliferation rate to convert a preneoplastic lesion into cancer.

Bioassays with laboratory animals such as rats and mice continue the most practical experimental procedure to study and identify chemical carcinogens. Although there are long-term carcinogenesis procedures that induce advanced carcinomas, for carcinogenicity testing purposes, models of cancer are frequently used as medium-term assays in which preneoplastic lesions such as papillomas in the skin, altered hepatocyte nodules in liver and polyps in colon are used as endpoint markers for determining quantitatively carcinogenic potential. Although mice models are useful for carcinogenicity studies, selection of host, susceptible or resistant animal strain, plays an important role for carcinogenicity evaluation and interpreting chemopreventive effect of substances in carcinogenesis studies [19] There is wide variety of available experimental models to induce organ specific cancer, and the most frequently assays in rodent are described in Table **1**.

Mouse Skin Tumor Assay

The widely used mouse skin tumor assay has allowed the understanding that cancer development is a multi-step process that at least includes three stages; initiation, promotion and progression (Fig. **2**). Initiation involves genetic changes by chemical genotoxic agents, for example, polycyclic aromatic hydrocarbons and alkylating agents such as N-nitrosamines. Tumor promoter substances such as esters of phorbol induce specific expansion of initiated skin cells to form visible premalignant lesions termed papillomas. The last stage involves progression of papillomas to malignant squamous cell carcinomas. Two positives markers for skin tumor progression are appearance of Gamma-Glutamyl Transpeptidase (GGT) and keratin 13, while negative markers are lack of expression of keratins 1 and 10 [21]. Progression of squamous cell carcinomas is characterized by cumulative chromosomal abnormalities including aneuploidies and trisomies of chromosomes 6 and 7. A frequent target gene of mutagens to skin cells is the oncogene *Hras1* [20]. Mutation of *Hras1* produces activation of the Epidermal Growth Factor Receptor (EGFR) and upregulation of the *fos* gene, thus AP-1 transcriptional activity has been associated with tumor malignant progression [22].

Induction of Oral Cavity Tumors

Oral tumors can be induced in rodents such as rats, mice and Syrian hamster by exposition to chemical carcinogens. These animal models intend to provide research tools for understanding development of human oral cancer. The protocol most frequently used is the 4-nitroquinoline N-oxide (4NQO) carcinogenesis model [25]. Animals are chronically exposed to this complete carcinogen in drinking water for 8 weeks or it can be directly applied by painting on specific region of oral cavity. This model is frequently used to evaluate anticarcinogenic effects of cancer chemopreventive substances [24]. Inflammation and lesions of oral cavity such as hyperkeratosis is produced after 4 weeks, preneoplastic lesions such as dysplastic hyperplasia or leukoplakias after 6 weeks and squamous cell carcinomas after 8 weeks. Although oral tumor is developed as a multistage process, the time-course of preneoplastic lesion development varies widely among experimental reports [25]. Other oral cavity tumor models resemble the initiation-promotion model used in skin tumor assays [26]; equally, initiation stage is performed by a single application of dimethylbenz(a)anthracene in SENCAR mice, the initiated cells can then be clonally expanded by chronic treatment with the promoter 12-O-tetradecanoylphorbol-13-acetate (TPA) [23]. Efficacy of this model to produce preneoplastic and malignant oral cavity lesions is comparable to the 4NQO carcinogenesis model.

Table 1: Organ-specific experimental models of chemical carcinogenesis in rodents

Target organ	Type of model	Initiator	Promoter	Neoplastic lesions	References
Skin	Initiation-promotion and multi-stage in mice	Polycyclic aromatic hydrocarbons; 7,12-Dimethylbenz(a)anthracene, Benzo[a]pyrene and N-nitrosamines	Ester of phorbol; 12-O-tetradecanoylphorbol-13-acetate (TPA)	squamous papillomas and carcinomas	[20-22]
Oral cavity	Chronic exposure and initiation-promotion in hamster, rats and mice	4-nitroquinoline N-oxide Dimethylbenz(a)anthracene	Benzoyl peroxide TPA	leukoplakias and Oral Squamous cell carcinomas	[23-26]
Stomach	Intermittent chronic exposure in rats and chemical initiation plus bacterial infection in Gerbil	Benzo[a]pyrene and N-Methyl-N'-Nitro-N-Nitrosoguanidine (MNNG) N-methyl-N-nitrosourea	Helicobacter pylori	Hyperplastic pyloric mucosa and adenocarcinomas	[27, 28]
Colon	Intermittent chronic exposure in rats and genetically altered APC Min Mice.	2-Amino-1-methyl-6-phenylimidazo[4,5-b]pyridine (PhIP), azoxymethane, 1,2-dimethylhydrazine		Aberrant crypt foci, colon polyps and colon carcinoma	[29-32]
Liver	Chronic exposition, initiation-promotion-progression and nutrients deficiency in rats	Aflatoxin B1, N-nitrosamines, N-diethylnitrosamine, nitrosomorpholine, 2-acetylaminofluorene pyridines	Phenobarbital, 2-acetylamino-fluorene	Altered hepatocyte foci, dysplastic nodules of hepatocytes and hepatocellular carcinoma	[33-36]
Lung	Intermittent chronic exposure in strain A mice.	Polycyclic aromatic hydrocarbons, nitrosamines, nitrosoureas, carbamates, aflatoxins, cigarette smoke 4-nitroquinoline N-oxide		Hyperplastic lesions, adenomas and carcinomas	[37-39]
Kidney	Initiation-promotion protocols in rats	N-nitrosomorpholine N-ethyl-N-hydroxyethylnitrosamine	Diphenylthiazole beta-cyclodextrin DL-serine basic lead acetate	Solid and Cystic adenomatous hyperplasias	[40, 41]

Induction of Stomach Tumors

Epidemiological studies of patients with gastric cancer have found that infection with *Helicobacter pylori* (*H. pylori*) is a definite biological stomach carcinogen. Stomach or gastric cancer can be induced experimentally in rodent models by chronic administration of genotoxic carcinogens such as N-methyl-N'-nitro-N-nitrosoguanidine (MNNG) and N-methyl-N-nitrosourea (MNU). Considering epidemiological data concerning *H. pylori* infection in etiology of gastric cancer Shimizu *et al.* performed a model that included *H. pylori* infection and chemical carcinogen treatment in Mongolian gerbils [42]. This model is generated by an initial treatment with MNNG for 10 weeks followed by inoculation with *H.pylori*. Those animals killed at week 50 developed adenocarcinomas in stomach [27]. Importantly, animals infected with *H. pylori* without chemical carcinogen treatment did not developed tumors, thus

H. pylori itself only causes chronic inflammation and acts as a promoter of stomach carcinogenesis in experimental models [28].

Induction of Tumors in Colon

There are two main rodent models for colon carcinogenesis, chemical carcinogenesis with azoxymethane and 1,2-dimethylhydrazine in rats and the APCMIN mice in which animals carrying a mutation in APC gene develop intestinal tumors spontaneously without need of carcinogen administration [30]. The preneoplastic lesion induced in both models corresponded to Aberrant Crypt Foci (ACF), these lesions can be quantitatively measured in short-term assays, thus animal models are frequently used as carcinogenicity test of xenobiotics, as well for study of chemopreventive efficacy of natural and synthetic compounds [29]. In long-term assays animals develop colon carcinomas [31]. This type of experimental induced lesion shows histological similarities to human colon cancer [32]. Histopathology of clinical cases in colon, has provided evidence of pretumoral lesions such as ACF and polyps that supports the concept of multistep tumor progression [43].

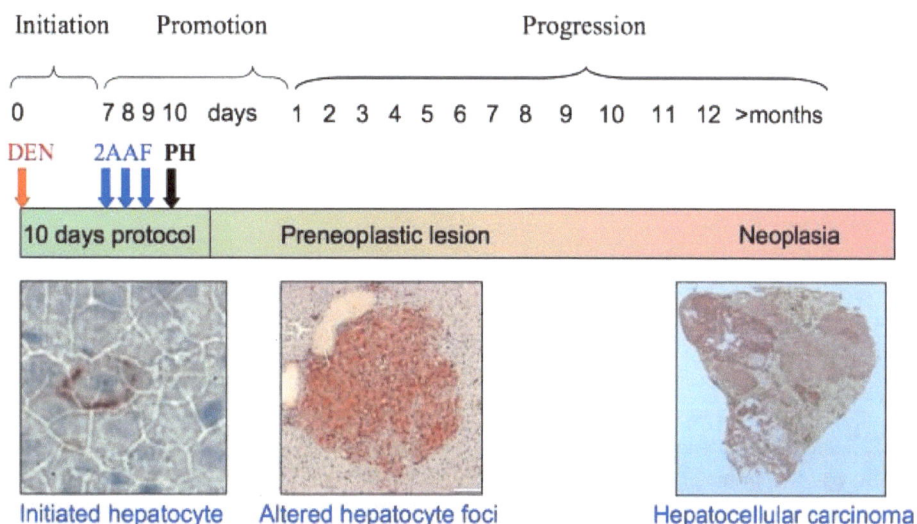

Figure 3: Lesions induced by chemical carcinogens in rat liver. A 10 day protocol to generate the resistant hepatocyte model was used; 1) initiated hepatocytes are induced by Diethylnitrosamine (DEN) treatment, 2) altered hepatocyte foci are promoted by 2-acetylaminofluorene (2AAF) treatment and a 70% Partial Hepatectomy (PH), 3) some preneoplastic lesions spontaneously progress to hepatocellular carcinoma after 9-12 months of initiating-promoting induction. Red color in the hepatic lesions corresponds to histological activity of the tumor marker Gamma Glutamyl Transpeptidase (GGT).

Rodent Models for Liver Cancer

Liver carcinogenesis models together with the mouse skin tumor assay have contributed to the concept of multistage carcinogenesis. One important feature in experimental liver carcinogenesis, either short- or long- term assays, is the great potential for metabolic activation of chemical carcinogens in this tissue. Carcinogenic hazard of chemicals that depend of metabolic activation can then be tested in liver models. Liver cells contain the broadest diversity of enzymes involved in xenobiotic metabolism including phase I detoxification enzymes such as Cyp450 members [44]. Other important feature of liver carcinogenesis is the possibility of early detection of carcinogen-induced lesions, from initiated hepatocytes to hepatocellular carcinomas, including intermediary preneoplastic lesions such as Altered Hepatocyte Foci (AHF) and hepatocyte dysplastic nodules (Fig. **3**). These hepatic lesions can be quantitatively measured after histological detection of enzymes abnormally overexpressed such as Gluthatione S-Transferase Pi (GSTP), Gamma Glutamyl Transpeptidase (GGT) and Glucose 6-Phosphate Dehydrogenase (G6PD). Due to the high potential of metabolic activation of carcinogens by liver, cancer of this organ, specifically hepatocellular carcinoma (HCC), can be induced with the most extensive variety of chemical carcinogens (> 220 substances in both rat and mouse) [17]. The most frequently carcinogen used in animal models is Diethylnitrosamine (DEN) which has demonstrated a strong genotoxic potential to hepatocytes [45], other liver carcinogens are N-nitrosomorpholine, aflatoxin B1, phenobarbital and 2-Acetylaminofluorene (2AAF). There are three types of models for chemical hepatocarcinogenesis in rats; 1) use of a single agent that must be a complete carcinogen by repeated administration or chronic exposure to animals, 2) use of more than 2 agents in initiation-promotion-progression protocols and 3) dietary methyl group deficiency, animals are fed with a diet lacking of methyl-group sources such as choline or methionine or folates develop liver cancer without added chemical carcinogens [34, 46]. For study of multistage carcinogenesis of liver; the Chronic Enzyme Induction (CEI) model [47] and the resistant hepatocyte (Solt & Farber) model [48] are the most studied. In the CEI model, AHFs are induced during carcinogen treatment by two steps; initiation with a genotoxic carcinogen such as DEN and promotion by chronically treatment with non-genotoxic agents such as the commonly used phenobarbital [33]. In the Solt & Farber model, preneoplastic lesions such as hepatocyte nodules are rapidly developed in synchrony, thus the main operational advantage of this model is the possibility to study sequential tumor development with a clear distinction of the three-stages of carcinogenesis. We have studied an alternative Solt & Farber model in which tumor induction was performed in a ten-day protocol (Fig. **3**), instead of 4 weeks in the original Solt & Farber model. This protocol induces Efficiently Hepatocellular Carcinomas (HCC) in liver by treatments with DEN, 2AAF and 70% Partial Hepatectomy (PH) to the rats [35, 49]. In early steps, the AHF and nodular lesions appear 4 weeks after initial induction; when one carcinogen is omitted the development of nodules does not occur [50]. Nodule induction is based in the two step initiation-promotion theory in which the DEN-initiated cells with a resistant phenotype are able to proliferate under a selective promotion provoked by the 2AAF/PH treatment. The histological phenotype of AHF and nodule developing using the Solt & Farber protocol has revealed striking similarities in experimental and human hepatocarcinogenesis. Consequently, nodular hepatocyte lesions, preceding HCC, represent the most prevalent form of hepatic preneoplasia observed in animals and humans [51].

Induction of Tumors in Lung

A frequent model for lung carcinogenesis studies in experimental animals is the lung cancer-susceptible strain A mice [37]. Although these animals develop lung tumors spontaneously during their lifetime, chemical carcinogens with epidemiological association to human lung cancer have shown to enhance tumor induction [39]. Classes of chemical that are strongly positive to this model are cigarette smoke compounds such as nitrosamines, nitrosoureas, hydrazines and polycyclic aromatic hydrocarbons [52]. Experimental induction of tumors in mice is performed by repeated intraperitoneal injections of a carcinogen. Depending on the time of tumor progression sacrificed animals exhibit hyperplastic lesions, lung adenomas and/or carcinomas. In addition to carcinogenicity testing of chemical substances on strain A mice, this model is commonly used for chemopreventive evaluation of carcinogenesis-inhibitors. Another model is the lung tumor induction with the carcinogen 4NQO to ICR mice, furthermore in this model it was shown that certain factors such as high fat diet [53], inhalation of sodium chloride mist [54] and Iron [55] enhances tumorigenesis in mice.

Induction of Tumors in Kidney

Renal tumors can be induced in rats subjected to chemical carcinogenesis protocols by administration of a combined treatment with N-nitrosomorpholine (NNM) and Diphenylthiazole (DPT) to rats; in this model cystic adenomatous lesions resemble microscopically renal cancer lesions in humans [40]. The protocol consists on chronic treatment with DPT from 39 to 48 weeks and NNM administration from week 4 to 7 after initial treatment with DPT; treatment with only one substance does not induce tumors. Another model induces renal adenomatous hyperplasias in rats and it has been performed as a protocol for tumor-promoter testing [41]. This includes dietary administration of N-ethyl-N-hydroxyethylnitrosamine for 2 weeks followed by unilateral nephrectomy at week 3 and treatment during 18 weeks with tumor promoting agents such as beta-cyclodextrin, DL-serine, basic lead acetate, trisodium nitrilotriacetate monohydrate and potassium bromate. This renal carcinogenesis model can be performed in a 20 weeks experiment.

Genetically Modified Animals: Transgenic and Knockout Mice Models

Research of molecular mechanism of tumor virology and the identification of gene-targets of chemical carcinogens, have allowed the discovery of certain genes (oncogenes) that can transform a normal cell into a cancer cell. In a normal cell condition, these genes, named proto-oncogenes, participate in biochemical pathways that communicate growth-stimulatory signals from extracellular space to a gene expression response resulting in cellular proliferation. Proto-oncogenes can be activated to oncogenes through genomic changes such as structural chromosome rearrangements including translocations, deletions and insertions, viral genome insertions that may result in gene amplification, and point mutations. These events can lead to a cellular behavior that results in neoplastic development. Overexpression or activation of oncogenes results in a mitogenic response through activation of cellular signal transduction pathways involved in cellular growth, differentiation, apoptosis, adhesion and migration. In addition to oncogenes, other genes relevant to cancer are tumor suppressor genes, these in contrast to oncogenes, limit cell proliferation and may induce apoptosis (cell death), thus, genetic changes can cause inactivation of tumor suppressor genes in cancer cells. Because both alleles of tumor suppressor genes must be inactivated for loss of their functions, Loss of Heterozygosity (LOH) in chromosomical region of tumor suppressor genes represents a relevant genotypic change that allows the development of a tumor.

Cellular functional roles of oncogenes and tumor suppressor genes have been successfully studied in genetically modified mice. Mouse models are generated by random or targeted integration of foreign DNA to mouse blastocyst (an early-stage embryo), DNA insertion to genome is done *via* homologous recombination resulting in a mouse germ line carrying a new DNA sequence, thus enabling the transmission of foreign DNA fragment to their descendents. A transgenic mouse is generated when the integrated DNA sequence is designed to be over-expressed. If the new DNA sequence corresponds to a deleted or inactive form of a gene a knockout mouse is produced. A constitutive inactivation of certain genes could be developmentally lethal and mouse embryos may die before birth. In this case and alternative is the generation of conditional knockout mice, in which the target gene inactivation is organ-specific or condition-specific.

 Cancer occurrence in mice under normal conditions is rare, hence, engineering specific cancer-inductor gene such as oncogene overexpression in transgenic mice and inactivation of tumor suppressor genes in knockout mice is an attractive method for studying molecular details of tumor development in an *in vivo* controlled environment. *In vivo* models allow research of tumor formation under physiological environment that include multicellular interaction in tissues, presence of endocrinous growth factors and inhibitors, and intact immune response. The first transgenic mouse that spontaneously developed tumors (termed oncomice) in brain and thymus, overexpressed the T-large antigen of the simian virus 40 (SV40) [56]. After this model several oncogenes were dominantly overexpressed in mice to produce cancer in different organs and tissues; endothelial cell tumors by polyoma virus middle T oncogene [57], lymphoid malignancy by *c-myc* oncogene [58], pancreatic neoplasia by *Ras* [59], mammary adenocarcinoma by *c-neu* [60], *c-Src* [61] and *AIB1* oncogenes [62] and bone tumors by *c-fos* [63]. Efficacy for tumor induction was determined by the capacity of a tissue specific promoter that drives oncogene expression. Because some researchers using a single oncogene transgenic mouse failed to induce tumors or tumor induction occurred with low efficiency, efforts have been made to increase dominant expression of oncogenes as crossing two transgenic strains produced double transgenic hybrids. These mice show enhanced oncogenic action with accelerated tumor development, thus, it is suggested that oncogenes could act cooperatively to induce cancer [64, 65].

Alternatively to the transgenic mice that overexpress oncogenes, the use of genetic germline engineering in mice to inactivate targeted genes has created a variety of animal models that encourage the study of tumor suppressor genes. The main example is the p53 deficient (-/-) mouse, which is viable and develops tumors rapidly (average of 4.5 months) when compared to heterozygous p53 (+/-) [66]. The knockout p53 mouse resembles the human Li-Fraumeni syndrome that increases susceptibility to cancer. The tumor suppressor gene p53 encodes a transcription factor protein involved in multiple cellular mechanisms; DNA repair, growth control through regulation of G1/S point of cell cycle and induction apoptosis. Thus, p53 plays a major role to preserve genome integrity, protection of cells from DNA damage and preventing neoplastic transformation [67]. The p53 mutations that produce functional inactivation have been detected in 50% of human tumors [68] demonstrating that loss of p53 activity is a frequent event in tumor development. Although more than 100 tumor suppressor genes have been described in cancer research [69], p53 and Retinoblastoma protein (Rb) remain as tumor suppressor genes that are of great importance in carcinogenesis [70]. Rb protein is closely associated to regulation of cell cycle progression; the hypophosphorylated state of Rb retains cells in G1 phase of cell cycle through interaction and inhibition of transcription factors such as E2F family, when Rb is phosphorylated as a consequence of growth factor stimulatory signals it releases the transcription factor E2F and the cell cycle can progress. Deregulation of the Rb pathway is frequent in human tumors [71]. Animal models for cancer research have been created in order to examine the role of Rb in tumorigenesis, due to its important function in cell cycle and cellular differentiation, the Rb knockout mice (homozygous disrupted gene) were nonviable because embryonic development was affected [72]. Interestingly the heterozygous deficient Rb mouse developed spontaneous adenocarcinomas in pituitary [73]. As expected a double knockout mouse, a combination of p53 deficiency with Rb heterozygosity, clearly predisposed the mice to acceleration of tumorigenesis, mainly the development of endocrine tumor types. Inactivation of both tumor suppressor genes p53 and Rb do cooperate in tumorigenesis [74].

Some genetically modified mice exhibit an increased susceptibility to chemical carcinogen-induced cancer, for example, lymphoma is induced by N-ethyl-N-nitrosourea (ENU) in pim-1 transgenic mice [75], urinary bladder carcinomas are induced by *p*-cresidine treatment in three lines of transgenic mice which express the v-Ha-*ras*, *c-myc,* or c-*neu* oncogenes [76]. The same transgenic mice lines exposed to the carcinogen reserpine can induce mammary gland adenocarcinomas. Also, potency of chemical hepatocarcinogens such as thioacetamide and N-OH acetylaminofluorene is increased for liver tumor formation in transgenic mice with high production of hepatic TGF-beta 1[77]. Considering this evidence, the potential use of transgenic mice has been proposed as a carcinogenicity test assay for identifying human chemical carcinogens [78]. Transgenic and knockout mice may offer advantages in shortening the time required for cancer bioassays and improving the accuracy of carcinogen identification; genotoxic and non-genotoxic carcinogens can be identified with increased sensitivity and specificity using diversity of genetically modified mice, for example, hemizygous p53$^{+/-}$ mice in which one allele of the p53 gene has been inactivated, the XPA$^{-/-}$ knockout mouse model in which both alleles of a nucleotide excision repair gene are absent, also the double knockout mice model XPA$^{-/-}$/p53$^{+/-}$ is also frequently used [78]. Moreover, the Tg.rasH2 transgenic mouse model which contain inserted multiple copies of human C-Ha-ras gene and the Tg.AC transgenic mouse model, carrying multiple copies of v-Ha-ras oncogen with a promoter of zeta-globulin, have developed malignant tumors in response to a number of genotoxic carcinogens and tumor promoters, but not to non-carcinogens chemicals [79].

The research focused on the use of genetically engineered mouse models of cancer is a still-growing field, with a clear objective to study mechanisms by which tumors develop in different organs, and to elucidate the roles of specific oncogenes and tumor suppressors. The Mouse Tumor Biology (MTB) database http://tumor.informatics.jax.org/mtbwi/index.do is an important list that systematically collects data concerning mice tumorigenesis and their genetic background. This database is the most extensive resource of mouse tumor pathobiology data currently available on the web; it includes mouse strains, transgenic and knockout mice, genes and mutations, tumor types, organs/tissues or cell types of tumor origin, pathology images, and references [80, 81].

IN VITRO MODELS FOR CANCER RESEARCH

For decades, culture of animal and human cells has been used as an important tool for cell biology, virology and cancer research. The growth, under laboratory conditions, of explants taken directly from an organ or tissue such as biopsy material is known as primary cell culture. Commonly, the primary culture contains a diversity of cell types with different properties to survive and proliferate under culture conditions. Most primary cell cultures from non-altered organs have limited lifespan, after certain number of cell divisions primary cells undergo senescence and stop cellular proliferation. In contrast some cultures derived from tumors of animal models and human patients are able to proliferate and multiply *in vitro*. Culture conditions vary widely for each cell type, frequently for mammalian cells, cell-incubators provide an appropriate temperature and gas composition (37 °C, 5% CO_2 content in air). The most interestingly factor for cell culture is the growth media, there is a diversity of cell-culture media; variations can be performed in their composition in relation to pH, biomolecules such as amino acids, nucleotides, glucose and growth factors. Culture media modification in *in vitro* models can be used to generate a vast number of experimental conditions, for example, addition of chemical carcinogens and/or drugs for *in vitro* testing. Cells can be grown in suspension or attached to specific surfaces forming cell monolayer cultures in two-dimension system, typically surface platforms are tissue culture-plastic or surfaces with extracellular matrix components such as collagen, fibronectin among others fibrous components. However, monolayer or suspension cultures have been subject to criticism because assays still reflect a highly artificial cellular environment that may not correspond to a tissue or organ situation, for example, a multicellular solid tumor. An *in vitro* alternative for cell culture mainly for immortalized cell lines is the three dimensional culture systems in which the multicellular tumor spheroid model is frequently used (Fig. **4**), this type of *in vitro* model has been considered as an intermediate complexity system between *in vivo* tumors and monolayer cultures [82].

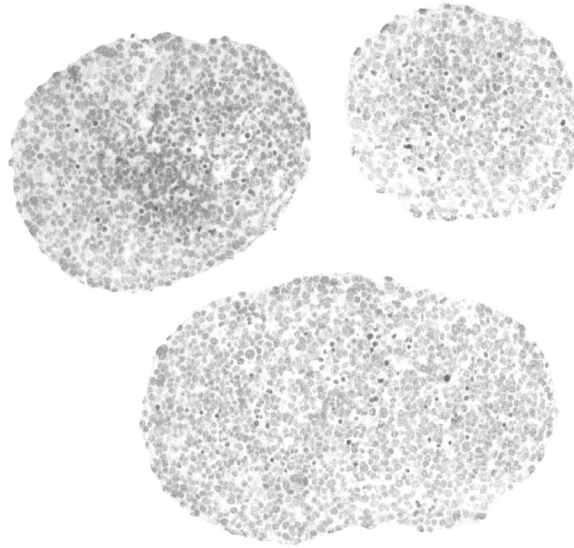

Figure 4: Section (5 μm) of 3 tumor spheroids formed by culturing HEK 293 cells. Courtesy of Magali Espinosa.

Immortal and Immortalized Cancer Cell Lines

Human and animal immortal cancer cell lines constitute an accessible set of biological models for cancer research. To produce a cancer cell line, cells are divided directly from tumor biopsies and placed into *in-vitro* culture conditions. If there is a successful culture, highly proliferating colonies of carcinoma cells population will emerge and propagate in culture dish. Most of cancer cell lines show an ability to grow autonomously with independence of stromal and extracellular matrix support, thus, immortal cancer cell lines are a selected subset of an advanced progression stage of tumor in which cell have acquired independence to survive and proliferate without stromal support. Some properties of cancer cell lines are; 1) ability to proliferate indefinitely, 2) anchorage independence, 3) loss of contact inhibition from other cells, 4) reduced requirements for mitogenic growth factors, 5) ability to generate high cellular density cultures, 6) high incorporation of glucose, 7) altered cellular morphology and 8) tumorigenicity in immunocompromised host mice. When cancer cell lines are implanted into nude mice lacking a functional immune system, they are able to proliferate and form tumors; this model is known as tumor xenografts experiment. However, cancer cell lines have been subject to criticism because they may represent selected clones adapted to an *in vitro* culture condition that are not representative of tumor origin. These clones acquire additional genetic abnormalities to be able to continue to grow *in vitro*. Furthermore, certain cancer cell lines are known to be contaminated by other cell lines and thus the origin of a cancer cell line is unclear. Even though, cancer cell lines are widely used in many biomedical research laboratories, when these cells are cultured under the right conditions, and by using the appropriate controls, several experiments may be performed [83]. Cancer cell lines are frequently used as *in vitro* model because they provide opportunities of genetic manipulation of cultured cells. Overexpression of specific genes such as oncogenes can be performed through DNA transfection studies; other example of genetic manipulation available in *in-vitro* models is gene knockdown that can be performed for example by using small interfering RNA [84]. Manipulation of gene expression, structure of proteins and genome integrity through molecular biology tools is highly accessible in cell culture and may provide important data with phenotypical association to human cancer.

Another approach, which has been shown to be of particular interest in the study of cancer progression, is the production of immortalized cell lines derived from healthy animal or human tissues. In this approach, transformed but not cancerous cells are produced by the introduction of the telomerase gene or viral genes to avoid senescence and apoptosis. Most of the protocols involve the transfection of the large T-antigen of SV40 or the E6/E7 genes of HPV. These viral proteins interfere with the p53 and Rb signaling cascades, resulting in an immortal phenotype that can be converted to full-blown cancerous phenotype with the introduction of additional oncogenes. Two of the advantages of this approach are the production of a more homogenous cell population and the possibility of assessing the participation of specific gene products in a temporal course that reflects more accurately the *in vivo* multi-step carcinogenic process.

Gene Overexpression Studies

One of the key advances of modern molecular biology is the possibility to introduce foreign DNA in cells to study the functions of genes and their products. Usually, a strong viral promoter is fused to the cDNA for the gene of interest with or without additional tag sequences and introduced into suitable cells. This can be accomplished by introducing naked DNA (transfection) or DNA packed in viral particles (infection). Transfection is an experimental procedure in which macromolecules such as DNA are incorporated into cells by chemical or biophysical methods. For introducing such molecules into cells, transient pores in the cell plasma membrane must be formed to allow the uptake and delivery of genetic material. Permeabilization of plasma membrane to these molecules can be induced by electroporation [85], using calcium phosphate [86], cationic lipid [87], ultrasound [88] and laser based methodologies [89]. Once foreign DNA has been introduced into cells, genes can be expressed in two types of modalities; 1) transient transfection which provide advantage due to fast expression of genes and transitory protein production and 2) stable transfection that ensures long-term, stable and defined gene and protein expression. For stable transfection, the introduced DNA must be incorporated into chromosomes or cellular genome. The type of vector used for stable transfection defines the integration efficiency, regulation of transgene expression and the selection conditions such as co-expression resistance towards a certain toxin. Gene transfection experiments in cultured cells have made possible to detect oncogenes in the DNA of various human tumor cells [90, 91]. Since a great part of oncogenes sequences have been cloned, their functional role can be explored in cultured cells; thus, signal transduction pathways can be explored when oncogenic members of cellular signaling are overexpressed in cells. Thus, the experimental option to integrate foreign genes into the genome of cells and their overexpression allows possibilities to analyze molecular events associated to neoplastic behavior of cells. The second approach is to pack the DNA of interest into viral particles, most commonly into adeno, retro or lentiviral systems. Due to safety concerns, the viral particles are packaged in permissive cells and are replication-deficient. The advantages of this approach are the ultimate efficiency of gene transduction, the higher reproducibility of the assays, the possible use in *in vivo* models and the possibility of transduce hard-to-transfect cells. The disadvantages are the higher cost and time needed to produce the viral particles, in addition to the obvious safety concerns.

Gene Knockdown by Small Interfering RNA

In vitro cell culture is a suitable model for depleting gene expression rate of specific genes through gene knockdown methodologies; one of the alternatives for gene silencing is RNA interference (RNAi) through the use of small interfering RNA (siRNA) technology. Natural siRNAs are short double strand RNA molecules (19 to 24 nucleotides) that are produced in a variety of organism; they interfere with the expression of specific genes as an intrinsic mechanism of transcript regulation. RNAi hybridize with target mRNA and block translation; alternatively RNAi may trigger the degradation of complementary mRNA, thus, production of an encoded protein is prevented. Furthermore, siRNA plays important roles in regulating cellular genome integrity through interference of viral genomes and transposon expression [92]. For gene expression manipulation purposes siRNA can be synthesized through molecular design against a specific mRNA [93], the outcome after siRNA transfection into cultured cells is the reduction or abolishment of gene expression. Similarly to transgenic overexpression, using appropriate plasmid vectors let perform stable transfection for siRNA [94]. In addition to the gene-silencing activity of siRNA and its potency for inactivate genes such as oncogenes or tumor suppressor genes for cancer research, the use of RNAi has created important expectations for the development of new target-specific anticancer drugs [95].

Cancer Stem Cells

A common characteristic of human solid tumors is the great heterogeneity among cellular types as well as histological and biological diversity, features of neoplastic cells. Cancer Stem Cells (CSC) are a tiny subpopulation of neoplastic cells that share several features when compared to normal stem cells such as cellular self-renewal and differentiation. An important feature of CSC is their high tumorigenic potential through derivation of neoplastic cells that form the bulk of the tumor. Thus, it has been proposed that CSC could be the cellular source of each tumor [96]. Other important characteristic of CSC is that they constitute a tumor reservoir with the capacity to regenerate or regrowth a tumor following unsuccessful treatment by tumor resection, chemotherapy or radiation, equal importance has been considered for the establishment of metastases [97]. Other feature of CSC is a phenotypical resistance not only to drugs but also to cellular insults such as oxidative stress; this has been associated to the high expression of multiple drug resistance transporter genes (ABC gene family) [98]. Origin of CSC is an interesting issue of current discussion and it has been proposed that multistage cancer development theories (initiation, promotion and progression) seen in chemical carcinogenesis models has a counterpart in CSC theory as follow; initiated cells → preneoplastic CSC → CSC → cancer [99]. This hypothesis has been sustained by the discovery of preneoplastic CSC that have the potential for both benign and malignant differentiation [100]. CSC have frequently been identified using specific markers for normal stem cells, including CD133, CD44, CD24, EpCAM, and ABCB5, however, when cancer subtypes are compared, presence of CSC markers is highly heterogeneous [101]. As a functional way to demonstrate tumorigenic potential of CSC, few cells are required (from 1 to 10) to form a new tumor in immunocompromised host mice ((NOD/SCID mice), while more than 1000 non-CSC malignant tumor cells must be inoculated to form a tumor by xenotransplantation assays, consequently frequency of CSC that can be isolated in human solid tumors has been estimated in a range of 0.1-0.0001 % [102]. The concept of CSC has significant implications in both clinical and basic cancer research, it has signified a new paradigm that allows scientist to rise new questions concerning; origin of cancer, carcinogenesis process, cellular targets of cancer-etiological agents, cell signaling of CSC, early detection, prevention and new strategies for cancer treatment. Cancer research of CSC is a promising area for discovery of molecular signatures and molecular targets for developing of new drugs specific for the cellular source of cancer.

CONCLUSIONS

The importance of *in vivo* and *in vitro* models for cancer research lies in the possibility of providing new knowledge and approaches for improved understanding of cancer biology and cancer treatment. Cancer remains as a complex group of diseases that kills thousands of humans around the entire world. Nevertheless there are new clinical approaches such as improved surgical methods and new chemotherapy agents that destroy proliferating cells; full elimination of tumor cells in advanced cancers is rare. Frequently after patient treatment, remaining cancer cells get back to renew more aggressive tumors. Reality is that cancer as a disease represents a complex biological scenario that encourages scientists to understand how cells work in an organism. The detailed study of altered cancer cells has provided a great amount of data that is helping researchers understand functions and homeostasis of normal cells. Although there is not a perfect cellular or animal model that can explain fully how cancer is developed in humans, the comprehensive analysis of them may be a more accurate approach to study human cancer and develop drugs that could be translated to human therapeutic applications.

ACKNOWLEDGEMENTS

Authors thank Dra. Irma Silva Zolezzi, Dra. Gisela Ceballos Cancino, Dra. Tatiana N. Olivares-Bañuelos and Biol. Roman García Ramirez for reviewing manuscript. Grant CONACyT (115431).

REFERENCES

[1]	Vidal M, Cagan RL. Drosophila models for cancer research. Curr Opin Genet Dev 2006; 16(1): 10-6.
[2]	Feitsma H, Cuppen E. Zebrafish as a cancer model. Mol Cancer Res 2008; 6(5): 685-94.
[3]	Calnek BW. Gordon Memorial Lecture. Chicken neoplasia--a model for cancer research. Br Poult Sci 1992; 33(1): 3-16.
[4]	Lapin BA. Use of nonhuman primates in cancer research. J Med Primatol 1982; 11(6): 327-41.
[5]	Porrello A, Cardelli P, Spugnini EP. Pet models in cancer research: general principles. J Exp Clin Cancer Res 2004; 23(2): 181-93.
[6]	Ames BN, Gold LS. The causes and prevention of cancer: the role of environment. Biotherapy 1998; 11(2-3): 205-20.
[7]	Clapp RW, Jacobs MM, Loechler EL. Environmental and occupational causes of cancer: new evidence 2005-2007. Rev Environ Health 2008; 23(1): 1-37.
[8]	Cogliano V, Straif K, Baan R, Grosse Y, Secretan B, El Ghissassi F. Smokeless tobacco and tobacco-related nitrosamines. Lancet Oncol 2004; 5(12): 708.
[9]	Katsusaburo Yamagiwa (1863-1930). CA Cancer J Clin 1977; 27(3): 172-3.
[10]	Rubin H. Synergistic mechanisms in carcinogenesis by polycyclic aromatic hydrocarbons and by tobacco smoke: a bio-historical perspective with updates. Carcinogenesis 2001; 22(12): 1903-30.
[11]	Javier RT, Butel JS. The history of tumor virology. Cancer Res 2008; 68(19): 7693-06.
[12]	Guengerich FP. Metabolic activation of carcinogens. Pharmacol Ther 1992; 54(1): 17-61.
[13]	van Schaik RH. CYP450 pharmacogenetics for personalizing cancer therapy. Drug Resist Updat 2008; 11(3): 77-98.

[14]   Silva Lima B, Van der Laan JW. Mechanisms of nongenotoxic carcinogenesis and assessment of the human hazard. Regul Toxicol Pharmacol 2000; 32(2): 135-43.

[15]   Sanchez-Perez Y, Carrasco-Legleu C, Garcia-Cuellar C, *et al.* Oxidative stress in carcinogenesis. Correlation between lipid peroxidation and induction of preneoplastic lesions in rat hepatocarcinogenesis. Cancer Lett 2005; 217(1): 25-32.

[16]   Gold LS, Manley NB, Slone TH, Rohrbach L, Garfinkel GB. Supplement to the Carcinogenic Potency Database (CPDB): results of animal bioassays published in the general literature through 1997 and by the National Toxicology Program in 1997-1998. Toxicol Sci 2005; 85(2): 747-808.

[17]   Gold LS, Manley NB, Slone TH, Ward JM. Compendium of chemical carcinogens by target organ: results of chronic bioassays in rats, mice, hamsters, dogs, and monkeys. Toxicol Pathol 2001; 29(6): 639-52.

[18]   Cogliano VJ. Use of carcinogenicity bioassays in the IARC monographs. Ann N Y Acad Sci 2006; 1076: 592-600.

[19]   Gordon T, Bosland M. Strain-dependent differences in susceptibility to lung cancer in inbred mice exposed to mainstream cigarette smoke. Cancer Lett 2008.

[20]   DiGiovanni J. Multistage carcinogenesis in mouse skin. Pharmacol Ther 1992; 54(1): 63-128.

[21]   Slaga TJ, Budunova IV, Gimenez-Conti IB, Aldaz CM. The mouse skin carcinogenesis model. J Investig Dermatol Symp Proc 1996; 1(2): 151-6.

[22]   Yuspa SH. The pathogenesis of squamous cell cancer: lessons learned from studies of skin carcinogenesis. J Dermatol Sci 1998; 17(1): 1-7.

[23]   Kim TW, Chen Q, Shen X, *et al.* Oral mucosal carcinogenesis in SENCAR mice. Anticancer Res 2002; 22(5): 2733-40.

[24]   Tanaka T, Makita H, Ohnishi M, *et al.* Chemoprevention of 4-nitroquinoline 1-oxide-induced oral carcinogenesis by dietary curcumin and hesperidin: comparison with the protective effect of beta-carotene. Cancer Res 1994; 54(17): 4653-9.

[25]   Vered M, Yarom N, Dayan D. 4NQO oral carcinogenesis: animal models, molecular markers and future expectations. Oral Oncol 2005; 41(4): 337-9.

[26]   Yang Y, Zhou ZT, Ge JP. Effect of genistein on DMBA-induced oral carcinogenesis in hamster. Carcinogenesis 2006; 27(3): 578-83.

[27]   Shimizu N, Inada K, Nakanishi H, *et al. Helicobacter pylori* infection enhances glandular stomach carcinogenesis in Mongolian gerbils treated with chemical carcinogens. Carcinogenesis 1999; 20(4): 669-76.

[28]   Tsukamoto T, Mizoshita T, Tatematsu M. Animal models of stomach carcinogenesis. Toxicol Pathol 2007; 35(5): 636-48.

[29]   Corpet DE, Pierre F. How good are rodent models of carcinogenesis in predicting efficacy in humans? A systematic review and meta-analysis of colon chemoprevention in rats, mice and men. Eur J Cancer 2005; 41(13): 1911-22.

[30]   Femia AP, Caderni G. Rodent models of colon carcinogenesis for the study of chemopreventive activity of natural products. Planta Med 2008; 74(13): 1602-7.

[31]   Maskens AP. Confirmation of the two-step nature of chemical carcinogenesis in the rat colon adenocarcinoma model. Cancer Res 1981; 41(3): 1240-5.

[32]   Sugimura T, Terada M. Experimental chemical carcinogenesis in the stomach and colon. Jpn J Clin Oncol 1998; 28(3): 163-7.

[33]   Pitot HC, Barsness L, Goldsworthy T, Kitagawa T. Biochemical characterisation of stages of hepatocarcinogenesis after a single dose of diethylnitrosamine. Nature 1978; 271(5644): 456-8.

[34]   Mikol YB, Hoover KL, Creasia D, Poirier LA. Hepatocarcinogenesis in rats fed methyl-deficient, amino acid-defined diets. Carcinogenesis 1983; 4(12): 1619-29.

[35]   Marche-Cova A, Fattel-Fazenda S, Rojas-Ochoa A, Arce-Popoca E, Villa-Trevino S. Follow-up of GST-P during hepatocarcinogenesis with DEN-2AAF in F344 rats. Arch Med Res 1995; 26 Spec No: S169-73.

[36]   Farber E, Sarma DS. Hepatocarcinogenesis: a dynamic cellular perspective. Lab Invest 1987; 56(1): 4-22.

[37]   Stoner GD, Adam-Rodwell G, Morse MA. Lung tumors in strain A mice: application for studies in cancer chemoprevention. J Cell Biochem Suppl 1993; 17F: 95-103.

[38]   Knaapen AM, Gungor N, Schins RP, Borm PJ, Van Schooten FJ. Neutrophils and respiratory tract DNA damage and mutagenesis: a review. Mutagenesis 2006; 21(4): 225-36.

[39]   Emmendoerffer A, Hecht M, Boeker T, Mueller M, Heinrich U. Role of inflammation in chemical-induced lung cancer. Toxicol Lett 2000; 112-113: 185-91.

[40]   Ito F, Toma H, Yamaguchi Y, Nakazawa H, Onitsuka S, Hashimoto Y. A rat model of chemical-induced polycystic kidney disease with multistage tumors. Nephron 1998; 79(1): 73-9.

[41]   Hiasa Y, Konishi N, Nakaoka S, *et al.* Possible application to medium-term organ bioassays for renal carcinogenesis modifiers in rats treated with N-ethyl-N-hydroxyethylnitrosamine and unilateral nephrectomy. Jpn J Cancer Res 1991; 82(12): 1385-90.

[42]   Shimizu N, Inada KI, Tsukamoto T, *et al.* New animal model of glandular stomach carcinogenesis in Mongolian gerbils infected with *Helicobacter pylori* and treated with a chemical carcinogen. J Gastroenterol 1999; 34 Suppl 11: 61-6.

[43]   Khare S, Chaudhary K, Bissonnette M, Carroll R. Aberrant crypt foci in colon cancer epidemiology. Methods Mol Biol 2009; 472: 373-86.

[44]   Pavek P, Dvorak Z. Xenobiotic-induced transcriptional regulation of xenobiotic metabolizing enzymes of the cytochrome P450 superfamily in human extrahepatic tissues. Curr Drug Metab 2008; 9(2): 129-43.

[45]   Perez-Carreon JI, Cruz-Jimenez G, Licea-Vega JA, Arce Popoca E, Fattel Fazenda S, Villa-Trevino S. Genotoxic and anti-genotoxic properties of *Calendula officinalis* extracts in rat liver cell cultures treated with diethylnitrosamine. Toxicol *In vitro* 2002; 16(3): 253-8.

[46]   Hoover KL, Lynch PH, Poirier LA. Profound postinitiation enhancement by short-term severe methionine, choline, vitamin B12, and folate deficiency of hepatocarcinogenesis in F344 rats given a single low-dose diethylnitrosamine injection. J Natl Cancer Inst 1984; 73(6): 1327-36.

[47]   Peraino C, Fry RJ, Staffeldt E. Reduction and enhancement by phenobarbital of hepatocarcinogenesis induced in the rat by 2-acetylaminofluorene. Cancer Res 1971; 31(10): 1506-12.

[48]   Solt DaF, Emmanuel. New principle for the analysis of chemical carcinogenesis. Nature 1976; 263: 701-3.

[49]   Perez-Carreon JI, Lopez-Garcia C, Fattel-Fazenda S, *et al.* Gene expression profile related to the progression of preneoplastic nodules toward hepatocellular carcinoma in rats. Neoplasia 2006; 8(5): 373-83.

[50]   Perez-Carreon JI, Dargent C, Merhi M, *et al.* Tumor promoting and co-carcinogenic effects in medium-term rat hepatocarcinogenesis are not modified by co-administration of 12 pesticides in mixture at acceptable daily intake. Food Chem Toxicol 2008.

[51]   Bannasch P, Haertel T, Su Q. Significance of hepatic preneoplasia in risk identification and early detection of neoplasia. Toxicol Pathol 2003; 31(1): 134-9.

[52]   Enzmann H, Iatropoulos M, Brunnemann KD, *et al.* Short- and intermediate-term carcinogenicity testing--a review. Part 2: available experimental models. Food Chem Toxicol 1998; 36(11): 997-1013.

[53]   Imaida K, Sato H, Okamiya H, Takahashi M, Hayashi Y. Enhancing effect of high fat diet on 4-nitroquinoline 1-oxide-induced pulmonary tumorigenesis in ICR male mice. Jpn J Cancer Res 1989; 80(6): 499-502.

[54]   Karube T, Katayama H, Takemoto K, Watanabe S. Induction of squamous metaplasia, dysplasia and carcinoma *in situ* of the mouse tracheal mucosa by inhalation of sodium chloride mist following subcutaneous injection of 4-nitroquinoline 1-oxide. Jpn J Cancer Res 1989; 80(8): 698-701.

[55]   Yano T, Obata Y, Ishikawa G, Ichikawa T. Enhancing effect of high dietary iron on lung tumorigenesis in mice. Cancer Lett 1994; 76(1): 57-62.

[56]   Brinster RL, Chen HY, Messing A, van Dyke T, Levine AJ, Palmiter RD. Transgenic mice harboring SV40 T-antigen genes develop characteristic brain tumors. Cell 1984; 37(2): 367-79.

[57]   Bautch VL, Toda S, Hassell JA, Hanahan D. Endothelial cell tumors develop in transgenic mice carrying polyoma virus middle T oncogene. Cell 1987; 51(4): 529-37.

[58]   Adams JM, Harris AW, Pinkert CA, *et al.* The c-myc oncogene driven by immunoglobulin enhancers induces lymphoid malignancy in transgenic mice. Nature 1985; 318(6046): 533-8.

[59]   Quaife CJ, Pinkert CA, Ornitz DM, Palmiter RD, Brinster RL. Pancreatic neoplasia induced by ras expression in acinar cells of transgenic mice. Cell 1987; 48(6): 1023-34.

[60]   Muller WJ, Sinn E, Pattengale PK, Wallace R, Leder P. Single-step induction of mammary adenocarcinoma in transgenic mice bearing the activated c-neu oncogene. Cell 1988; 54(1): 105-15.

[61]   Guy CT, Muthuswamy SK, Cardiff RD, Soriano P, Muller WJ. Activation of the c-Src tyrosine kinase is required for the induction of mammary tumors in transgenic mice. Genes Dev 1994; 8(1): 23-32.

[62]   Torres-Arzayus MI, Font de Mora J, Yuan J, *et al.* High tumor incidence and activation of the PI3K/AKT pathway in transgenic mice define AIB1 as an oncogene. Cancer Cell 2004; 6(3): 263-74.

[63]   Ruther U, Komitowski D, Schubert FR, Wagner EF. c-fos expression induces bone tumors in transgenic mice. Oncogene 1989; 4(7): 861-5.

[64]   Sinn E, Muller W, Pattengale P, Tepler I, Wallace R, Leder P. Coexpression of MMTV/v-Ha-ras and MMTV/c-myc genes in transgenic mice: synergistic action of oncogenes *in vivo*. Cell 1987; 49(4): 465-75.

[65]   Sandgren EP, Quaife CJ, Pinkert CA, Palmiter RD, Brinster RL. Oncogene-induced liver neoplasia in transgenic mice. Oncogene 1989; 4(6): 715-24.

[66]   Donehower LA, Harvey M, Slagle BL, *et al.* Mice deficient for p53 are developmentally normal but susceptible to spontaneous tumors. Nature 1992; 356(6366): 215-21.

[67]   Cadwell C, Zambetti GP. The effects of wild-type p53 tumor suppressor activity and mutant p53 gain-of-function on cell growth. Gene 2001; 277(1-2): 15-30.

[68]   Soussi T, Lozano G. p53 mutation heterogeneity in cancer. Biochem Biophys Res Commun 2005; 331(3): 834-42.

[69] Yang Y, Fu LM. TSGDB: a database system for tumor suppressor genes. Bioinformatics 2003; 19(17): 2311-2.

[70] Sherr CJ, McCormick F. The RB and p53 pathways in cancer. Cancer Cell 2002; 2(2): 103-12.

[71] Kaelin WG, Jr. Alterations in G1/S cell-cycle control contributing to carcinogenesis. Ann N Y Acad Sci 1997; 833: 29-33.

[72] Lee EY, Chang CY, Hu N, *et al.* Mice deficient for Rb are nonviable and show defects in neurogenesis and haematopoiesis. Nature 1992; 359(6393): 288-94.

[73] Hu N, Gutsmann A, Herbert DC, Bradley A, Lee WH, Lee EY. Heterozygous Rb-1 delta 20/+mice are predisposed to tumors of the pituitary gland with a nearly complete penetrance. Oncogene 1994; 9(4): 1021-7.

[74] Harvey M, Vogel H, Lee EY, Bradley A, Donehower LA. Mice deficient in both p53 and Rb develop tumors primarily of endocrine origin. Cancer Res 1995; 55(5): 1146-51.

[75] Breuer M, Slebos R, Verbeek S, van Lohuizen M, Wientjens E, Berns A. Very high frequency of lymphoma induction by a chemical carcinogen in pim-1 transgenic mice. Nature 1989; 340(6228): 61-3.

[76] Tennant RW, Rao GN, Russfield A, Seilkop S, Braun AG. Chemical effects in transgenic mice bearing oncogenes expressed in mammary tissue. Carcinogenesis 1993; 14(1): 29-35.

[77] Schnur J, Nagy P, Sebestyen A, Schaff Z, Thorgeirsson SS. Chemical hepatocarcinogenesis in transgenic mice overexpressing mature TGF beta-1 in liver. Eur J Cancer 1999; 35(13): 1842-5.

[78] Cohen SM, Robinson D, MacDonald J. Alternative models for carcinogenicity testing. Toxicol Sci 2001; 64(1): 14-9.

[79] Tennant RW, French JE, Spalding JW. Identifying chemical carcinogens and assessing potential risk in short-term bioassays using transgenic mouse models. Environ Health Perspect 1995; 103(10): 942-50.

[80] Begley DA, Krupke DM, Vincent MJ, Sundberg JP, Bult CJ, Eppig JT. Mouse Tumor Biology Database (MTB): status update and future directions. Nucleic Acids Res 2007; 35(Database issue): D638-42.

[81] Krupke DM, Begley DA, Sundberg JP, Bult CJ, Eppig JT. The Mouse Tumor Biology database. Nat Rev Cancer 2008; 8(6): 459-65.

[82] Kunz-Schughart LA. Multicellular tumor spheroids: intermediates between monolayer culture and *in vivo* tumor. Cell Biol Int 1999; 23(3): 157-61.

[83] Masters JR. Human cancer cell lines: fact and fantasy. Nat Rev Mol Cell Biol 2000; 1(3): 233-6.

[84] Gopalakrishnan B, Wolff J. siRNA and DNA transfer to cultured cells. Methods Mol Biol 2009; 480: 31-52.

[85] Potter H. Transfection by electroporation. Curr Protoc Immunol 2001; Chapter 10: Unit 10 5.

[86] Kingston RE, Chen CA, Okayama H. Calcium phosphate transfection. Curr Protoc Immunol 2001; Chapter 10: Unit 10 3.

[87] Selden RF. Transfection using DEAE-dextran. Curr Protoc Immunol 2001;Chapter 10:Unit 10 4.

[88] Rome C, Deckers R, Moonen CT. The use of ultrasound in transfection and transgene expression. Handb Exp Pharmacol 2008(185 Pt 2): 225-43.

[89] Yao CP, Zhang ZX, Rahmanzadeh R, Huettmann G. Laser-based gene transfection and gene therapy. IEEE Trans Nanobioscience 2008; 7(2): 111-9.

[90] Weinberg RA. Oncogenes and the molecular biology of cancer. J Cell Biol 1983; 97(6): 1661-2.

[91] Wynford-Thomas D. Oncogenes and anti-oncogenes; the molecular basis of tumor behaviour. J Pathol 1991; 165(3): 187-201.

[92] Bagasra O, Prilliman KR. RNA interference: the molecular immune system. J Mol Histol 2004; 35(6): 545-53.

[93] Peek AS, Behlke MA. Design of active small interfering RNAs. Curr Opin Mol Ther 2007; 9(2): 110-8.

[94] Zentilin L, Giacca M. *In vivo* transfer and expression of genes coding for short interfering RNAs. Curr Pharm Biotechnol 2004; 5(4): 341-7.

[95] Hokaiwado N, Takeshita F, Banas A, Ochiya T. RNAi-based drug discovery and its application to therapeutics. IDrugs 2008; 11(4): 274-8.

[96] Tomasson MH. Cancer stem cells: A guide for skeptics. J Cell Biochem 2009.

[97] Yi SY, Nan KJ. Tumor-initiating stem cells in liver cancer. Cancer Biol Ther 2008; 7(3): 325-30.

[98] Kuo MT. Redox regulation of multidrug resistance in cancer chemotherapy: molecular mechanisms and therapeutic opportunities. Antioxid Redox Signal 2009; 11(1): 99-133.

[99] Gao JX. Cancer stem cells: the lessons from pre-cancerous stem cells. J Cell Mol Med 2008; 12(1): 67-96.

[100] Chen L, Shen R, Ye Y, *et al.* Precancerous stem cells have the potential for both benign and malignant differentiation. PLoS ONE 2007; 2(3): e293.

[101] Visvader JE, Lindeman GJ. Cancer stem cells in solid tumors: accumulating evidence and unresolved questions. Nat Rev Cancer 2008; 8(10): 755-68.

[102] Quintana E, Shackleton M, Sabel MS, Fullen DR, Johnson TM, Morrison SJ. Efficient tumor formation by single human melanoma cells. Nature 2008; 456(7222): 593-8.

CHAPTER 9

Molecular Diagnosis and Prognosis

M. Verónica Ponce-Castañeda[1,*] and Lourdes Cabrera-Muñoz[2]

[1]*Unidad de Investigación Médica en Enfermedades Infecciosas, Hospital de Pediatría, CMN SXXI, IMSS, México D.F.* [2]*Departamento de Patología, Hospital Infantil de México Federico Gómez*

Abstract: Detection of DNA and RNA alterations and proteins associated with cancer are used as indicators or biomarkers for specific tumor traits that help in cancer diagnosis and patient management. Molecular diagnosis in cancer is a new discipline that incorporates genomic and proteomic information related to malignant, pre-malignant and normal tissues from which clinically useful cancer biomarkers are expected to be identified. The goal is to find and clinically validate biomarkers associated with cancer risk, early detection, phenotypic tumor aggressivity, tumor staging, or biomarkers associated to prognosis such as response to treatment, disease recurrence and survival. Challenges for achieving this goal arise from a need of significant economic investment, as well as a multidisciplinary approach and the inherent molecular complexity of cancer itself.

Keywords: Cancer biomarkers, PCR, antigens, chromosomal translocations, RT-PCR, immunohistochemistry, oncogenomics, oncoproteomics.

INTRODUCTION

Although our understanding of cancer molecular pathogenesis during the last forty years has advanced significantly, the most important aspect of cancer diagnosis for most tumor types is made by a pathologist based on microscopic examination of a tumor biopsy. In the majority of solid tumors cases a pathologist also participates in staging the tumor to define the cancer as localized or metastatic disease. A biomarker is a characteristic that is measured objectively as an indicator of normal or pathogenic processes [1]. Tumor biomarkers thus are molecules produced by the tumor cells, but most of these molecules are also produced by non tumor tissues, and therefore tumor biomarkers are not diagnostic of cancer. However some cancer biomarkers usually detected in the tumor or body fluids, have clinical value because they can complement histopathologic diagnosis, helping in tumor staging and selection of therapy.

Emergence of global analyses of gene expresssion and the human genome project are expanding our knowledge of the molecular pathogenesis of cancer [2-4]. These technologies have yielded long lists of disease associated genes and proteins with potential utility as biomarkers. The development of biomarkers will provide new tools that can be used in a wide variety of clinical settings impacting many aspects of cancer field. As molecular bases of the malignant phenotype are uncovered and specific tumors characterized, additional biomarkers are becoming incorporated into routine diagnostic criteria and algorhythms.

Few clinically validated cancer biomarkers are available. These are listed in Table **1**. The only tumor biomarker detected in serum with a wide physician acceptance as a tool for screening is the protein Prostate Specific Antigen (PSA). PSA is used in the identification and monitoring of prostate carcinoma, one of the most common tumors in males older than 50 years. The other cancer biomarker of wide use for screening is the Papanicolau smear to detect cervical cancer, a serious public health problem especially in less industrialized countries.

Some biomarkers have proven very useful in the clinical setting. For example, identification of estrogen and progesterone receptors in breast cancer predict a better prognosis and are indicative of likely response to tamoxifen therapy [5]. Prominent biomarkers that are themselves molecular targets for relatively new treatments with monoclonal antibodies, are CD20 in B-cell non-Hodgkin's lymphomas [6, 7], HER2/Neu in

---

*Address correspondence to M. Verónica Ponce-Castañeda:** Unidad de Investigación Médica en Enfermedades Infecciosas, Hospital de Pediatría, CMN SXXI, IMSS, México D.F.; E-mail: vponce@ifc.unam.mx

Javier Camacho (Ed)

breast cancer and EGFR for metastatic colon carcinoma [8] [9]. Expression of these biomarkers in tumor specimens indicates treatment with corresponding monoclonal antibodies (rituximab, trastuzumab and cetuximab respectively), because tumor cells that express these molecules will likely respond to those treatments. CD20, HER2 and EGFR are membrane proteins expressed or overexpressed mainly on tumor cells, and the above mentioned monoclonal antibodies directed against these proteins, mediate cytotoxic effects depleting tumor cells and thus improving survival

Table 1: Cancer biomarkers currently in clinical use

CANCER BIOMARKER	USE
Alpha Fetoprotein (AFP)	Detection in serum for staging in non seminomatous testicular cancer
Human Chorionic Gonadotropin- Beta (BHCG)	Detection in serum for staging in testicular cancer, and for non-seminomatous germ cell tumors
CA19-9	Detection in serum for monitoring pancreatic cancer
CA125	Detection in serum for monitoring ovarian cancer
Papanicolau	Screening and detection of cervical cancer
Epidermal Growth Factor Receptor (EGFR)	Detection in tumor for selection of therapy
c-KIT	Detection in gastrointestinal tumor for selection of therapy
Thyroglobulin	Detection in serum for monitoring Thyroid cancer
PSA	Detection in serum for screening and monitoring of prostate cancer
CA 15-3	Detection in serum for monitoring breast cancer
CA27-29	Detection in serum for monitoring breast cancer
Estrogen and Progesterone Receceptor	Detection in tumor for selection of hormonal therapy
HER/NEU2	Detection in tumor for prognosis and selection of therapy
NMP22	Detection in urine for monitoring in bladder cancer
Fibrin/FDP	Detection in urine for monitoring bladder cancer
BTA	Detection in urine for monitoring bladder cancer

Another pair of biomarkers able to identify patients whose tumors will respond to treatment with tyrosine kinase inhibitor imatinib (Gleevec), are identification of the BCR-ABL translocation in Chronic Myeloid Leukemia (CML) and expression of c-KIT protein in Gastrointestinal Stromal Tumors (GIST). In CML the Philadelphia chromosome [t(9;22)] was identified as a chromosomal translocation that leads to a fusion gene and chimeric protein BCR-ABL. This fusion gene codifies a continuously active tyrosine kinase enzyme that drives tumor cell proliferation. The search for a specific inhibitor for this kinase, led to the development of imatinib, a selective compound that inhibits enzymatic function of ABL but is also an inhibitor of c-KIT another tyrosine kinase enzyme involved in cell proliferation too and expressed in GIST. Thus both tumor types respond to imatinib because this molecule exerts its effects decreasing the activity of these enzymes causing regression or destruction of the malignant process [10]. These examples illustrate how basic research on tumor biology and biochemistry led to identification of a molecular therapeutic target and a cancer biomarker itself.

From the diagnostic point of view, the goal of molecular analyses and the search for biomarkers in tumor tissues are aimed at specific histopathological diagnostic needs and also at solving important clinical problems. For example the recurrent chromosomal translocations identified in many hematologic malignancies and more recently in sarcomas, help providing additional molecular criteria to subclassify diseases [11, 12]. These molecular criteria are translated in to more accurate diagnosis and treatments in disease entities that sometimes are difficult to distinguish in morphological terms. From other point of view, new discoveries made by research aimed to understand the biology of tumors had provided information with clinical implications that can be used as biomarkers or diagnostic tests. For example the discovery of germ line mutations in the BRCA1 gene associated with familial breast and ovarian carcinoma, allows screening of individuals and identifying family members at higher risk in affected families before the disease develops. Once individuals are identified, they can be monitored closely, increasing the possibilities to detect tumors in earlier stages, when treatment usually has better success. Although familial breast cancer constitutes approximately 10% of all breast cases [13], cost-benefit considerations limit the wider use of this cancer biomarker.

STRATEGIES TO SEARCH AND VALIDATE CANCER BIOMARKERS

Some key points are important in the search and validation of cancer biomarkers. Technological advances and development of new tools in genomics and bioinformatics are enabling the study of cellular and global alterations associated with specific tumors and this may allow discovery of novel biomarkers. The search for cancer biomarkers beyond tumor tissues has been focused on blood and urine in order to identifying and developing minimally invasive tests for cancer biomarkers associated with tumors or clinicaly relevant events. Blood or body fluid components that can provide cancer evidence of malignancy and thus be useful as biomarkers include: circulating tumor cells, DNA, RNA proteins and metabolites. Other important aspects in cancer biomarker research are the technical developments that allow the analysis of massive amounts of expressed genes such as expression microarrays, oncoproteomics and mass spectrometry [14-16]. These technologies have permitted the analysis of thousands of tumor and blood proteins, and have made the search for protein cancer biomarkers a very active research field. Many proteins from tumors, blood and other body fluids have been explored and found to be potential cancer biomarkers. Despite this, very few cancer biomarkers have proven useful in the clinical setting. Clinical validation is a crucial aspect of biomarker development, because in order to prove the utility of a cancer biomarker, prospective studies and prolonged follow up are needed [17]. Rigorous assessment of the relationships between a biomarker and a clinical or epidemiological parameter must be demonstrated. Thus to establish a consistent and reliable link between a biomarker and early detection, disease relapse, response to treatment, or survival, individuals at risk or patients must be enrolled in prospective well controlled clinical cohorts. Additionally, tissues (tumor and blood for example) must be obtained handled according to established protocols in order to allow potential biomarkers to be measured [18, 19]. Study populations have to be powered taking into account the clinical or epidemiological parameter to be studied, the prevalence of the outcome of interest such that an appropriate number of individuals will be included and the clinical outcomes or events will occur during the proposed follow up. All of these aspects imply the need for a multi-disciplinary approach, frequently with multi-institutional involvement, cost-benefits considerations, and also challenging organizational structures [18].

For any cancer biomarker or group of biomarkers to be useful, two critical criteria must be fulfilled: high sensitivity and high specificity. Sensitivity for an early detection biomarker for example, refers to the percentage of people affected by a tumor that will be correctly identified by the biomarker. Thus 100% sensitivity for a biomarker means that all affected persons will be identified with the biomarker. In contrast if a biomarker is not very sensitive there will be many false negative results and thus many persons with the targeted outcome (having cancer) will be undetected by the biomarker. Specificity refers to percentage of non affected people that will be correctly identified as free of disease, therefore 100% specificity for a biomarker means that all people not affected by the tumor, will be correctly classified when the test result is negative. If a biomarker has a low specificity measuring it will yield many false positive results and thus there will be many people testing positive even though they are free of disease. Markers of early detection or risk assessment must be highly specific and sensitive in order to be useful for cancer screening purposes. However, different combinations of sensitivity and specificity are required of any given biomarker assay, depending on the intended application of the biomarker.

METHODS MOST COMMONLY USED IN CANCER MOLECULAR DIAGNOSIS

The single most flexible and sensitive method used in cancer molecular pathology is the Polymerase Chain Reaction (PCR). For most tumor specimens the amount of material available for analysis is limited, and this technique is particularly useful because it permits a many-fold (10^6) amplification of a given DNA segment from complex genetic material in a few hours. It is a powerful enzymatic technique that uses thermo stable DNA polymerases to synthesize DNA copies, using a mixture of four deoxynucleotides (dATP, dTTP, dCTP, dGTP) the molecular building blocks of DNA. PCR also uses a pair of oligonucleotides commonly known as primers, whose sequences are complementary to the flanking regions of DNA to be copied and that prime the enzyme in order to begin DNA synthesis. The enzymatic reaction is based on the ability of DNA polymerase to use single strand DNA and a short segment of double stranded DNA as a template to add complimentary nucleotides and thus complete the synthesis of a new double stranded DNA. In order to do this, DNA must first be denatured or "melted" into single strands, which is achieved by heating the solution to disrupt hydrogen bonds that maintain DNA's double stranded structure. Subsequent lowering of the temperature allows the annealing of the primers to their complementary target sequences and the thermo stable DNA polymerase to begin double stranded DNA synthesis [20]. The use of thermo stable DNA polymerase allows repeating the cycle of denaturing and synthesis as long as reagents are available in the chemical reaction. Repeating this cycle 25 -30 times results in replication of the DNA region of interest from 10^7 to 10^{11} times, making the amplified products easily detectable. Since the cycles are performed in an automated thermocycler, the whole process can be accomplished in a few hours. Gel electrophoresis is the method most commonly used to analyze PCR products. Using agarose or polyacrylamide gel electrophoresis allows visualization and analysis of amplified DNA fragments.

In general through the use of PCR, DNA mutation analyses, identification of chromosomal translocations and identification of DNA or RNA from oncogenic microorganism are the most informative biomarkers in molecular diagnosis of cancer. The most common method used for detecting point mutations is real time PCR, a kinetic monitoring of DNA amplification during PCR. Accumulation rate of the PCR product is directly proportional to the quantity of starting target DNA or RNA sequences and thus can also be used for gene expression analyses. In order to detect more complex mutations Single Strand Conformation Polymorphism (SSCP) is used in combination with DNA sequencing [21-23]. SSCP builds on the principle that migration of single stranded DNA on non denaturing polyacrylamide gels is sequence- dependent, and conformation of single stranded DNA molecules can be altered by point mutations, small deletions or insertions changing the mobility of single strand bands on a gel when compared with a normal or known DNA. Other molecular techniques such as Southern blots are used for detection of bigger deletions (*e.g.* loss of heterozygozity), Reverse Transcriptase coupled to PCR and Fluorescent *in Situ* Hybridization (FISH) are the most common methods used for detection of chromosomal translocations. Other assays used in cancer research that might have clinical implications, include DNA methylation assays, telomerase activity and microsatellite determinations.

HEMATO ONCOLOGY

The field in which most relevant clinical advances had been achieved in molecular diagnosis is hemato-oncology, because gene fusions that result from chromosomal translocations are useful diagnostic markers and potential therapeutic targets. Recurrent chromosomal translocations in leukemias and lymphomas were first identified using cytogenetic techniques that allowed visualization of chromosomes [24]. Molecular characterization of these genetic alterations lead to increasing understanding of molecular pathogenesis and identification of numerous genes involved in cancer development [25]. Detailed molecular analysis of recurrent chromosomal breakpoints revealed that in general these rearrangements can have two consequences: leading either to fusion of coding regions from two different genes frequently transcription factors, or leading to a juxtaposition of the coding region from one gene juxtaposed to the regulatory elements (enhancer/promoter) from another gene -usually the T cell receptor- or heavy chain immunoglobulin locus, Fig. **1** [26].

Fusion genes frequently involve transcription factors that are transcribed into mRNA and in turn produce novel fusion proteins with altered functional properties. Juxtaposition or relocation of a coding gene produces aberrant expression of the relocated gene. Table **2** lists the most common chromosomal translocations found in hematologic malignancies.

From the diagnostic point of view these molecular genetic events are significant because they are recurrent, highly specific and have diagnostic implications. Many translocations involving fusion genes are detectable using PCR strategies in which RNA is first isolated from tumor specimens, using Reverse Transcriptase enzyme, RNA is converted in to cDNA and mRNA fusion transcripts can be detected using PCR with specific primers targeting the sequences of the fusion genes involved in the breakpoints. Amplified DNA can be detected in agarose or polyacrylamide gel electrophoresis as mentioned before [20].

Two outstanding examples that illustrate the clinical relevance of chromosomal translocations as biomarkers are: RT-PCR detection of [t (9;22)] in CML patients, and detection of [t (15;17)] in Acute Myelogenous Leukemia (AML) patients. Those patients testing positive for the translocations are candidates to be treated with imatinib and to all trans retinoic acid respectively which are specific targeted therapies directed towards the chimeric products of the corresponding chromosomal translocations, the tyrosine kinase fusion (BCR-ABL) and a Retinoic Acid Receptor Fusion (PML-RARA) [27-29]. Even though these diseases represent only a small subset of leukemia patients, the response to treatment results in complete remission in a high proportion of cases, and thus cytogenetic and molecular genetic findings are now an important factor helping in determining chemotherapy regimes for most patients with acute leukemia.

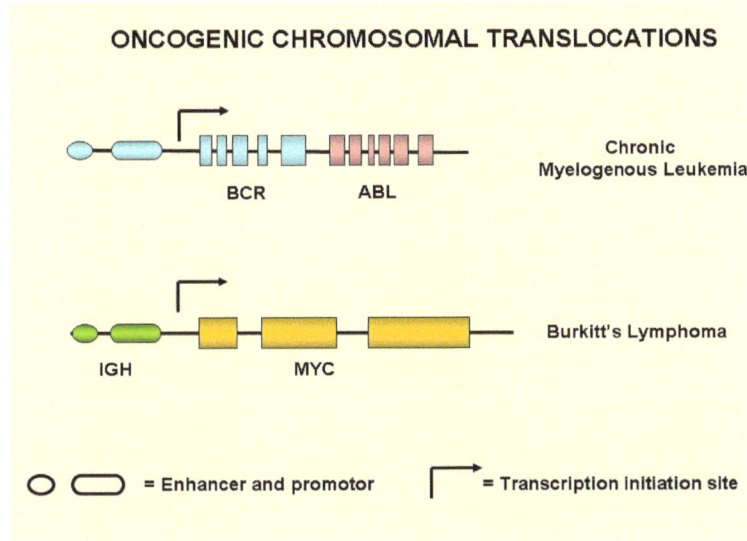

Figure 1: Two types of functional alterations derive from chromosomal translocations. Juxtaposition of different coding regions as in CML or juxtaposition of enhancer / promoter elements to oncogenes as in Burkitt's lymphoma.

Table 2: Recurrent chromosomal translocations identified in hematologic malignancies

Tumor	Translocation	Genes Involved
B CELL LYMPHOMAS		
Difuse large B cell lymphoma	t(3;14) t(14;15) t(1;22) t(1 ;14)	IGH, BCL6, BCL2, BCL8, FCGRIIb, MUC, NfkB2
Follicular lymphoma	t(14;18)	BCL2
Burkitt's lymphoma	t(8;14)	c-MYC
Mantle cell lymphoma	t(11;14)	BCL1
Lymphoplasmacytoid lymphoma	t(9;14)	PAX5
MALT lymphoma	t(11;18)	API1-MALT1
MYELOID LEUKEMIAS		
Chronic myelogenous leukemia	t(9;22)	BCR-ABL
Acute myelogenous leukemia M2	t(8;21)	AML1-ETO
Acute myelomonocytic leukemia M4	inv(16)	NYH11-CBFB
Acute promyelocytic leukemia M3	t(15;17)	PML-RARA
B CELL LEUKEMIAS		
Acute lymphoblastic leukemia (Ph+)	t(9;22)	BCR-ABL
Pre-B Acute lymphoblastic leukemia	t(1;19) t(12;21)	PBX1-E2A, TEL-AML1
T CELL LEUKEMIAS - LYMPHOMAS		
Pre-T Acute lymphoblastic leukemia	t(4 ;11)	NUP98-RAP1GDS1
Anaplastic large cell lymphoma	t(2;5)	NPM-ALK

Diagnosis of hematologic specimens is based first on morphology and use of immunophenotyping and karyotyping. Even though hundreds of recurrent chromosomal rearrangements have been reported in hematologic malignancies, molecular analysis of chromosomal rearrangements is most useful in only a small number of cases, as mentioned before detection of [t (9;22)] in CML and [t (15;17)] in AML is critical and a first step for starting therapy. Search for chromosomal translocations is a useful strategy also when morphologic criteria are inconclusive. Notably besides helping in the diagnosis of difficult cases, molecular detection of chromosomal translocations is a useful and powerful tool in detection of minimal residual disease. Microscopic evaluation of tumor cells in a normal cell background is successful when they are in a relation of at least 1 per 100. PCR based detection of a specific chromosomal fusion product can increase the sensitivity of detection to 1 in 10^7 to 1 in 10^{10} cells significantly broadening microscopic detection [30]. Minimal residual disease diagnosis is clinically relevant for evaluation of treatment in patients with acute lymphoblastic leukemia, by analysis of junctional regions of rearranged immunoglobulin and T cell receptor genes. The technique is complex because the junctional region of each tumor has to be identified before the patient specific assays can be designed for monitoring [31, 32]. These assays have very significant impact in various clinical settings including staging, response to treatment and early relapse.

Table 3: Recurrent chromosomal translocations identified in sarcomas

Tumor	Translocation	Genes Involved
Ewing's sarcoma /	t(11;22)	EWS-FLI1
Peripheral neuroectodermal	t(21;22)	EWS-ERG
tumor	t(7;22)	EWS-ETV1
	t(17,22)	EWS-E1AF
	t(2;22)	EWS-FEV
Synovial sarcoma	t(X;18)	SYT-SSX1
	t(X;18)	SYT-SSX2
	t(X;18)	SYT-SSX4
Alveolar rhabdomyosarcoma	t(2;13)	PAX3-FKHR
	t(1;13)	PAX7-FKHR
Alveolar soft tissuee sarcoma	t(X;17)	ASPL-TFE3
Desmoplastic small round cells tumors	t(11;22)	EWS-WT1
Dermatofibrosarcoma protuberans	t(17;22)	COL1A-PDGFB
Congenital fibrosarcoma	t(12;15)	ETV6-NTRK3
Endometrial stromal sarcoma	t(7;17)	JAZF1-JJAZ1
Myxoid round cell liposarcoma	t(12;16)	TLS-CHOP
	t(12;22)	EWS-CHOP

SARCOMAS

Sarcomas are malignant tumors arising from soft tissues and together with hematologic malignancies represent 10% of all forms of human cancers. Sarcomas are a rare group of tumors with significant morphologic variation and are often difficult to classify. During the last twenty years in a significant group of sarcomas listed in Table **3**, specific and recurrent chromosomal translocations have been identified [33]. These structural chromosomal alterations produce fusion genes involved in pathogenesis and from the point of view of molecular diagnostics comprise useful biomarkers for the diagnosis, as well as detection of minimal residual disease [34]. Similarly to some hematologic chromosomal translocations, fusion genes in sarcomas involve fusion of transcription factors with novel and altered functions, however in contrast to those translocations seen in hematologic malignancies, translocations in sarcomas include the occurrence of alternative variants. The alternative variants share in one of the breakpoints the same gene of the most common variant, but the other component of the breakpoint involves a different gene creating genetic heterogeneity, as is the case of EWS-FLI1 translocation found in Ewing's sarcoma, in which other partners genes of EWS have been described like ERG, ETV1, E1AF and others. In general however, the variant locus is structurally and functionally related to the gene involved in the most common variant [35]. Clinical and pathologic features have been associated with chromosomal fusion variants suggesting that molecular heterogeneity may contribute to phenotypic heterogeneity of these tumors [11] .

CARCINOMAS

Carcinomas account for almost 80% of all human cancers and the number of clinically relevant molecular analyses for these tumors is very limited. Multiple types of genetic alterations have been described and multiple models of oncogenesis proposed. Cytogenetic analyses of different carcinomas show more complex patterns of numerical and structural chromosomal aberrations than those described in hematologic neoplasias, including aneuploidy, polyploidy, insertions, deletions, loss of heterozygocity and point mutations in multiple individual genes, depending on the tumor type [36]. Not all the abnormalities described in carcinomas have been involved in cancer development, and more likely a proportion of such alterations might drive oncogenesis and a proportion might not have oncogenic consequences [37]. Although recurrent chromosomal translocations were thought to occur exclusively in hematologic malignancies, a limited but growing number of epithelial chromosomal translocations in common carcinomas such as thyroid, renal, and prostate among others have been reported recently and are listed in Table **4** [38, 39]. Chromosomal translocations in epithelial tumors constitute only 10% of all chromosomal translocations described, and this disproportion might be more reflective of technical limitations than of their lack of a causal role in carcinomatous carcinogenesis [40]. For a comprehensive list of translocations, genes and cytogenetics in cancer see:

http://cgap.nci.nih.gov/Chromosomes

http://atlasgeneticsoncology.org//index.html

It is expected that novel technological developments such as massive parallel sequencing or gene expression analysis tools such as cancer outlier profile analysis [39], will facilitate the discovery of more chromosomal translocations in carcinomas in the upcoming years.

Table 4: Recurrent chromosomal translocations identified in carcinomas

Tumor	Translocation	Genes involved
Secretory breast carcinoma	t(12;15)	ETV6-NTRK3
Thyroid papillary carcinoma	t(10 ;1)	RET-NTRK1
Follicular thyroid carcinoma	t(2;3)	PAX8-PPARγ
Papillary renal carcinoma	t(X;1)	PRCC-TFE3
Malignant salivary gland tumor	t(3;8)	CTNNB1-PLAG1
Head and neck tumor, midline carcinomas	t(15;19)	BRD4-NUT
Lung adenocarcinoma	t(2;inv2)	EML4-ALK
Prostate cancer	t(21;21)	TMPRSS2-ERG
	t(21;7)	TMPRSS2-ETV1
	t(21;17)	TMPRSS2-ETV4

Another important source of cancer biomarkers in carcinomas has been derived from microarray gene expression analysis specifically in primary breast cancer, through identification of "signatures" associated to clinical outcomes like development of metastasis or survival and thus with prognostic value [41, 42]. From this analysis, a multiparameter gene expression test has been developed with the potential of helping to identify newly diagnosed patients at highest and lowest risk of breast cancer recurrence, though their full clinical utility has yet to be established, and results need to be interpreted with caution. A more significant impact on populations at large from this type of studies might be achieved, if it becomes possible to arrive at a reduced number or even single-marker-test ideally detectable in paraffin tissues using immunohistochemistry with the same predictive value as those gene expression "signatures" based on RNA analyses.

CONCLUSIONS

Technological advances during the last decades have made it possible to uncover the molecular basis of cancer and from this knowledge some examples of remarkable clinical success has been achieved. During this process molecular cancer biomarkers are slowly being developed, translating knowledge into clinical applications that help cancer diagnosis and contribute to better-informed clinical decisions. Emergence of global analyses of gene expression and proteins has yielded long lists of disease-associated molecules, broadening our understanding of tumor biology. Organizing the complex and heterogenous molecular information related to tumor histopathological phenotypes and clinical outcomes into corresponding temporal dimensions is a challenging but attainable goal for molecular pathology for the years to come.

REFERENCES

[1]   Prentice RL. Surrogate and mediating endpoints: current status and future directions. J Natl Cancer Inst 2009; 101(4): 216-7.

[2]   Nevins JR, Potti A. Mining gene expression profiles: expression signatures as cancer phenotypes. Nat Rev Genet 2007; 8(8): 601-9.

[3]   Lapointe J, Li C, Higgins JP, *et al.* Gene expression profiling identifies clinically relevant subtypes of prostate cancer. Proc Natl Acad Sci USA, 2004; 101(3): 811-6.

[4]   Alizadeh AA, Eisen MB, Davis RE. Distinct types of diffuse large B-cell lymphoma identified by gene expression profiling. Nature 2000; 403(6769): 503-11.

[5]   Harris L, Fritsche H, Mennel R. American Society of Clinical Oncology 2007 update of recommendations for the use of tumor markers in breast cancer. J Clin Oncol 2007; 25(33): 5287-312.

[6]   Maloney DG. Immunotherapy for non-Hodgkin's lymphoma: monoclonal antibodies and vaccines. J Clin Oncol 2005; 23(26): 6421-8.

[7]   Fanale MA, Younes A. Monoclonal antibodies in the treatment of non-Hodgkin's lymphoma. Drugs 2007; 67(3): 333-50.

[8]   Van Cutsem E, Köhne CH, Hitre E, *et al.* Cetuximab and chemotherapy as initial treatment for metastatic colorectal cancer. N Engl J Med 2009; 360(14): 1408-17.

[9]   Ross JS, Schenkein DP, Pietrusko R, *et al.* Targeted therapies for cancer 2004. Am J Clin Pathol 2004; 122(4): 598-609.

[10]   Deininger, M.W. and B.J. Druker. Specific targeted therapy of chronic myelogenous leukemia with imatinib. Pharmacol Rev 2003; 55(3): 401-23.

[11]   Kelly KM, Womer RB, Sorensen PH, Xiong QB, Barr FG. Common and variant gene fusions predict distinct clinical phenotypes in rhabdomyosarcoma. J Clin Oncol 1997; 15(5): 1831-6.

[12]   Nambiar, M, Kari V, Raghavan SC. Chromosomal translocations in cancer. Biochim Biophys Acta 2008; 1786(2): 139-52.

[13]   Loman N, Johannsson O, Kristoffersson U, Olsson H, Borg A. Family history of breast and ovarian cancers and BRCA1 and BRCA2 mutations in a population-based series of early-onset breast cancer. J Natl Cancer Inst 2001; 93(16): 1215-23.

[14]   Coe BP, Chari R, Lockwood WW, Lam WL. Evolving strategies for global gene expression analysis of cancer. J Cell Physiol 2008; 217(3): 590-7.

[15]   Garcia-Escudero R, Paramio JM. Gene expression profiling as a tool for basic analysis and clinical application of human cancer. Mol Carcinog 2008; 47(8): 573-9.

[16]   Cho WC, Cheng CH. Oncoproteomics: current trends and future perspectives. Expert Rev Proteomics 2007; 4(3): 401-10.

[17]   Rifai N, Gillette MA, Carr SA. Protein biomarker discovery and validation: the long and uncertain path to clinical utility. Nat Biotechnol 2006; 24(8): 971-83.

[18]   Ludwig JA, Weinstein JN. Biomarkers in cancer staging, prognosis and treatment selection. Nat Rev Cancer 2005; 5(11): 845-56.

[19]   Sawyers CL. The cancer biomarker problem. Nature 2008; 452(7187): 548-52.

[20]   Maniatis T, Fritsch EF, Sambrook J. Molecular Cloning: A Laboratory Manual. 1982, Cold Spring Harbor NY: Cold Spring Harbor Laboratory.

[21]   Orita M, Suzuki Y, Sekiya T, Hayashi K. Rapid and sensitive detection of point mutations and DNA polymorphisms using the polymerase chain reaction. Genomics 1989; 5(4): 874-9.

[22]   Orita M, Iwahana H, Kanazawa H, Hayashi K, Sekiya T. Detection of polymorphisms of human DNA by gel electrophoresis as single-strand conformation polymorphisms. Proc Natl Acad Sci USA 1989; 86(8): 2766-70.

[23]   Murray V. Improved double-stranded DNA sequencing using the linear polymerase chain reaction. Nucleic Acids Res 1989; 17(21): 8889.

[24]   Raimondi SC. Current status of cytogenetic research in childhood acute lymphoblastic leukemia. Blood 1993; 81(9): 2237-51.

[25]   Rowley JD. The role of chromosome translocations in leukemogenesis. Semin Hematol, 1999; 36(4 Suppl 7): 59-72.

[26]   Rabbitts TH. Commonality but diversity in cancer gene fusions. Cell 2009; 137(3): 391-5.

[27]   Maurer J, Janssen JW, Thiel E, *et al.* Detection of chimeric BCR-ABL genes in acute lymphoblastic leukaemia by the polymerase chain reaction. Lancet 1991; 337(8749): 1055-8.

[28]   Kawasaki ES, Clark SS, Coyne MY, *et al.* Diagnosis of chronic myeloid and acute lymphocytic leukemias by detection of leukemia-specific mRNA sequences amplified *in vitro.* Proc Natl Acad Sci USA 1988; 85(15): 5698-702.

[29]   Castaigne S, Balitrand N, de Thé H, *et al.* A PML/retinoic acid receptor alpha fusion transcript is constantly detected by RNA-based polymerase chain reaction in acute promyelocytic leukemia. Blood 1992; 79(12): 3110-5.

[30]   Neale GA, Coustan-Smith E, Stow P, *et al.* Comparative analysis of flow cytometry and polymerase chain reaction for the detection of minimal residual disease in childhood acute lymphoblastic leukemia. Leukemia 2004; 18(5): 934-8.

[31]   van Dongen JJ, Langerak AW, Brüggemann M, *et al.* Design and standardization of PCR primers and protocols for detection of clonal immunoglobulin and T-cell receptor gene recombinations in suspect lymphoproliferations: report of the BIOMED-2 Concerted Action BMH4-CT98-3936. Leukemia 2003; 17(12): 2257-317.

[32]   van der Velden VH, Cazzaniga G, Schrauder A *et al.* Analysis of minimal residual disease by Ig/TCR gene rearrangements: guidelines for interpretation of real-time quantitative PCR data. Leukemia 2007; 21(4): 604-11.

[33]   Leonard DGB. Diagnostic Molecular Pathology. Major Problems in Pathology. 2003, Philadelphia, PA: Saunders.

[34]   Fredericks WJ, Galili N, Mukhopadhyay S *et al.* The PAX3-FKHR fusion protein created by the t(2;13) translocation in alveolar rhabdomyosarcomas is a more potent transcriptional activator than PAX3. Mol Cell Biol 1995; 15(3): 1522-35.

[35]   Davis RJ, Barr FG. Fusion genes resulting from alternative chromosomal translocations are overexpressed by gene-specific mechanisms in alveolar rhabdomyosarcoma. Proc Natl Acad Sci USA 1997; 94(15): 8047-51.

[36]   Aplan PD. Causes of oncogenic chromosomal translocation. Trends Genet 2006; 22(1): 46-55.

[37]   Stratton MR, Campbell PJ, Futreal PA. The cancer genome. Nature 2009; 458(7239): 719-24.

[38]   Aman P. Fusion genes in solid tumors. Semin Cancer Biol 1999; 9(4): 303-18.

[39]   Tomlins SA. Recurrent fusion of TMPRSS2 and ETS transcription factor genes in prostate cancer. Science 2005; 310: 644-8.

[40]   Kumar-Sinha C, Tomlins SA, Chinnaiyan AM. Evidence of recurrent gene fusions in common epithelial tumors. Trends Mol Med 2006; 12(11): 529-36.

[41]   van 't Veer LJ, Dai H, van de Vijver MJ, *et al.* Gene expression profiling predicts clinical outcome of breast cancer. Nature 2002; 415(6871): 530-6.

[42]   Karlsson E, Delle U, Danielsson A, *et al.* Gene expression variation to predict 10-year survival in lymph-node-negative breast cancer. BMC Cancer 2008; 8: 254.

CHAPTER 10

Chemotherapy and Design of New Antineoplastic Compounds

Claudia Rivera-Guevara, María Elena Bravo-Gómez and Lena Ruiz-Azuara[*]

Departamento de Química Inorgánica y Nuclear, Laboratorio de Química Inorgánica Medicinal, Facultad de Química, Universidad Nacional Autónoma de México, Av. Universidad 3000, Ciudad Universitaria, México D.F. 04510, Mexico

Abstract: The successful use of chemotherapy in the treatment of several diseases has been one of the great drug development stories of the last century. Motivated by this, we present here an overview of the various steps required to develop a new drug treatment. An introductory view of the field of medicinal chemistry is provided as an example to a broad discipline that has successfully designed procedures that are routinely used for drug development. A detailed view of the subfield of bioinorganic medicinal chemistry is then presented which describes the research and development involved in the design of new metal-based drugs. A specific example of the development of the CASIOPEINAS® family compounds, a set of copper based molecules is used to illustrate the wide range of strict scientific procedures involved from initial design to the final registration of the drug.

Keywords: Medicinal chemistry, chemotherapy, drug design, drug develop, drug testing, bioinorganic chemistry, metal compounds, copper compounds, antineoplastic, casiopeínas®.

INTRODUCTION

Paul Erhlich coined the term "chemotherapy" for the use of a known chemical that treated parasites. From 1903 to 1915 he devoted most of his time to the development of chemotherapeutic agents, using similar procedures to those used nowadays to identify anticancer drugs [1]. He emphasized the value of animal models, using diseased specimens to study the effects of drug treatment. Around 1900 such models existed only for infectious diseases, shortly after mice were infected with tubercle bacillus and pneumococci, mice and rats with trypanosomes, and rabbits with syphilis. With the development of organic chemistry and the support of the pharmaceutical industry, Erhlich was able to synthesize a large series of arsenic compounds, finding that number 606th was active, not only against trypanosome infections, but also against rabbit syphilis. This drug was called salvarsan (the savior of mankind) and was the first man-made chemical found to be effective in the fight of human parasitic diseases.

The use of chemotherapy for cancer started as a treatment for metastases. The ability to cure cancer depends of course on many variables due to its own etiology. The need for chemotherapy arose out of the appreciation that cancer was not a localized process, thus not amenable to control by the commonly used regional procedures [2]. The hypothesis that chemical compounds might be effectively used in the treatment of cancer was not received with great enthusiasm despite the successful use of synthetic chemicals and natural products against parasitic, common bacterial infections and tuberculosis. It is important to highlight that there are two types of drugs used in the treatment of any disease, those that suppress the symptoms but fail to remove the cause at the heart of the disease and those that cure [3]. The use of drugs against malaria was considered as the beginning of curative drug therapy but despite its success the possibility that chemotherapy could cure cancer was taken with great pessimism [4].

Paul Erhlich, in opposition to all efforts, at the start of the 20th century began a research program in drug development for cancer treatment. Not only was he a visionary but also approached research with defiance, as clearly illustrated by the banner above the entrance of his laboratory that read *"Abandone all hope all you who enter here"*. His research investments paid off in 1898, when he discovered the first alkylating agent although it took nearly 50 years before it was successfully applied to the treatment of neoplastic diseases in humans [1].

[*]**Address correspondence to Lena Ruiz-Azuara:** Departamento de Química Inorgánica y Nuclear, Laboratorio de Química Inorgánica Medicinal, Facultad de Química, Universidad Nacional Autónoma de México, Av. Universidad 3000, Ciudad Universitaria, México D.F. 04510; e-mail: ruizazuara@gmail.com

The research of cancer treatment dramatically evolved at the turn of the century as a result of three fundamental works. The first was the development of cancer surgery leading Halsted, in 1894, to propose the use of *en-block* resection as part of cancer treatment, particularly in a radical mastectomy. Around the same time, Roentgen, with the discovery of X-ray radiation, gave physicians an alternative method for treating localized cancer. The third advance had its roots in the work of Paul Erhlich, who used rodent models for infectious diseases and gave George Clowes from Roswell Park Memorial Institute in Buffalo, the foundations to develop in the early 1900's inbred rodent lines that could carry transplanted tumors [1]. These models and others have since then served as the testing ground for potential cancer chemotherapy agents. Alkylating agents were developed as a result of the secret gas warfare program in both world wars. During this time, several observations were made for particular agents that caused marrow and lymphoid hypoplasia, which led to the use of these chemicals to treat lymphomas, although later the remission of tumors was observed. Recently, the work of Farber on the effect of folic acid on leukemic cell growth in children with lymphoblastic leukemia and the development of the antifols as cancer drugs has firmly illustrated the potential of chemotherapy in the treatment of cancer [2]

MEDICINAL CHEMISTRY

The search for new drugs in the context of chemotherapy help developed the field of medicinal chemistry, a discipline centered on the design and synthesis of novel drugs [5].

In medicinal chemistry the drugs are defined as low molecular weight chemicals that interact with macromolecular targets in the body. A benefic effect is then produced depending primarily on the level of the dose, administration route and schedule. These drugs are, in general, classified according to their pharmacological effect, the particular biochemical process they affect, the type of structures they formed, or the molecular target with which they interact [5].

In order to understand how drugs operate it is necessary to first learn how they interact with the molecular target in the body (pharmacodynamics) and how they are capable of reaching it (pharmacokinetics). It is also important to keep in mind that a drug currently on the market is the result of a long process, which requires huge time commitment and substantial financial investment. The journey from inception to production can be divided into three stages: drug design, drug testing and finally drug development. It is to these three different processes that we now turn our attention.

I. Drug Discovery

Most medicinal chemistry projects start by identifying a drug target. Specific tests are performed and several proposed targets are discussed based on their chemical properties, searching primarily for a compound with the desired biological properties. Once an active compound is identified, new molecular modifications are performed in order to improve its properties (drug design).

Before any medicinal chemistry project can get underway, a lead compound is required. A lead compound will be identified based on some particular property that is considered to be therapeutically useful. Compound identification is the starting point when designing a new drug. Lead compounds can be obtained from natural or synthetic sources and maybe designed using computer modeling or NMR studies [Nuclear Magnetic Resonance].

Lead Compounds from Natural Sources

The natural world provides us with an unlimited source of potentially effective lead compounds. Evolution has resulted in the selection of potent biologically active structures, which serve a wide range of purposes in nature. Many such compounds are secondary metabolites, which are produced in mature organisms. Natural sources provide highly diverse and structurally unique lead compounds. However, it takes time to isolate them from their natural source, and the lead compounds are often complex in structure to be easily synthesized. A few examples of commonly used compounds derived from natural sources are given below.

Flora: Plants and trees are a traditional source of biologically active compounds, which routinely serve as lead compounds, or as medicines in their own right. A few examples are taxanes [6], vinca-alkaloids [7], and campothecynes [8]. Historical records (Ethnobotanics) often provide clues as to which plants are worth studying; however, many plant species in ecologically diverse areas have never been analyzed at all [9, 10].

Animals: Venoms and toxins are a source of useful lead compounds. Their potency often indicates strong interactions with important molecular targets in the body. Studying those interactions has proven very useful in designing drugs that will effectively target specific molecular sites [11, 12].

Microorganisms: Microorganisms have provided metabolites that are useful antibiotics but have also been used as lead compounds for the development of other antibacterial agents. Fungal metabolites have also been used. For example, penicillin [13], cephalosporin [14], ergometrine [15] and the statins [16] are well known fungal secondary metabolites known to have a wide spectrum of biological activities and are commonly employed in treatments in various fields of medicine.

Marine Chemistry: Many biologically active compounds have been isolated from fish, coral, sponges, and marine microorganisms. Marine chemistry is a promising source of new lead compounds, primary due to their unexplored nature. The cone shell venom peptides (conotoxins) [17], for example, have been recently used to effectively treat neuropathic pain.

Human Biochemistry: Neurotransmitters, hormones, and enzyme substrates are all potential lead compounds [18]. A rational design inspired by human biochemistry has led to synthesize drugs for diverse therapeutic uses. One famous example is triamcinolone, a synthetic corticosteroid used to treat several medical conditions, such as rheumatoid arthritis.

Lead Compounds from Synthetic Sources

Synthetic compounds may prove useful as lead compounds, regardless of whether they are synthesized with a therapeutic aim or not. Generaly are molecules with some similarity to an active one.

Combinatorial Synthesis: This method involves the automated or semi-automated synthesis of compounds using solid phase synthetic techniques. Far more compounds can be synthesized in a particular time period using this method than by conventional synthetic ones and so the odds of finding a lead compound are greatly increased.

Compound Data Banks/Libraries: Pharmaceutical companies have synthesized a number of compounds and synthetic intermediates over the years. These are stored, and referred to, as compound Banks or libraries. Such storages are not just for historical purposes but serve as useful databases for potential lead compounds. Pharmaceutical companies, for example, are constantly coming up with potentially new targets as a result of studying the various genome projects that are mapping the DNA of humans and other organisms. Once a new target is discovered, a search for a lead compound that will have some affinity with the specific target has to be made. Many compounds that have been synthesized in the past have been proven to have affinity with specific targets and are thus worth studying. The advantage in using compound Banks is that they provide us with a broad source of readily available structures that can be quickly tested on a new target. The disadvantage is that they often lack structural diversity since companies often synthesize hundreds if not thousands of compounds based solely on the structure of one primary lead compound.

II. Drug Design

Once a lead compound is identified, analogs are synthesized and tested in order to identify structural features that are important for the initially observed activity (pharmacophore). These features are retained during the design of analogs with often improved pharmacodynamic and pharmacokinetic properties. Cisplatin, cisplatinum, or cis-diamminedichloroplatinum (II) (CDDP) is the first members of a class of inorganic anti-cancer drugs. Analogs were then subsequently designed with the aim of reducing the adverse effects of the lead compound, while retaining or improving its therapeutic properties: carboplatin and oxaliplatin [19].

The Pharmacophore

The pharmacophore of drugs defines the important functional groups required for binding or activity, and their relative positions or active conformation, which defines the topography adopted by a drug when it binds to a target site. Detailed knowledge of the active conformation is vital before the pharmacophore of a specific drug can be defined.

Target-based Pharmacophores: If the structure of the binding site is known, it is possible to define a pharmacophore based on the amino acid residues present in the binding site. Molecular modeling can be used to define what types of groups are required to bind to the available amino acids and where should they be positioned.

Pharmacophore and Substructure Searches: Novel lead compounds are always in demand, whether they are intended for a specific drug target that has just been discovered, or for an established target that has had several other drugs designed to interact with it. In the latter case, it is common for a pharmaceutical company and their competitors to make literally thousands of analogs of an established lead compound and to relentlessly investigate the particular structural class of compounds at hand. Eventually, there comes a time when progress through this route becomes difficult. Alternatively, a competitor may have impeded further investigation in the field through the establishment of various patents. In such circumstances, the search for a new lead compound having a totally different kind of structure that will interact with the same target provides the only way forward. If such a structure is found, it then allows the company to devise novel alternatives that avoid similarities with currently existing groups of compounds.

Binding Interactions in Drugs Design

Drugs normally bind to their targets by using intermolecular bonding forces such as ionic bonding, hydrogen bonding, Van der Waals interactions, and dipole-dipole interactions although some drugs may form covalent bonds (Table **1**).

Functional Groups as Binding Groups

Functional groups are important in binding drugs to a specific target. Preparing analogs can test the relevance of a functional group to a specific binding. The analog can then be tested to see whether activity has been increased or lost. Some strategies to design specific structures within binding groups or to figure out whether a functional group is crucial or not for molecular recognition are cited in Table **1**; many other functional groups (miscellaneous groups) are present in drugs for reasons other than binding. For example, some functional groups are used to modify the electronic properties of a drug while others are used as metabolic blockers or conformational restraints (Table **2**).

Table 1: Chemical interaction in drug design

Weak Interactions	Strong Interactions
Hydrogen bonding: Hydrogen bonding results from interactions between an electrophilic hydrogen on one molecule (the hydrogen bond donor) and an electronegative atom (the hydrogen bond acceptor) on another. The interaction is weaker than that of an ionic bond, but is still important in drug-target interactions.	**Covalent bonds:** Some drugs form covalent bonds to their targets. Alkylating agents react with nucleophilic groups such as serine, cysteine and guanine leading to the formation of a covalent bond and the irreversible inhibition of the target. Some enzyme inhibitors undergo a normal enzyme-catalyzed mechanism and form a reaction intermediate which is covalently linked to the active site.
Van der Waals interactions: Van der Waals interactions are weak interactions that occur between hydrophobic groups such as aromatic rings and alkyl chains. They arise due to the random fluctuations in electron density leading to transient regions that are electron rich or electron poor.	**Ionic bonding:** Ionic bonds are formed between groups of opposite charge and are important for many drug-target interactions. Many of the body's own chemical messengers interact through ionic bonding.
Dipole-dipole interactions: Dipole-dipole moments may be important in orientating a molecule when it enters a specific binding site. The dipole moment of the drug may align itself with localized dipole moments present in the binding site. If the alignment is such that the binding groups are correctly positioned, then the drug is more likely to bind and subsequently induce activity.	

Bioinorganic Chemistry

The discipline of bioinorganic chemistry aims to elucidate the mechanisms by which metal ions (usually transition metals) aid biological processes [20, 21]. As a consequence of this knowledge, inorganic chemistry offers many opportunities for medicinal chemistry. As a result of advances in bioinorganic chemistry, the discovery of metal-based drugs has moved from chance discovery, as it was the case of antineoplastic drug CDDP, to rational drug design, as in the case of Fosrenol, which was approved by FDA in 2004 for the treatment of hyperphosphatemia [22].

Metal ions exhibit interesting reactivity and spectroscopic properties as well as diverse binding modes and a great variety of geometries. Carbon, the most widely used element in drug design today, can only generate a fairly limited number of geometries. Despite its simplicity, Carbon has allowed the design of an incredible large number of different molecules bearing effective therapeutic properties.

By contrast, metal ions can create either labile or inert bonds with coordination numbers ranging from one to twelve, and with numerous geometries. This simple fact suggests that metal ions can be used to construct therapeutic molecules whose shapes and structures would be impossible if not extremely difficult to replicate using carbon-based compounds. The judicious choice of ligands provides molecular reconnaissance as well as adequate tuning of reactivity and solubility properties, thus resulting in a very broad spectrum of therapeutic uses.

Table 2: Functional groups in drugs design

Hydrogen bond	*Alcohols and phenols:* Alcohols and phenols are capable of acting as hydrogen bond donors or acceptors. The functional groups can be converted to ethers or esters to determine whether they can act as such. *Ketones and aldehydes:* A carbonyl group can interact by dipole-dipole interactions or as a hydrogen bond acceptor. Reduction to an alcohol and its subsequent conversion to an ether or ester could be used to test whether the group is important or not. *Esters:* Esters could act as hydrogen bond acceptors. However, they are usually present in drugs to 'mask' polar groups such as alcohols, phenols or carboxylic acids. *Amides:* Amides could interact with binding sites by acting as hydrogen bond donors or acceptors. Hydrolysis of the amide is easy to carry out in this case, but will likely split the drug in two if the amide is a vital part of the skeletal backbone. N-methylation of a secondary amide could also provide information regarding its importance as a binding group.
Hydrophobic interactions	*Alkenes and aromatic rings*: Alkenes and aromatic rings are planar hydrophobic groups that are likely to interact by van der Waals interactions with hydrophobic pockets or planar regions in the binding site. Reducing either group would result in a bulkier group that is unlikely to interact efficiently. *Alkyl groups*: Alkyl groups can act as important binding groups if they form van der Waals interactions with hydrophobic regions present in the binding site. Varying the size of the groups helps determining the extension of the hydrophobic region.
Ionic interactions	*Carboxylic acids*: Carboxylic acids can interact with binding sites by either ionic bonding or as hydrogen bond donors or acceptors. Conversion of a carboxylic acid to an ester could prevent ionic or hydrogen bond donor interactions. The steric bulk of the ester may also hinder the ability of the group for acting as a hydrogen bond acceptor. *Amines:* Amines may be ionized or unionized. In an ionized form, they could interact with carboxylate groups. In a unionized state, they can interact as hydrogen bond donors or acceptors. Conversion to an amide is expected to disrupt their bonding ability. *Quaternary ammonium salts*: Quaternary ammonium salts can interact with negatively charged carboxylate groups through ionic bonding. Alternatively can interact with aromatic rings by induced dipole interactions. The importance of such interactions could be explores by synthesizing analogs where the quaternary ammonium group is replaced with an amine or an amide.
Covalent bonding	*Alkyl halides:* Alkyl halides are reactive groups that can interact with nucleophiles present in proteins and nucleic acids. Nucleophilic substitution results in a covalent bond between the macromolecule and the drug. Alkyl fluorides are nonreactive. Fluorine is often introduced to affect the electronic properties of the drug, or as a metabolic blocker. *Thiols:* Thiols are often found in drugs that interact with zinc metalloproteinases. The thiol groups can form a strong bond to the zinc ion. Methylation or oxidation of the thiol group usually causes a dramatic fall in activity.

Structure-Activity Relationships

The goal of medicinal chemists is to create molecules with a specific set of desired properties. However, the lack of deterministic procedures and inherent empiricism, which is at the core of new drug discovery, has made drug discovery an extremely challenging process. Both trial and error synthesis of compounds and their random screening for activity has proved to be extremely time consuming and not cost effective.

Table 3: Representative list of common descriptors used in quantitative structure–property relationship

Solubility	**Topological**
Molar solubility (S)	Wiener index (W)
Mole fraction solubility (X)	Randic indices
Activity coefficients (Log gw)	Kier and Hall connectivity indices (*X*)
Hildebrand solubility parameters (dH)	Kier shape index
	Kier flexibility index
Lipophilic	Balaban index (J)
Log Po/w	Information content (IC) indices
Log D	Kappa shape indices
Rm (TLC)	Topological complexities
Log k9, LogKw (RPLC)	Eccentric connectivity index
Hansch substituent	Detour index
constant (p)	
Rekker's fragmental	**Geometrical**
constant (f)	Principle moments of inertia
	Molecular volume
Electronic	Molecular surface area
Ionization constant (pKa)	Shadow indices
Hammett constant (d)	Solvent accessible molecular surface area
Taft polar constant (d*)	Gravitation index
Taft inductive and resonance components (d1, dR)	
Dipole moments	**Electrostatic**
Hydrogen bonding parameters	Maximum and minimum partial charges in the molecule
	Polarity parameters
Steric	Charged partial surface area (CPSA) descriptors
Taft steric parameter (Es)	
Molar refractivity (MR)	**Quantum-Chemical**
Parachor	Charge distribution-related descriptors
Charton steric parameter (y)	HOMO-LUMO energies
van der Waal's parameters	Orbital electron densities
	Superdelocalizabilities
Constitutional	Atom–atom polarizabilities
Total number of atoms	Molecular polarizabilities
Number of individual types of atoms	Quantum molecular energies
Total number of bonds	
Number of individual types of bonds	**Miscellaneous**
Number of rings	Chemical shifts: 1H, 13C (dppm)
Molecular weight	IR frequencies (v)
Average atomic weight	Surface tension

Structure-based design, as a result, has now been accepted as a rational approach for the generation of new pharmaceuticals, where analogs of a lead compound are synthesized and tested to see how structural variations affect their activity. This procedure is usually implemented by creating either Structure-Activity Relationships (SAR) or Quantitative Structure-Activity Relationships (QSAR). The first one relies on the principle of similarity, and the second one, aims to derive a quantitative mathematical model of the activity. In both cases, the results aim to identify groups that are important to binding interactions and promote activity.

The conclusions drawn from SAR studies are sensitive on the test procedures that are used. *In vitro* testing can help determine the key structural features required for binding interactions as well as the cellular effects resulting from them. *In vivo* tests can help elucidate the structural features that are responsible for the overall physiological activity. These tests take pharmacokinetics into account as well as the effectiveness of binding.

QSAR involve the construction of a mathematical formalism, which relates the biological activity of compounds with their physicochemical properties.

There are several methods used to perform QSAR studies, which are based mainly on the number and type of structural modifications. Traditional QSAR studies are carried out on a range of analogs sharing a common skeleton but having different substituents.

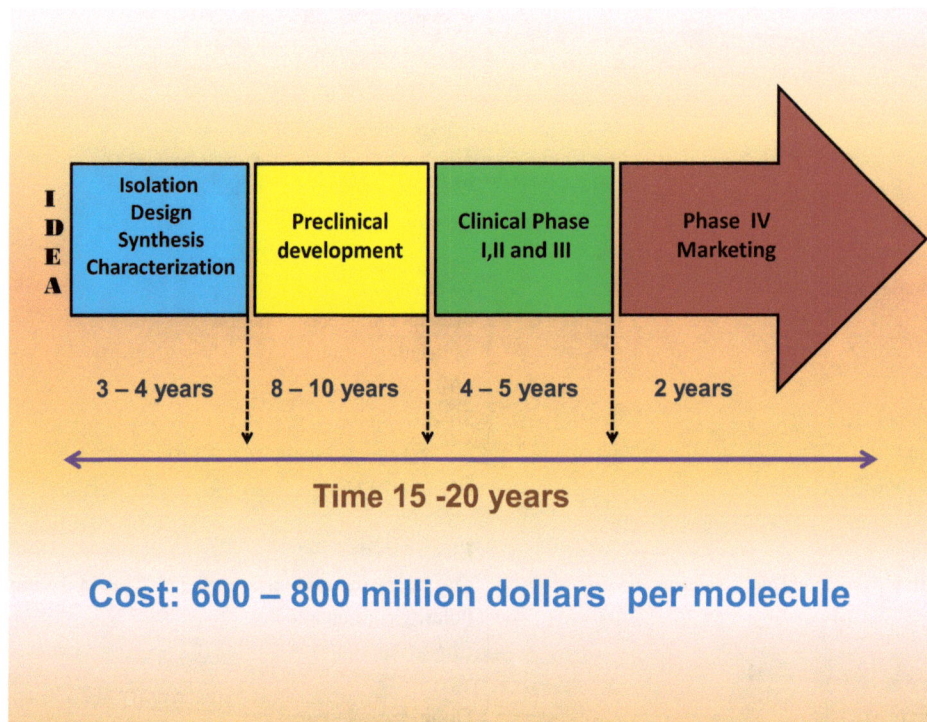

Figure 1: General diagram illustrating a typical drug development procedure.

Classical QSAR methods describe structure-activity relationships in terms of physicochemical parameters and steric properties (Hansch analysis, extrathermodynamic approach), certain structural features (Free Wilson analysis) or both (mixed approach). An initial QSAR equation relates biological activity to one or two physical properties. This equation can then be expanded by adding relationships to other physical features (Table **3**). 3D QSAR methods, especially Comparative Molecular Field Analysis (CoMFA), take into account three-dimensional structures and the binding modes of protein ligands. 3D QSAR is not restricted to compounds having the same skeleton and can be used for molecules sharing a common pharmacophore, or for molecules that bind to the same site.

III. Drug Testing and Development

New drugs should always be patented as quickly as possible. Pre-clinical trials are then carried out later to assess the properties and safety of the newly developed drug. If these prove satisfactory, clinical trials are subsequently carried out (Fig. **1**).

The development of a large-scale synthesis proceeds in parallel to the biological testing. Regulatory authorities are then finally responsible for approving drugs for clinical trials and the market place [23, 24].

Testing A Lead Compound

In order to search for lead compounds, a suitable test is required. This could involve, for example, a test that helps reveal a specific effect. It could be a physiological effect on a tissue preparation, organ or test animal, a cellular effect resulting from the interaction of a lead compound with a particular target (such as a receptor or an enzyme) or, alternatively, it could be a molecular effect, such as the binding of a compound with a receptor. In the last two situations, the molecular target can be important to a particular disease state, and in such cases, the lead compound may not have the desired physiological activity at all. For example, there have been several instances where the natural agonist for a receptor was used as the lead compound for an antagonist. Here the crucial property for the lead compound was that it should be recognizable and bound to the binding site of the target receptor. The lead compound was then modified to bind as an antagonist rather than as an agonist. For example, the chemical messenger histamine was used as the lead compound in developing the anti-ulcer agent cimetidine. Histamine is an agonist that activates histamine receptors in the stomach wall to increase gastric acid release. Cimetidine acts as an antagonist at these receptors, thus reducing the levels of gastric acid released and allowing the body to heal from the ulcer.

Biological Testing Drugs

Relevant tests are required to test the activity and selectivity of compounds against specific targets. *In vivo* tests involve the use of live animals, whereas *in vitro* tests do not. *In vitro* tests are more suitable for routine testing. However, they are incapable in assessing how effectively a drug might reach its target in a living organism. They also usually cannot predict how the drug will act after it is metabolized. The test can then give negative results for drugs, which need to be metabolized in order to become the biological active compound (prodrugs). In addition, they are also incapable in predicting whether the metabolite might be toxic or not. *In vivo* tests are thus important in demonstrating the physiological effects of a drug.

In vitro **tests:** *In vitro* tests can be carried out on isolated enzymes, cells, tissues and organs; sometimes they can employ physical methods in order to detect the binding ability to proteins, DNA or other biomolecules, in particular when this binding triggers a biological response. Some representative examples of *in vitro* tests are cited bellow:

a) **Enzyme inhibition:** Enzyme kinetics can be used to determine whether a drug is acting as a competitive or noncompetitive inhibitor. The strength of an inhibitor is measured by its IC_{50} value, which is the concentration of the inhibitor required to reduce enzyme activity by 50% [25, 26].

b) **Receptor studies:** Receptor studies are carried out using cells, tissue cultures, tissue preparations or isolated organs. Both affinity and efficacy can be measured. Affinity is the strength by which compounds bind to the receptor. Affinity can be measured using radio ligand labeling techniques. The extent to which the test compound inhibits the binding of a radio ligand is measured and its position within the Scatchard plot reveals whether the test compound prevents radio ligand binding competitively or noncompetitively [27]. In this case, the IC_{50} value for the test compound is the concentration of compound that prevents 50% of the radioactive ligand being bound.

Efficacy is the strength of cellular or biochemical response resulting from receptor binding. Drugs with a strong affinity do not necessarily have a strong efficacy. Cells and tissue cultures are useful for studying the biochemical effects of receptor activation, while tissue preparations and organs are useful for measuring certain physiological effects. Efficacy is thus a measure of the biochemical or physiological effect resulting from the binding of a drug to its target, and measures the maximum effect a drug can produce. Its potency is defined as the concentration of agonist required to produce 50% of the maximum possible effect. Schield analysis is then used to determine the dissociation constant (K_d) of a competitive antagonist.

c) **Microbiological testing:** Antibacterial agents are tested *in vitro* by studying how effectively they kill or inhibit the growth of bacterial strains [28]. *In vivo* tests measure how effectively the agent clears up an infection in a test animal.

d) **High throughput screening:** High throughput screening involves the rapid screening of compounds on an automated, small-scale basis. Genetically engineered cells are normally used so that any effect arising from the interaction of a drug with an enzyme or receptor is easily discernable. In this case, the desired effect can be accurately measured [29].

e) **Testing by NMR spectroscopy:** Nuclear Magnetic Resonance (NMR) spectroscopy can detect whether or not a specific compound binds to a target protein [30]. Spectra are calculated such that molecules with short relaxation times (*i.e.* large molecules) are not detected if the test compound binds to the protein, its signatures in the spectrum will then not be observed.

f) **Other specific *in vitro* tests**: When an interaction with a specific biomolecule is directly related to the biological effect, physical methods can then be employed as screening tests. For some chemotherapeutic agents employed as antineoplastic drugs, the interaction with DNA is usually a required step in the action mode [31]. Interaction with DNA can be measured using by a broad range of techniques that use covalent and no-covalent bindings. Useful examples of these techniques are spectroscopic titration, thermal denaturation, DNA viscosity measuremnts, molecular fluorescence, Atomic Force Microscopy (AFM) and in the case of metal complexes the metallation of DNA measured by atomic absortion techniques.

Another example of a physical method employed as a screening test is the inhibition of hemozoin formation. This process is essential for the survival of malaria parasite and it is found to be absent in the host. In consequence, it is an attractive drug target for antimalarian drugs such as quinolines, which bind to free heme preventing the formation of hemozoin disposal products produced by malaria parasites thus leading to a clear toxic response [32]. The formation of beta-hematin (hemozoin) can be monitored by IR spectrum or UV spectrum by the interaction method in the n-octanol/acetate buffer interface.

Testing drugs *in vivo*: *In vivo* testing is essential to establish whether a candidate drug can reach its intended target in a living organism, have the desired physiological effect, and have no undesirable side effects. Both normal and transgenic animals (animals that have been genetically modified) are used for *in vivo* tests and it is important to understand any biochemical differences between species when carrying out these tests. Two important parameters that can be obtained using *in vivo* tests are drug potency and therapeutic ratio/index [33].

a) **Drug potency:** Drug potency is the concentration of drug required to produce 50% of the maximum desired effect.

b) **Therapeutic ratio/index:** The therapeutic ratio (or index) compares the dose level of a drug required to produce a desired effect in 50% of a sample test (ED_{50}) versus the dose level that is lethal to 50% of the sample (LD_{50}).

Preclinical Testing

Once a molecule with promising biological properties is selected for development, it is necessary to perform several tests before reaching clinical testing. The preclinical testing stage has as a first goal to understand the safety properties of the drug in order to allowsafe human studies. The preclinical testing includes toxicity testing, pharmacokinetics, pharmacodynamics and drug metabolism studies. Usually two species are required, the most used are canine and murine models but the selection of the species must be based on which correlates better with the effects on humans.

Toxicity Studies

The aim of these studies is to evaluate the side effects that could be generated by a new compound. Due to the ethical constraints on performing toxicity tests in humans, relevant safety assessment has been studied in laboratory animals, although extrapolation of risk assessment from animals to human is still challenging. Toxicity tests are classified in two types according to the duration of the study and the type of side effects.

a) **Short-term toxicology:** These tests, acute or sub-acute, are carried out on animals to identify what dose levels lead to toxic effects with a single dose or during short periods of exposition. The results are used to determine safe dose levels for clinical trials.

b) **Long-term toxicology:** these tests are carried out to test a drug searching for chronic toxicity such as carcinogenicity, mutagenicity, reproduction abnormalities and toxicity to specific organs that are targeted by that drug.

Drug Metabolism Studies

Pharmacokinetics studies of a novel compound are an important part of the corpus of knowledge required to understand the safety and efficacy. They are also essential to guarantee effective duration of action and help selection of the appropriate route of administration. In a drug discovery program, accurate pharmacokinetic and metabolic data of the drug must be available as early as the results of *in vitro* biological screening are ready.

An understanding of the kinetics of active metabolite formation is important not only for predicting the therapeutic outcome, but it is also necessary for assessing toxic effects of metabolites arising from the novel compounds. Many of the currently available drugs have one or more metabolites with biological activity, whether pharmacological or toxic. The specific metabolite may differ in distribution and clearance from the parent drug. One common method for studying the metabolism of a drug is the labeling study, in which radio labeled drugs are used to detect any drug metabolites formed. The isotopes that are commonly used for labeling studies are heavy isotopes such as deuterium and carbon-13, and radioactive isotopes such as tritium and carbon-14. A labeling synthesis should be designed so that the isotopic label is incorporated as late as possible into the synthesis.

Formulation Studies

Formulation studies are carried out to establish a particular dosage preparation, such as a pill or capsule, which will be consistent in its properties and will contain a specific level of the drug. Pharmacokinetics knowledge is necessary to select the adequate formulation of a drug and usually these studies are performed simultaneously. In the other hand, the stability of a drug preparation must be studied under various conditions of temperature, humidity and light. Containers must be used which do not interact with the preparation. Stability tests help to establish the shield life of the preparation, and the storage conditions that should be used.

Clinical Trials

Clinical trials are carried out to test the therapeutic effects of new drugs and to ensure that they have no unacceptable side effects. Safety and efficacy are the main goals and trials are conducted anywhere between one and four phases. Depending on the type of drug and stage of development, healthy volunteers or patients are enrolled (Fig. **2**).

The number of patients is increased as the various clinical phases are implemented, therefore the cost is considerable and a sponsor, usually the government or a pharmaceutical industry, is required.

Phase I: These trials are normally carried out on healthy volunteers to establish dosing levels, and to carry out pharmacokinetic studies although therapeutic effects are usually not tested. Special groups of volunteers may be tested if the drug is likely to be targeted specifically to that population. Drugs with strong side effects as those designed to treat cancer can be tested in terminal phase patients in order to establish secure dose levels.

Phase II: These studies are carried out on patients suffering from the disease that the drug was intended to treat. One group of patients receives the drug and another group receives a placebo or a conventional drug. Neither patient nor doctor knows which patient receives the placebo or the drug. Different dose levels and strategies are then used on different groups to establish the best dosing regimen. These studies demonstrate whether or not the drug is therapeutically useful and whether or not it produces any appreciable side effects.

Phase III: These studies similar to phase II studies but are carried out on a larger number of patients in order to increase statistical validity, both for the drug's efficacy and its safety.

Phase IV: These studies continue after the drug has been marketing. They are designed to study the effects of long-term use and to identify any rare side effects that may arise, better known as pharmacovigilancy.

DRUG DEVELOPMENT FOR NEW ANTINEOPLASTIC COMPOUNDS

I. Metal Compound in Chemotherapy

Currently there are about 48 anticancer drugs registered for clinical use worldwide, but thousands of experimental drugs have been synthesized or extracted from natural products. Only 3 out of 48 are metal based drugs (cisplatin

(CDDP), carboplatin and oxaliplatin) [34]. Recently, however, several metal-containing agents (gallium, germanium, tin and bismuth), early-transition metals complexes (titanium, vanadium, niobium, molybdenum and rhenium) and late-transition metal complexes (ruthenium, rhodium, iridium, copper and gold) have all shown to have some potential for chemotherapy.

The most prominent discovery in metal-containing therapeutics is the cisplatin (*cis*-diamminedichloroplatinum(II), *cis*-DDP, CDDP). Over the years, researchers have dedicated huge efforts to design analogues which surpass the pharmacological properties of platinum compounds in use such as carboplatin and oxaliplatin [35, 36]. Despite such efforts, many antitumor compounds with high activity level and promising properties have failed to reach the clinic phases. This is because of their deficient physicochemical properties and unsuccessful pharmaceutical implementations as well as the complexity in controlling their selective toxicity or pharmacological properties.

Four decades of research in this field have only produced a small number of clinically applied compounds, most often developed through serendipity, as CDDP, rather than through rational chemical design. However, the medicinal inorganic chemistry has acquired in recent years enough knowledge to make significant advances in the field, moving from serendipity to rational drug design through a variety of approaches. Several research groups have started to search new anticancer metal-based drugs mainly focusing on those of platinum, especially analogs of cisplatin, and on DNA targeting [37]. Recent progress in the field of cell biology and cancer research has also allowed the discovery of receptors and growth factors that are up-regulated in cancer cells and can be exploited as new targets for anticancer drug design. These employ thiol containing proteins and redox processes [22] as alternative targets in order to activate the drugs selectively in the tumor by using either cellular processes or by controlled external activation such as light activation [38, 39].

II. Copper Compounds Design

The cytotoxic activity of a metal complex, which is closely related to its antitumor activity, is controlled by the identity of a metal, its oxidation state and the properties of its coordination ligands. However, in many cases only one of them dominates. Gianferrara *et al.* [40] have, for example, suggested a categorization of metal anticancer compounds that is independent of the nature of its bio-target(s) and is based solely on the role of the metal. Their classification scheme is based on the mode of action of the metal and gives rise to five different classes:

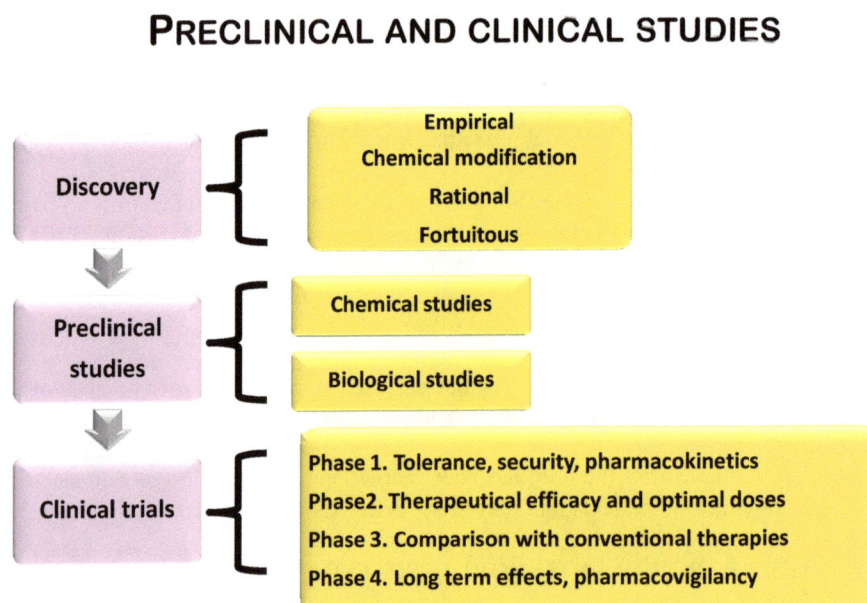

Figure 2: A drug development diagram is shown in which the various clinical phases are detailed.

i. The metal has a functional role, *i.e.* it must bind to the biological target as CDDP.

ii. The metal has a specific structural role, *i.e.* it is instrumental in determining the shape of the compound. In this case, binding to the biological target occurs through non-covalent interactions [41], as the inhibitor of glycogen synthase kinase 3b [Ru(Cp)(CO)].

iii. The metal is a carrier for active ligands that are delivered *in vivo* such as Cu(II) complexes of Non-Steroidal Antiinflammatorydrugs (NSAIDs) [42].

iv. The metal compound is a catalyst, *i.e.* organometallic half-sandwich Ru(II) compounds [(η^6-arene)-Ru(azpy)I]+ (azpy = *N,N*-dimethylphenyl-azopyridine, arene = *p*-cymene or biphenyl) [43].

v. The metal compound is photoactive and behaves as a photo-sensitizer, *i.e.* strong photo-oxidants $[Ru(L)_3]^{2+}$ or $[Os(L)_3]^{2+}$ complexes acting with a good π-acceptor polyazaaromatic L Ligands [44, 45].

The elements mentioned above have been used extensively in the synthesis and characterization of a series of compounds designed with specific structural characteristics that are likely to lead to antitumor activity. In this specific case, Copper was chosen as the preferred metal because is an essential element in several physiological functions. This argument was used to justify the design of new antitumoral compounds which could diminish toxic effects, besides chelates were used that favor the cis-configuration around the metal ion. Finally the mixed chelates should present different degree of hydrophobicity to favor the absorption and distribution properties. A more in depth review of metal compounds for cancer chemotherapy can be found in [46].

III: The Proposal for a New Antineoplastic: Casiopeínas®

The mixed chelate copper(II) complexes, whose general formula is described by [Cu(N-N)(O-O)]NO$_3$ or [Cu(N-N)(O-N)]NO$_3$, have been patented and registered under the name of CASIOPEINAS® [47-49]. CASIOPEINAS® have been fully characterized by analytical methods and their structures have been resolved by X-ray diffraction techniques [50-58] (Fig. 3). The chemical and structural data reported so far show that the copper (II) center in this type of ternary complexes is placed in a slightly distorted square planar geometry [52-55, 57, 58].

In these compounds, the selected ligands were substituted: 2,2'-bipyridines (bpy) and 1,10-phenanthrolines (phen), they both are nitrogen-donor bidentate ligands with a relatively high affinity [59-61] with copper. Their extended aromatic ring system allows these ligands to bind to DNA by intercalative and non-intercalative interactions either as free ligands or in metal complexes [62-64]. L-amino acids were chosen as secondary ligands based on their affinity with (bpy) and (phen) copper(II) complexes [60, 61] as well as for their low toxicity. Finally, salal and acac ligands have also good affinity with (phen)copper(II) complexes [60, 65] and might help modulate the redox properties of the metal center.

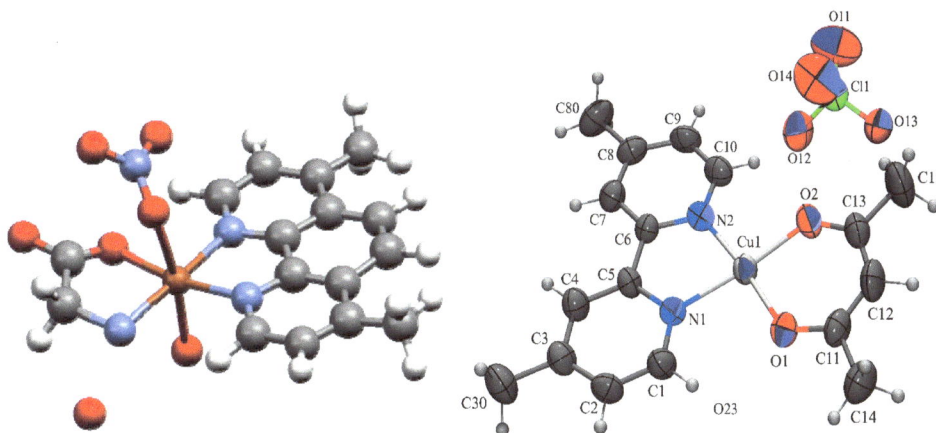

Figure 3: Structures of casiopeína IIgly and casiopeína III-ia.

Stability formation constants for mixed-ligand complexes with 1,10-phenanthroline as primary ligand show an enhancement compared to statistical expectations when the secondary ligand is an O-O donor[60]. There is no experimental data for stability constants of ternary Cu complexes with substituted phenanthrolines due, to their low solubility and there is some data for [Cu(phen)(gly)]NO$_3$ K =7.69 and [Cu(phen)(acac)]NO$_3$ K =8.1[59].

The effect on the strength of the interaction between Cu(x-phen) and oxygen donor bidentate ligands caused by the substituent on the phenanthroline was, however, studied by Gasque *et al.* [65] through the variations on the Cu-O stretching frequencies and their relationship with phenanthroline pKa. The study suggests that an increase in phenanthroline basicity weakness Cu-O bonds in this type of compounds.

The higher stability of these compounds also correlates well with local softness providing an explanation of the particular reactive behavior [66, 67].

IV. Casiopeínas Testing

Structure-Activity Relationships

 The structure-activity relationship analysis has generated several considerations concerning the antitumor potential activity of this type of copper(II) complexes. Our hypothesis is that the nature, number and position of the substituents on the diimine ligands as well as the modification of α-L-amino acidate (or O-O donor) have a crucial effect either on the selectivity or on the degree of biological activity shown by the ternary copper(II) complexes (Table **4**). This effect could be due to the modification of physicochemical properties of the complexes, such as the redox behavior of metal center or the water solubility of the complex [66].

Table 4: Antiproliferative activity on human tumor cell lines tested *in vitro*: IC50 (μM) on HeLa, SiHa, MCF-7 and HCT-15. Values are given as the mean of 3 independent experiments ± SE

No	Compound	IC50			
		HeLa	**SiHa**	**MCF-7**	**HCT-15**
1	[Cu(2,2'-bipyridine)(acetylacetonate)]NO$_3$	42 ± 3.1	40.5 ± 2.0	103.7 ± 9.6	67.3 ± 1.6
2	[Cu(4,4'-dimethyl-2,2'-bipyridine)(acetylacetonate)]NO$_3$, Cas III ia	18.2 ± 2.7	14.5 ± 1.5	15.9 ± 1.8	40.5 ± 4.6
3	[Cu(1,10-phenanthroline)(acetylacetonate)]NO$_3$,	10.7 ± 0.9	6.8 ± 0.9	8.1 ± 0.5	7.3 ± 0.7
4	[Cu(4-methyl-1,10-phenanthroline)(acetylacetonate)]NO$_3$	1.6 ± 0.1	3.4 ± 0.5	5.6 ± 0.7	6.0 ± 0.9
5	[Cu(5-methyl-1,10-phenanthroline)(acetylacetonate)]NO$_3$	6.2 ± 0.7	3.2 ± 0.2	4.4 ± 0.5	2.6 ± 0.4
6	[Cu(4,7-dimethyl-1,10-phenanthroline)(acetylacetonate)]NO$_3$	1.4 ± 0.1	0.96 ± 0.09	4.9 ± 0.6	2.1 ± 0.1
7	[Cu(5,6-dimethyl-1,10-phenanthroline)(acetylacetonate)]NO$_3$	3.4 ± 0.5	1.7 ± 0.2	3.9 ± 0.4	1.9 ± 0.3
8	[Cu(3,4,7,8-tetramethyl-1,1-phenanthroline)(acetylacetonate)]NO$_3$	1.9 ± 0.2	1.2 ± 0.1	2.2 ± 0.3	1.4 ± 0.2
9	[Cu(5-phenyl-1,10-phenanthroline)(acetylacetonate)]NO$_3$	3.9 ± 0.3	3.0 ± 0.3	3.9 ± 0.4	2.5 ± 0.3
10	[Cu(4,7-diphenyl-1,10-phenanthroline)(acetylacetonate)]NO$_3$,	4.2 ± 0.6	3.2 ± 0.5	2.2 ± 0.3	3.2 ± 0.4
11	[Cu(5-chloro-1,10-phenanthroline)(acetylacetonate)]NO$_3$	4.5 ± 0.5	8.8 ± 0.6	9.8 ± 0.5	12.9 ± 0.5
12	[Cu(5-nitro-1,10-phenanthroline)(acetylacetonate)]NO$_3$	21.3 ± 2.6	10.2 ± 1.1	14.7 ± 1.4	35.0 ± 2.4
13	[Cu(1,10-phenanthroline)(glycinate)]NO$_3$	13.9 ± 1.3	27.3 ± 2.2	9.6 ± 1.1	21.2 ± 2.5
14	[Cu(4-methyl-1,10-phenanthroline)(glycinate)]NO$_3$	8.7 ± 0.7	10.2 ± 1.0	7.7 ± 0.6	5.1 ± 0.5
15	[Cu(5-methyl-1,10-phenanthroline)(glycinate)]NO$_3$	6.2 ± 0.6	5.7 ± 0.6	4.7 ± 0.2	3.7 ± 0.4
16	[Cu(4,7-dimethyl-1,10-phenanthroline)(glycinate)]NO$_3$, Cas IIgly	5.5 ± 0.7	5.5 ± 0.8	4.6 ± 0.4	2.0 ± 0.2
17	[Cu(5,6-dimethyl-1,10-phenanthroline)(glycinate)]NO$_3$	5.3 ± 0.1	3.1 ± 0.3	4.4 ± 0.3	2.1 ± 0.1
18	[Cu(3,4,7,8-tetramethyl-1,10-phenanthroline)(glycinate)]NO$_3$	1.8 ± 0.0	1.4 ± 0.2	2.6 ± 0.2	1.8 ± 0.4

Table 4: cont....

19	[Cu(4,7-diphenyl-1,10-phenanthroline)(glycinate)]NO$_3$	5.1 ± 0.2	6.6 ± 0.9	4.1 ± 0.4	7.6 ± 0.7
20	[Cu(5-chloro-1,10-phenanthroline)(glycinate)]NO$_3$	14.3 ± 0.5	13.9 ± 1.3	23.2 ± 2.3	22.3 ± 1.6
21	[Cu(5-nitro-1,10-phenanthroline)(glycinate)]NO$_3$	44.8 ± 1.5	17.9 ± 2.2	28.64 ± 3.4	47.3 ± 6.5
	CDDP	5.1 ± 0.4	5.4 ± 0.5	5.6 ± 0.8	21.8 ± 2.4

According to QSAR studies, the presence of the central fused aromatic ring in the phen containing complexes is necessary to preserve the antiproliferative activity. IC$_{50}$ has a strong relationship with the half-wave potential (E$_{1/2}$) of the copper center. In these studies, the most active complexes are found to be those that are the weaker oxidants. The change of secondary ligand from *acac* to *gly* has less influence on biological activity than the alterations on the diimine ligand [66].

In Vitro and *In Vivo* Testing

These compounds have been tested in several models *in vitro*, as *in vivo*, showing antiproliferative [66], cytotoxic [68], cytostatic [69], genotoxic [68-70] and antitumor activities [71, 72] with promising results. It is important to note that the antiproliferative activity has also been observed on cisplatin resistant murine cell lines without the ability to induce apoptosis between cisplatin sensitive and resistant cells [73].

The antitumor activity *in vivo* has been tested mainly on murine model (L1210, S180. B16 and Lw1) where ILS (increase life span) is determined according to National Cancer Institute screening panel finding promising results (Fig. **4**). Additionally, some of these compounds have been tested *in vivo* in murine glioma C6 [72] and xenograft tumor models as colon carcinoma HCT-15 [71].

Every study has shown promising results and has revealed that the substitution on diimina ligand and the changes on secondary ligand as well, modify the magnitude of the biological activity [66, 67].

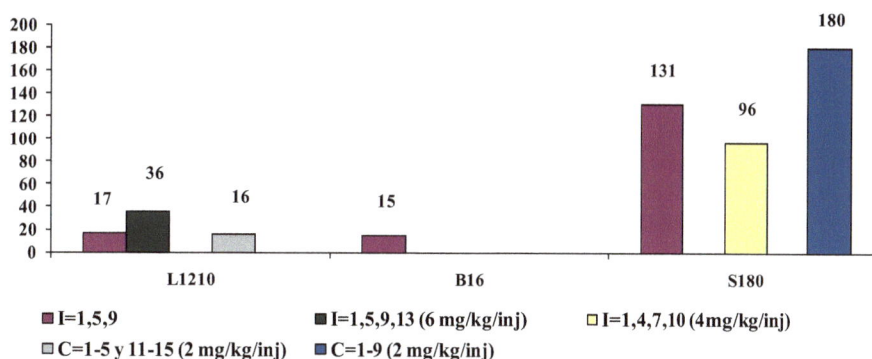

Figure 4: Increase life span with Casiopeína IIgly *i.p.* Administration on murine models. Sarcoma S180 (S180), Melanoma B16 (B16), and Leukemia L1210 (L1210). I: intermittent dose days and C: chronic dose day.

Mechanism of Action

The mode of action of Casiopeínas® has not been totally elucidated and remains the subject of several studies although there is evidence suggesting that these compounds might act by at least three different modes of activity: (i) catalytic ROS generation, (ii) mitochondrial toxicity and (iii) direct interaction with DNA.

Casiopeínas® are able to inhibit cell proliferation in tumor models as medulloblastoma [74], HCT-15 [71] and murine glioma C6 [72] as well as produce cell dose-dependent death by apoptosis dependent or independent on caspase activation [71-73]. This effect might be the result of one or several signals that could be mediated by the generation of ROS [68], by the observed mitochondrial toxicity [72, 75, 76], or by both, and might play, alone or cooperatively, an important role in the regulation of cell death induced by this type of complexes.

Mitochondrial toxicity is considered a possible therapeutic target and an effective strategy in cancer therapy [77]. Inhibition of respiration and ATP synthesis was observed in mitochondria after the administration of these copper complexes. The damage is observed in several different mitochondrial sites in a dose dependent manner, compromising the energy dependent processes in the cells [78]. Casiopeína II-gly inhibits enzyme that have important roles in the normal mitochondrial functions [75, 76]. In high doses these compounds induce the stimulation of basal respiration. This is followed by strong inhibition that correlates with mitochondrial swelling, which in turn depends on potassium channel activation and subsequent cytochrome c releasing [76]. This final event is an apoptotic signal that activates caspase 9 and apoptosis protease activating factor-1 [78]. Casiopeínas also cause the loss of mitochondrial membrane potential in medulloblastoma [75] and glioma C6 cells [72].

Casiopeínas IIgly and III-ia, in addition, inhibit the rates of state 3 and uncoupled respiration in mitochondria, the first one being about 10 times more potent than the second one [76]. This observed inhibition is consistent with QSAR studies on antiproliferative activity [66]. Mitochondria from liver, kidney and hepatoma AS-30D showed a similar sensitivity towards CasIIgly, whereas heart mitochondria are found to be more resistant [76]. These results suggest that Casiopeínas disrupt several different mitochondrial sites, bringing about inhibition of respiration and ATP synthesis, which could compromise energy dependent processes such as cellular duplication.

Some researchers, on the other hand, have observed that the inhibition of cell proliferation [68, 72] and DNA degradation [68, 72, 79] in the presence of reducing agents are simultaneous to ROS generation. Lipid peroxidation [72] and reduced glutathione depletion [80] have been observed as a result of casiopeínas administration. These effects suggest that oxidation of DNA and other cellular components could also be the stress signal that triggers cell death by apoptosis.

Other results have shown that there is also the possibility of direct interaction of complexes with DNA by intercalative and non-intercalative interactions as expected for these complexes due to the planar aromatic moiety of their diimine ligands [62, 63, 81].

Another study has reported that the activation of Poly(ADP-ribose) polymerase -1 (PARP-1) resulting from DNA damage, induces a high Apoptosis Inductor Factor Release (AIF) and its nuclear translocation leads to cell death through a caspase-independent mode [74]. This could explain the observations on murine glioma C6 [72] and human ovarian carcinoma CH1 [73] where the apoptosis was observed to take place by caspases-independent mechanisms.

The Casiopeinas tested have shown significant biological activity on tumoral cell line HCT-15 [71], which has inactive p53. It is well known that cellular lines with inactive p53 are resistant to mitochondrial drugs [82], also it has been demonstrated that DNA damage induced by some chemotherapeutics enhances the apoptotic function of p73, which selectively activates the transcription of proapoptotic target genes [83].

Cas IIgly (**16**) is found to induce a dramatic drop in intracellular levels of GSH in human lung cancer H157 and A549 cells, and is able to use GSH as source of free electrons to catalyze the Fenton reaction. In both cell lines, the toxicity of Cas IIgly (2.5-5 μM) was potentiated by the GSH synthesis inhibitor L-buthionine sulfoximine (BSO) and reduced by the catalytic antioxidant manganese(III) meso-tetrakis(N,N'- diethylimidazolium-2-yl) porphyrin (MnTDE-1,3-IP5+), thus playing an important role in oxidative stress [84].

Cas IIgly also caused an over-production of Reactive Oxygen Species (ROS) in the mitochondria and a depolarization of the mitochondrial membrane. Moreover, Cas IIgly produced mitochondrial DNA damage that resulted in an imbalance of the expression of the apoproteins of the mitochondrial respiratory chain, which also can contribute to increase ROS production. These results suggest that Cas IIgly initiates multiple possible sources of ROS overproduction leading to mitochondrial dysfunction and cell death.

The cellular targets of casiopeínas could be others in addition to mitochondria and DNA. The administration *in vivo* of complexes of this family produces severe damage in erythrocytes, which is expressed as hemolytic anemia [85]. This has lead us to think that DNA interactions or energy disruptions on mitochondria are not required at certain dose level to trigger a cytotoxic response. In this case, ROS generation might be the key signal in these cells since the observed haemolytic response its similar to that provoked by copper(II) salts.

In summary, at the molecular level, the evidence strongly suggests that damage to several biological targets appear to be mediated by a large number of heterogeneous mechanisms, working simultaneously.

Metabolism Studies

Pharmacokinetic studies have been essential in the preclinical tests of Casiopeínas in order to obtain important information such as the half-life, stability, and protein binding potential.

The pharmacokinetic behavior of Casiopeína III ia was evaluated in rats using HPLC techniques. This method, validated for concentrations ranging from 5 to 100 mg/ml, showed good repeatability and accuracy as well as low limits of quantification and detection. The recovery of Casiopeina III ia (**2**) was found to be reproducible, steady and sufficiently sensitive to perform protein binding by equilibrium dialysis [86].

For the HPLC method, validation in rats with Casiopeína II gly has proved to be useful, fast, sensitive, simple and reliable, and it was validated for concentrations ranging from 2.5 to 50 mg/ml. In addition, the method had successful repeatability and accuracy. The recovery of Casiopeina IIgly was also reproducible and steady over the entire calibration range [87].

Casiopeína II gly was also evaluated in beagle dogs demonstrating to have good precision, accuracy, an acceptable recovery and low limits of quantification and detection. Pharmacokinetics parameters such as clearance and half life were obtained and demonstrated to have a high elimination rate, and also showed similar results to those reported in rat assay [88].

Toxicity

Cytotoxicity raises a concern about casiopeína selectivity towards tumor cells; that is the reason why several comparative studies have been performed in different cell lines both normal and transformed ones. Casiopeína II-gly has shown *in vitro* inhibition on HeLa and hepatoma AS-30D cell lines, without disrupting the viability of non tumor cell lines as lymphocytes at equivalent level doses [78].

Opposite to this effect, inhibition of cell respiration and the loss of mitochondrial potential are similar in liver, kidney and AS-30 D cells employing 1-10 nmol (mg protein)$^{-1}$ *in vitro* concentrations [76], which leads us to conclude that adverse reactions could exist after administration of these complexes *in vivo*. Regardless of the *in vivo* toxicity in mice and rats, these compounds have a LD 50 higher than cisplatin and show different degrees of toxicity as result of changes in their structures with a strong relationship with cytotoxicity [66].

Casiopeína III-ia at *i.p.* doses of 6.74 μmol/kg and 13.5 μmol/kg q.d. 4x 6, causes adhesions and inflammation at the peritoneal surface of mice nu/nu, the latter due to chronic irritation. On the other hand, the IV administration of casiopeína II-gly causes hemolytic anemia accompanied by leukocytosis and neutrophilia, an inflammation response to the increased erythrocyte destruction and morphological changes in the spleen [84, 89]. All hematological effects are dose-dependent and reversible after 15 days with a single dose of 5 mg/kg. The type of damage is compatible with ROS and it is similar to that produced by toxicity associated to copper [85].

The principal adverse effects of these complexes are respiratory and cardiovascular toxicity. Casiopeina II-gly and casiopeína III-ia induce diminution of cardiac work and O_2 consumption in isolated perfused rat hearts with glucose plus octanoate. The half-maximal inhibitory concentrations are 4 and 4.6 μM, respectively. These effects are attributable to the strong inhibition of the energetic metabolism mentioned above. Remarkably, Casiopeínas are less toxic than adriamycin, a well-known potent cardiotoxic and antineoplastic drug, which has a wide clinical use [75].

The 99 lethal dose (DL$_{99}$) in an acute toxicity study in dogs was calculated to be 200 mg/m^2 for Casiopeína III-ia and 160 mg/m^2 for casiopeína II-gly [90]. At these high doses both compounds cause tachypnoea, drop in arterial blood pressure, tachycardia followed by bradycardia and finally cardiac arrest no later than 25 minutes after administration. Probably the lung edema is caused by a joined toxicity to the lung capillary bed, and particularly to the heart.

The analysis by transmission electron microscopy shows structural disarrangement of cardiac muscle fibers, swelling and loss of mitochondrial crests [90]. The same effects have been observed on mitochondrion of HCT-15 cells *in vitro* [71].

CONCLUSIONS

The development of a new drug represents a formidable task, since it requires several years of work and a large collaborative effort of various research groups. One of the purposes of Medicinal Chemistry is, however, to develop and test alternative therapeutic options as well as to understand their mechanisms of action with the aim of improving current treatments so as to better the patients' quality of life. The key objectives are to follow the appropriate steps to drug discover and continue to develop new chemotherapeutic agents.

The role of bioinorganic chemistry in both, the development of medicinal inorganic agents and in the understanding of the underlying mechanisms of action, clearly indicates that the field of 'metals in medicine' will continue to make important contributions to the advancement of human health in the 21st century.

One of the most promising designs in the field of copper-based antitumor agents is the group of complexes named casiopeínas®. These compounds can act by a set of miscellaneous mechanisms in addition to DNA binding, providing, at least in principle, a new class of chemotherapeutic with a broad spectrum of activity.

ACKNOWLEDGEMENTS

The authors would like to thank CONACyT (14622) and Instituto Ciencia y Tecnología D.F. for the scholarship. Besides several works presented, were partially supported by CONACyT (87-806), PAPIIT (IN227110) and PICSA (10-61).

REFERENCES

[1]   Marshall EK. Historical perspectives in chemotherapy, in advances in chemotherapy. In: Goldin A, Hawking IF, ed. New York: Academic Press 1964.

[2]   DeVita VT Jr. The evolution of therapeutic research in cancer. N Engl J Med 1978; 298 (16): 907-10.

[3]   DeVita VT Jr., Bleickardt EW. National Oncology Forum: perspectives for the year 2000. Cancer J 2001; 7 Suppl 1: S2-13.

[4]   Hempelmann E, Tcsarowicz I, Oleksyn BJ. [From onions to artemisinin. Brief history of malaria chemotherapy]. Pharm Unserer Zeit 2009; 38(6): 500-7.

[5]   Graham L P. An introduction to medicinal chemistry. New York: Oxford University 2005.

[6]   Araque Arroyo P, Ubago Perez R, Cancela Diez B, Fernandez Feijoo MA, Hernandez Magdalena J, Calleja Hernandez MA. Controversies in the management of adjuvant breast cancer with taxanes: Review of the current literature. Cancer Treat Rev 2010.

[7]   Ferrari S, Palmerini E, Alberghini M, *et al.* Vincristine, doxorubicin, cyclophosfamide, actinomycin D, ifosfamide, and etoposide in adult and pediatric patients with nonmetastatic Ewing sarcoma. Final results of a monoinstitutional study. Tumori 2010; 96(2): 213-8.

[8]   Lima P, Dos Santos LV, Sasse EC, Lima CS, Sasse AD. Camptothecins Compared with Etoposide in Combination with Platinum Analog in Extensive Stage Small Cell Lung Cancer: Systematic Review with Meta-Analysis. J Thorac Oncol 2010; 25.

[9]   Mehta RG, Murillo G, Naithani R, Peng X. Cancer chemoprevention by natural products: how far have we come? Pharm Res 2010; 27(6): 950-61.

[10]   Gullett NP, Ruhul Amin AR, Bayraktar S, *et al.* Cancer prevention with natural compounds. Semin Oncol 2010; 37(3): 258-81.

[11]   Park JH, Kim KH, Kim SJ, Lee WR, Lee KG, Park KK. Bee venom protects hepatocytes from tumor necrosis factor-alpha and actinomycin D. Arch Pharm Res 2010; 33(2): 215-23.

[12]   D'Suze G, Rosales A, Salazar V, Sevcik C. Apoptogenic peptides from Tityus discrepans scorpion venom acting against the SKBR3 breast cancer cell line. Toxicon 2010; 56(8): 1497-505.

[13]   Wennergren G and Lagercrantz H. "One sometimes finds what one is not looking for" (Sir Alexander Fleming): the most important medical discovery of the 20th century. Acta Paediatr 2007; 96(1): 141-4.

[14]   Bo G.Giuseppe. Brotzu and the discovery of cephalosporins. Clin Microbiol Infect 2000; 6 : 6-9.

[15]   Lee M R. The history of ergot of rye (Claviceps purpurea) II: 1900-1940. J R Coll Physicians Edinb 2009; 39(4): 365-9.

[16]   Stossel, T.P., The discovery of statins. Cell 2008; 134(6): 903-5.

[17] Livett BG. Sandall DW, Keays D, *et al.* Therapeutic applications of conotoxins that target the neuronal nicotinic acetylcholine receptor. Toxicon 2006; 48(7): 810-29.

[18] Bernstein S. Historic reflection on steroids: Lederle and personal aspects. Steroids 1992; 57(8): 392-402.

[19] Ruiz-Azuara L, Bravo-Gómez ME. New Approaches the treatment of cancer. In: Mejia M, Navarro S. Metals in cancer treatment: Nova Sciences Publishers 2010.

[20] Lippard SJ. Bioinorganic chemistry: a maturing frontier. Science 1993; 261(5122): 699-700.

[21] Lippard SJ and Berg JM. Principles of Bioinorganic Chemistry. Mill Valley, California: University Science Books, 1994.

[22] Fricker SP. Metal based drugs: from serendipity to design. Dalton Trans 2007(43): p. 4903-17.

[23] McKee AE, Farrell AT, Pazdur R, Woodcock J. The role of the U.S. Food and Drug Administration review process: clinical trial endpoints in oncology. Oncologist 2010; 15: 13-8.

[24] Kwitkowski VE, Prowell TM, Ibrahim A, *et al.* FDA approval summary: temsirolimus as treatment for advanced renal cell carcinoma. Oncologist 2010; 15(4): 428-35.

[25] Kinoshita M, Kodera Y, Hibi K, *et al.* Gene expression profile of 5-fluorouracil metabolic enzymes in primary colorectal cancer: potential as predictive parameters for response to fluorouracil-based chemotherapy. Anticancer Res 2007; 27(2): 851-6.

[26] Frankfurt OS, Krishan A. Apoptosis enzyme-linked immunosorbent assay distinguishes anticancer drugs from toxic chemicals and predicts drug synergism. Chem Biol Interact 2003; 145(1): 89-99.

[27] Naik PK, Dubey A, Soni K, Kumar R, Singh H. The binding modes and binding affinities of epipodophyllotoxin derivatives with human topoisomerase IIalpha. J Mol Graph Model 2010; 26.

[28] Mekonen M, Abate E, Aseffa A, *et al.* Identification of drug susceptibility pattern and mycobacterial species in sputum smear positive pulmonary tuberculosis patients with and without HIV co-infection in north west Ethiopia. Ethiop Med J 2010; 48(3): 203-10.

[29] Gridling M, Stark N, Madlener S, *et al. In vitro* anti-cancer activity of two ethno-pharmacological healing plants from Guatemala Pluchea odorata and Phlebodium decumanum. Int J Oncol 2009; 34(4): 1117-28.

[30] Cerdan R, Collin D, Lenouvel F, Felenbok B, Guittet E. The Aspergillus nidulans transcription factor AlcR forms a stable complex with its half-site DNA: a NMR study. FEBS Lett 1997; 408(2): 235-40.

[31] Rao R, Patra AK, Chetana PR. DNA binding and oxidative cleavage activity of ternary (L-proline)copper (II) complexes of heterocyclic bases. Polyhedron 2007; 26: 5331-8.

[32] Hempelmann E, Tesarowicz I, Oleksyn BJ. [From onions to artemisinin. Brief history of malaria chemotherapy]. Pharm Unserer Zeit 2009; 38(6): 500-7.

[33] Jayant RD, McShane MJ, Srivastava R. *In vitro* and *in vivo* evaluation of anti-inflammatory agents using nanoengineered alginate carriers: Towards localized implant inflammation suppression. Int J Pharm 2010; 2.

[34] Kelland L. The resurgence of platinum-based cancer chemotherapy. Nat Rev Cancer 2007; 7(8): 573-84.

[35] Lippert B. 30 Years of Cisplatin-Chemistry and Biochemistry of a Leading Anticancer Drug. Verlag Helvetica Chimica Acta, Wiley-VCH: Zürich 1999.

[36] Kelland LR, and Farrell N. Platinum-Based Drugs in Cancer Therapy, Humana Press Inc 2000.

[37] Clarke M J, and Sadler P, eds. Metallopharmaceuticals. Vol. 1, Springer: Dublin, 1999.

[38] Van Rijt SH, and Sadler PJ. Current applications and future potential for bioinorganic chemistry in the development of anticancer drugs. Drug Discov Today 2009.

[39] Ronconi L and Sadler PJ. Using coordination chemistry to design new medicines. Coordin Chem Rev 2007; 251: 1633-48.

[40] Gianferrara T, Bratsos I, Alessio E. A categorization of metal anticancer compounds based on their mode of action. Dalton Trans 2009; 7(37): 7588-98.

[41] Smalley KS, Contractor R, Haass NK, *et al.* An organometallic protein kinase inhibitor pharmacologically activates p53 and induces apoptosis in human melanoma cells. Cancer Res 2007; 67(1): 209-17.

[42] Dillon CT, Hambley TW, Kennedy BJ, Lay PA, Weder JE and Zhou Q. Copper and zinc complexes as antiinflammatory drugs. Met Ions Biol Syst 2004; 41: 253-77.

[43] Dougan SJ, Habtemariam A, McHale SE, Parsons S, Sadler PJ. Catalytic organometallic anticancer complexes. Proc Natl Acad Sci USA 2008; 105(33): 11628-33.

[44] Lecomte JP, Kirsch-De Mesmaeker A, Feeney, MM, Kelly JM. Ruthenium(II) complexes with 1,4,5,8,9,12-hexaazatriphenylene and 1,4,5,8-tetraazaphenanthrene ligands: key role played by electron transfer in DNA cleavage and adduct formation. Inorg. Chem 1995; 34: 6481-6491.

[45] Moucheron, C, Kirsch-De Mesmaeker A, Choua S. Photophysics of Ru(phen)2(PHEHAT)2+: A Novel "Light Switch" for DNA and Photo-oxidant for Mononucleotides. Inorg. Chem 1997; 36(4): 584–592.

[46] Ruiz-Azuara L, Bravo-Gomez ME. Copper Compounds in Cancer Chemotherapy. Curr Med Chem 2010; 17(31): 3606-15.

[47]   Ruiz-Azuara L. Preparation of new mixed copper aminoacidate complexes from phenylate phenathrolines to be used as "anticancerigenic" agents. 07/628,628: Re 35,458. 1992, USA

[48]   Ruiz-Azuara L. Process to obtain new mixed copper aminoacidate complexes from phenylatephenanthroline to be used as anticancerigenic agents. 07/628,843: RE 35,458, Feb. 18 (1997). 1992, United States Patent.

[49]   Ruiz-Azuara L. Copper amino acidate diimine nitrate compounds and their methyl derivatives and a process for preparing them. 07/628,628: 5,576,326. 1996, United States Patent.

[50]   Solans X, Ruiz-Ramírez L, Gasque L, Briansó JL. Structure of (1,10-phenanthroline) (salicylaldehydato)copper (II) nitrate. Acta Cryst C 1987; 43: 428-30.

[51]   Solans X, Ruiz-Ramirez L, Martinez A, Gasque L, Brianso JL. Structures of chloro(glycinato)(1,10-phenanthroline)copper(II) monohydrate (I) and aqua(1,10-phenanthroline)(L-phenylalaninato)copper(II) nitrate monohydrate (II). Acta Crystallogr C 1988; 44 (Pt 4): 628-31.

[52]   Solans X, Ruíz-Ramírez L, Martínez A, Gasque L, y Moreno-Esparza R. Mixed chelate complexes. III. Structures of (L-alaninato)(aqua)(2,2'-bipyridine)copper(II) nitrate monohydrate and aqua(2,2'-bipyridine)(L-tyrosinato)copper(II) chloride trihydrate. Acta Cryst C 1992; 48: 1785-8.

[53]   Solans X, Ruíz-Ramírez L, Martínez A, Gasque L, Moreno-Esparza R. Mixed chelate complexes. II. Structures of L-alaninato(aqua)(4,7-diphenyl-1,10-phenanthroline)copper(II) nitrite monohydrate and aqua(4,7-dimethyl-1,10-phenanthroline)(glycinato)(nitrato)copper(II) monohydrate. Acta Cryst C 1993; 49: 890-893.

[54]   Alvarez-Larena A, Briansó-Penalva, JL, Piniella JF, Moreno-Esparza R, Ruiz-Ramírez L, Ferrer-Sueta G. Aqua (glycinato) (3,4,7,8-tetramethyl-1,10-phenanthroline)copper(II) Nitrate. Acta Cryst. C 1995; 51: 852-854.

[55]   Gasque L, Moreno-Esparza R, Ruiz-Ramírez L Medina-Dickinson G. Aqua (4,7-diphenyl-1,10-phenanthroline) (salicylaldehydato)copper(II) nitrate monohydrate. Acta Cryst. C 1999; 55: 1065-1067.

[56]   Gasque L, Moreno-Esparza R, Ruiz-Ramírez L, Medina-Dickinson G. (5,6-Dimethyl-1,10-phenanthroline) (nitrato) (salicylaldehydato) copper (II). Acta Cryst. C 1999; 55: 1063-5.

[57]   Moreno-Esparza R, Molins E, Briansó-Penalva JL, Ruiz-Ramírez L, Redón R. Aqua(1,10-phenanthroline)(L-serinato)copper(II) Nitrate. Acta Cryst. C 1995; 51: 1505-8.

[58]   Venkatraman R, Zubkowski JD,Valente E J. Aqua(1,10-phenanthroline)(L-prolinato)copper(II) nitrate monohydrate. Acta Cryst C 1999; 55: 1241-1243.

[59]   McBryde WAE, Brisbin DA, Irving H. The stability of metal complexes of 1,10-phenanthroline and its analogues. Part III. 5-Methyl-1,10-phenanthroline. J Chem Soc 1962; 5245-53.

[60]   Gasque L, Moreno-Esparza R, Ruiz-Ramírez L. Stability of Ternary Copper and Nickel Complexes with 1,10-phenanthroline. J of Inorg Biochem 1992; 48: 121-7.

[61]   Kwik WL, Ang KP and Chen G. Complexes of (2,2'-bipyridyl) copper(II) and (1,10-phenanthroline) copper(II) with some amino acids. J Inorg Nucl Chem 1980; 42(2): 303-13.

[62]   Ruili Huang AW, Covell DG. Anticancer metal compounds in NCI's tumor-screening database: putative mode of action. Biochemical Pharmacology 2005; 69: 1009-39.

[63]   Chikira M, Tomizawa Y, Fukita D, *et al.* DNA-fiber EPR study of the orientation of Cu (II) complexes of 1,10-phenanthroline and its derivatives bound to DNA: mono(phenanthroline)-copper(II) and its ternary complexes with amino acids. J Inorg Biochem 2002; 89(3-4): 163-73.

[64]   Rao R, Patra AK. and Chetana PR. DNA binding and oxidative cleavage activity of ternary (L-proline) copper (II) complexes of heterocyclic bases. Polyhedron, 2007; 26: 5331-8.

[65]   Gasque L, Medina G, Ruiz-Ramirez L, Moreno-Esparza R. Cu-O stretching frequency correlation with phenanthroline pKa values in mixed copper complexes. Inorg Chim Acta 1999; 288: 106-11.

[66]   Bravo-Gomez ME, Garcia-Ramos JC, Gracia-Mora I, Ruiz-Azuara L. Antiproliferative activity and QSAR study of copper(II) mixed chelate [Cu(N-N)(acetylacetonato)]NO3 and [Cu(N-N)(glycinato)] NO3 complexes, (Casiopeinas). J Inorg Biochem 2009; 103(2): 299-309.

[67]   Martinez A, Salcedo R, Sansores LE, Medina G, Gasque L. A density functional study of the reactivity and stability of mixed copper complexes. Is hardness the reason? Inorg Chem 2001; 40(2): 301-6.

[68]   Alemon-Medina R, Brena-Valle M, Munoz-Sanchez JL, Gracia-Mora, MI, Ruiz-Azuara L. Induction of oxidative damage by copper-based antineoplastic drugs (Casiopeinas). Cancer Chemother Pharmacol 2007; 60(2): 219-28.

[69]   Sánchez-Bartéz F. Thesis Maestro en Ciencias Químicas "Determinación de la capacidad genotóxica, citotóxica y citostática de las Casiopeínas Igli, IIgli y III-ia en linfocitos, médula ósea de ratón y linfocitos humanos en cultivo.". Asesor: Ruiz-Azuara, L. Universidad Nacional Autónoma de México, 2006.

[70]   Ruiz-Ramírez L, de la Rosa ME, Gracia-Mora I, *et al.* Casiopeinas, metal-based drugs a new class of antineoplastic and genotoxic compounds. J of Inorg Biochem 1995; 59(2-3): 207.

[71] Carvallo-Chaigneau F, Trejo-Solis C, Gomez-Ruiz C, *et al.* Casiopeina III-ia induces apoptosis in HCT-15 cells *in vitro* through caspase-dependent mechanisms and has antitumor effect *in vivo*. Biometals 2008; 21(1): 17-28.

[72] Trejo-Solis C, Palencia G, Zuniga S, *et al.* Cas IIgly induces apoptosis in glioma C6 cells *in vitro* and *in vivo* through caspase-dependent and caspase-independent mechanisms. Neoplasia 2005; 7(6): 563-74.

[73] De Vizcaya-Ruiz A, Rivero-Muller A, Ruiz-Ramirez, *et al.* Induction of apoptosis by a novel copper-based anticancer compound, casiopeina II, in L1210 murine leukaemia and CH1 human ovarian carcinoma cells. Toxicol *In Vitro* 2000; 14(1): 1-5.

[74] Mejia C, and Ruiz-Azuara L. Casiopeinas IIgly and IIIia Induce Apoptosis in Medulloblastoma Cells. Pathol Oncol Res 2008.

[75] Hernandez-Esquivel L, Marin-Hernandez A, Pavon N, Carvajal K, Moreno-Sanchez R. Cardiotoxicity of copper-based antineoplastic drugs casiopeinas is related to inhibition of energy metabolism. Toxicol Appl Pharmacol 2006; 212(1): 79-88.

[76] Marin-Hernandez A, Gracia-Mora I, Ruiz-Ramirez L, Moreno-Sanchez R. Toxic effects of copper-based antineoplastic drugs (Casiopeinas) on mitochondrial functions. Biochem Pharmacol 2003; 65(12): 1979-89.

[77] Dias N and Bailly C. Drugs targeting mitochondrial functions to control tumor cell growth. Biochem Pharmacol 2005; 70(1): 1-12.

[78] Rodriguez-Enriquez S, Vital-Gonzalez PA, Flores-Rodriguez FL, *et al.* Control of cellular proliferation by modulation of oxidative phosphorylation in human and rodent fast-growing tumor cells. Toxicol Appl Pharmacol 2006; 215(2): 208-17.

[79] Rivero-Mulle, A, De Vizcaya-Ruiz A, Plant N, Ruiz L and Dobrota M. Mixed chelate copper complex, Casiopeina IIgly, binds and degrades nucleic acids: a mechanism of cytotoxicity. Chem Biol Interact 2007; 165(3): 189-99.

[80] Alemon-Medina R, Munoz-Sanchez JL, Ruiz-Azuara L, Gracia-Mora I. Casiopeina IIgly induced cytotoxicity to HeLa cells depletes the levels of reduced glutathione and is prevented by dimethyl sulfoxide. Toxicol *In Vitro* 2008; 22(3): 710-5.

[81] Moreno-Esparza R, Escalante-Tovar S and Ruiz-Ramirez L. DNA-planar copper complexes interaction, - stacking vs H bond. Acta Cryst A 2002; 18.

[82] Bunz F, Hwang PM, Torrance C, *et al.* Disruption of p53 in human cancer cells alters the responses to therapeutic agents. J Clin Invest 1999; 104(3): 263-9.

[83] Costanzo A., Merlo P, Pediconi N, *et al.* DNA damage-dependent acetylation of p73 dictates the selective activation of apoptotic target genes. Mol Cell 2002; 9(1): 175-86.

[84] Kachadourian R, Brechbuhl HM, Ruiz-Azuara L, Gracia-Mora I, Day BJ. Casiopeina IIgly-induced oxidative stress and mitochondrial dysfunction in human lung cancer A549 and H157 cells. Toxicology 2010; 268(3): 176-83. [71].

[85] De Vizcaya-Ruiz A, Rivero-Muller A, Ruiz-Ramirez L, Howarth JA, Dobrota, M. Hematotoxicity response in rats by the novel copper-based anticancer agent: casiopeina II. Toxicology 2003; 194(1-2): 103-13.

[86] Fuentes-Noriega I, Ruiz-Ramirez L, Tovar Tovar A, Rico-Morales H, Gracia-Mora I. Development and validation of a liquid chromatographic method for Casiopeina IIIi in rat plasma. J Chromatogr B Analyt Technol Biomed Life Sci 2002; 772(1): 115-21.

[87] Reyes L, Fuentes-Noriega I, Ruiz-Ramirez L, Macias L. Development and validation of a liquid chromatographic method for Casiopeina IIgly in rat plasma. J Chromatogr B Analyt Technol Biomed Life Sci 2003; 791(1-2): 111-6.

[88] Cañas-Alonso RC, Fuentes-Noriega I, Ruiz-Azuara L. Pharmacokinetics of casiopeína iigly in beagle dog: a copper based compound with antineoplastic activity. JBABM 2010; 2(2): 028-34

[89] Asano R, Kaseda M, y Hokari S. [The effect of copper and copper. o-phenanthroline complex on cattle erythrocytes.]. Nippon Juigaku Zasshi 1983; 45(1): 77-83.

[90] Leal-Garcia M, Garcia-Ortuno L, Ruiz-Azuara L, Gracia-Mora I, Luna-Delvillar J, Sumano H. Assessment of acute respiratory and cardiovascular toxicity of casiopeinas in anaesthetized dogs. Basic Clin Pharmacol Toxicol 2007; 101(3): 151-8.

CHAPTER 11

Mechanisms of Therapy Resistance in Cancer

Iván Restrepo, Cindy Sharon Ortiz and Javier Camacho[*]

Department of Pharmacology, Centro de Investigación y de Estudios Avanzados del Instituto Politécnico Nacional, Avenida Instituto Politécnico Nacional 2508, México D. F. 07360, México

Abstract. The effects of many anticancer drugs are unfortunately masked by drug resistance developed by several tumors. This represents a strong and major challenge in cancer research. Drug resistance is due to several factors, including membrane transporters taking out drugs from the cell, molecular mechanisms repairing or inhibiting the damage caused by the drugs, mutations in anticancer drug targets, or even anatomic structures affecting either drug penetration or elimination. Here we will review the molecular aspects of therapy resistance mechanisms. Research on the inhibition of proteins involved in drug resistance or design of new anticancer drugs overcoming such mechanisms with no doubt will result in a major advancement in cancer treatment.

Keywords: Drug resistance, multidrug resistance, ABC transporters, tamoxifen, antibodies, EGFR mutations.

INTRODUCTION

The response of tumor cells to drugs can be defined by a number of molecular mechanisms, from the penetration of the substance into the cell to cell death or arrest at any stage of the cell cycle. Chemotherapeutic resistance appears as a consequence of extrinsic and intrinsic factors, including cellular mechanisms that repair or inhibit the damage caused by drugs, or anatomic structures that affect drug penetration or increase its elimination [1]. Fig. **1** summarizes some of the most common mechanisms of therapy resistance displayed by cancer cells.

MULTI DRUG RESISTANCE

Multi Drug Resistance (MDR) is a system of protection of the cell against numerous compounds, including drugs with different mechanisms of intracellular activity. In general, this mechanism of resistance produces decreased intracellular drug concentrations by increasing its elimination, which occurs as a consequence of the activation of glycoprotein Gp170 which is coded by the MDR1 and MDR2 genes. Transport proteins of the ABC family determine MDR of tumor cells, some of them operating as the first step of action of the toxic substance at the stage of drug penetration through the cell membrane and its intracellular accumulation [1]. It is important to consider that the MDR phenotype is multifactorial and cancer cells are able to overcome the effects of chemosensitizers through diverse mechanisms to combat drug-induced cytotoxicity [2]. Some soluble factors including cytokines, hormones, and growth factors, as well as interactions between tumor cells and extracellular matrix molecules or adjacent cells, may play a significant role in the pathogenesis and progression of human cancers; these same factors may also contribute to the survival of cancer cells after initial therapy, allowing resistant cells to proliferate and acquire multiple mechanisms of drug resistance [2].

Many cancers are characterized by an initial sensitivity to chemotherapy and later an acquired resistance to therapy that invariably leads to patient relapse through the expansion of a MDR population of cancer cells. *In vitro* studies have led to the identification of four classes of acquired MDR [2]:

o   reduced drug accumulation.

o   alterations in drug targets.

o   increased repair of drug-induced damage.

o   inhibition of apoptotic signaling pathways.

*Address correspondence to Javier Camacho: Department of Pharmacology, Centro de Investigación y de Estudios Avanzados del Instituto Politécnico Nacional, Avenida Instituto Politécnico Nacional 2508, México D. F. 07360, México; E-mail: fcamacho@cinvestav.mx

The observation of acquired drug resistance, taken together with the clinical observation that acquired mechanisms of MDR develop only after prolonged treatment, suggests that there might be initial antiapoptotic mechanisms that promote cell survival [2].

Reduced intracellular drug accumulation has been associated with overexpression of the ATP-binding cassette transporter, *Pgp/MDR-1* and related drug transporters, including MDR proteins 1, and breast cancer resistance proteins [2]. ATP Binding Cassette proteins (ABC) have a wide variety of substrates and are characterized by the presence of an ATP-binding domain of specific structure and are present in all living organisms [3]. This family of proteins reduces drug accumulation including vincristine, doxorubicin, and taxol; interestingly, lung resistance protein has also been associated with drug resistance *via* a redistribution of doxorubicin from the nucleus to cytoplasm without overall changes in total cellular drug accumulation [2]. In humans, there are 49 members in the ABC transporter superfamily, which is divided into seven subfamilies (ABCA, ABCB, ABCC, ABCD, ABCE, ABCF, and ABCG). Several are known to efflux anticancer drugs and thereby cause drug resistance when overexpressed in model cancer cell lines [3]. Diverse studies have been used to determine which ABC transporters are involved in MDR. Studying the expression of ABC transporters using real time RT-PCR has shown the reliable correlation between expression of several ABC proteins and decreased cell sensitivity to different drugs, and it was also shown that no less than 30 ABC proteins can stimulate a decrease in drug sensitivity in tumor cells [1]. The use of microchips to compare transcription of the ABC transporter-encoding genes in cell lines resistant and sensitive to antitumor drugs showed that 28 transporters can define resistance to some drugs. They can be regulated at different levels such as transcription and translation; the *MDR1* gene transcription is activated by very different factors-antitumor drugs, ultraviolet radiation, inducers of differentiation, phorbol esters, carcinogens, etc [1]. Various signal cascades are involved in the regulation of ABC proteins. The effects of retinoids are achieved due to their interaction with nuclear receptors of the RAR family, mainly RARα; overexpression of the RARα gene in cells of solid tumors and some hemoblastoses enhance constitutive expression of the *MDR1* gene. Ras mutations are found in approximately 25-30% of all human tumors, and interestingly Raf-mediated signal pathway may be involved in regulation of *MDR1* gene transcription [1].

DRUG TARGET ALTERATIONS

Modifications of drug targets are best characterized by alterations in the expression and function of DNA topoisomerases. Topoisomerase II family members are targets for several classes of chemotherapeutic drugs, including anthracylines, anthracenediones, and epipodphyllotoxins; the genotoxic nature of these compounds lies in the stabilization of DNA-topoisomerase II complexes after DNA cleavage, resulting in the accumulation of DNA double-strand breaks. Resistance to these topoisomerase II inhibitors has been shown to result from decreased levels of topoisomerase II expression and decreased enzymatic activity arising from mutations in specific domains of this protein [2]. Many classes of chemotherapeutic drugs elicit their cytotoxic effects by damaging DNA. A likely mechanism of MDR is increased rates or levels of DNA repair; *i.e.*, DNA repair enzyme MGMT catalyzes the removal of methyl adducts of the O^6 of guanine resulting from treatment with nitrosoureas and levels of MGMT enzymatic activity have been shown to correlate with sensitivity to nitrosourea-mediated cell death, suggesting that MGMT may be an important effector of drug resistance. Some chemotherapeutic drugs use physiological apoptotic pathways to mediate cell death. Bcl-2 family of proteins has been demonstrated to play a major role in the regulation of programmed cell death and has recently been shown to correlate with acquired MDR [2]. Matrix independent growth is a major step in cellular transformation leading to cancer because transformed cells lose the requirement for adhesion, and it is also proposed that cancer cells use the antiapoptotic effects of matrix adhesion for survival. Particularly, integrin ligation has been demonstrated to protect tumor cells from a number of apoptotic stimuli. Several mechanisms of Cell Adhesion-Mediated Drug Resistance (CAMDR) have been identified, and these mechanisms of *de novo* drug resistance could be classified under four general categories: 1) decreased cellular proliferation, 2) alterations in drug target, 3) decreased apoptosis and, 4) integrin signaling cascades and cytoskeletal rearrangements [2].

Tyrosine Kinase Inhibitors (TKI)

The ErbB family of receptor tyrosine kinases include EGFR, ErbB2 (Her2/Neu), ErbB3 (Her3), and ErbB4 (Her4), which are overexpressed in a variety of human solid tumors [4]. These receptors lead to subsequent activation of intracellular signaling cascades such as the PI3K/Akt, Raf/MEK/Erk, and STAT signaling pathways [5]. Activation of the ErbB molecules correlates strongly with the pathogenesis and poor prognosis of many forms of cancer, and targeting the ErbB receptors has been intensely pursued as an important cancer therapeutic strategy. Anti-ErbB antibodies generally lead to disruption of the normal dimeric state of the transforming receptor complex, inhibiting kinase activity as well as causing downregulation of the expression of the receptor on the cell surface [4]. Although both of these two ErbB-targeted approaches have shown clinical promise, an increasing body of evidence indicates that patients initially responsive to ErbB targeted therapies may suffer from recurrence and develop tumors refractory to the original treatment, and a large percentage of ErbB positive cancers demonstrate a predisposition to resistance to ErbB targeted therapeutics [4]. Acquired resistance to EGFR tyrosine kinases inhibitors occurs in non-small cell lung cancer patients who initially respond to treatment but whose cancer then progresses. This acquired resistance has been associated with the development of a secondary mutation in EGFR, analogous to those observed in BCR-Abl and KIT in imatinib resistant chronic myelogenous leukemia and gastrointestinal stromal cell tumors, respectively. Initial studies have identified the T790M mutation in approximately 50% of cancers with acquired resistance to EGFR TKIs. Previous experiments have demonstrated that continued activation of the PI3K network is sufficient to confer resistance to EGFR TKIs [5]. Additionally the loss of inhibitory elements of the PI3K pathway, as PTEN and SIRP1, could participate in the resistance to EGFR inhibitors [4]. EGFR can form heterodimers with other members of their family like Her2 and then initiate a kinase signaling cascade that could inhibit apoptosis and stimulate cell proliferation mediated *via* PI3K /Akt and Erk1/2 MAPK [6]. Gefitinib reduced the phosphorylation levels of EGFR, ErbB3, and Erk in human squamous carcinoma A431 cells, accompanied by activation of the signaling events mediated by the IGF-1 receptor such as phosphorylation of IRS-1 and the interaction of IRS-1 with PI3K. Loss of IGFBPs and activation of IGF-IR signaling may contribute to resistance to EGFR-targeted TKIs and simultaneous inhibition of EGFR and IGF-IR may effectively prevent recurrence in human cancers characterized by overexpression of EGFR [4]. Following clinical treatments with TKIs some patients develop resistance though diverse mechanisms; one of them is associated with the acquisition of the T790M mutation in the EGFR kinase domain creating a steric hindrance that limits the binding of the TKIs [4]. Amplification of MET, an RTK, was identified as another mechanism of acquired resistance; MET amplification causes resistance because it phosphorylates ErbB-3, which in turn activates PI3K. Additionally, by immunoprecipitating PI3K it has been determined that its signaling is maintained in the resistant cells by an activated IGFIR pathway and interestingly, a combination of an EGFR and an IGFIR inhibitor was sufficient to reverse the resistant phenotype [5]. Gastrointestinal Stromal Tumor (GIST) is commonly associated with activating mutations in the KIT receptor tyrosine kinase. Imatinib mesylate is an oral agent that specifically inhibits the BCR-ABL and ABL tyrosine kinases as well as the KIT and PDGFR receptor tyrosine kinases. Imatinib was used in the treatment of chronic myelogenous leukemia and was tested in the metastatic or unresectable GIST and was found to induce a partial response or stable disease. Primary resistance to imatinib occurs in about 15% of the patients. In up to 90% of the cases, GISTs have activating mutations in either the KIT or PDGFRA receptor tyrosine kinases; mutations tend to be single amino acid substitutions in the KIT kinase domains and occur particularly in exon 17. Such mutations were not observed in non-resistant, or primary resistant tumors. In CML, second site mutation in BCR-ABL is the predominant mechanism of imatinib resistance [7].

Hormone Resistance

Tumor resistance to hormonal agents frequently develops over time and presents a major impediment to the long-term effectiveness of such treatments. One of the most common hormonal-related treatments is the use of the selective estrogen receptor modulator tamoxifen. Most of the actions of estrogens and antiestrogens are mediated by the Estrogen Receptor (ER). Resistance would clearly result from loss of the steroid receptor protein, which could also be the consequence of mutant or variant receptors defective in hormone binding or in subsequent gene transcriptional regulation. Mutant receptors may be constitutively active without hormones or may recognize antiestrogens as estrogens, the latter resulting in tamoxifen-stimulated growth [8]. Estrogen-occupied ER-α normally enhances cell proliferation, at least in part by increasing the production of some growth factors and proto-oncogene proteins. Hormone resistance in such cells may result in a constitutive growth factor or oncogene protein production, attributable for example to altered hormone-response elements in growth factor genes or proto-oncogene mutations [8]. Proliferation and properties of estrogen receptor-positive cells can be influenced by factors produced by surrounding, estrogen receptor-negative cells; one can envision that overproduction of growth factors or oncogene products by adjacent estrogen receptor-negative breast cancer cells or by other surrounding cells (*e.g.*, stromal cells) may result in stimulation of proliferation or invasiveness *via* mechanisms that are not effectively antagonized by anti-estrogens [8]. PI3K and MAPK activated by EGFR family members are important for ER signaling in some tumors, as they phosphorylate and activate ER or its co-regulators, increase transcriptional activation potential and enhance cell proliferation. In addition it is possible that in tumors expressing both receptors (Her2 and ER), cell proliferation could be increased and may contribute to hormonal therapy resistance [6]. Gene expression profile studies have identified a set of breast cancer antiestrogen resistance genes suggesting the profile has a predictive value in breast cancer patients [9]. In addition, pharmacokinetics changes may include deficient uptake or retention of the hormone or antiestrogen by the cancer cell or an active system promoting the efflux of the hormonal agent. Alterations may include cellular metabolism of the antiestrogen to biologically inactive forms or to estrogenic forms [8].

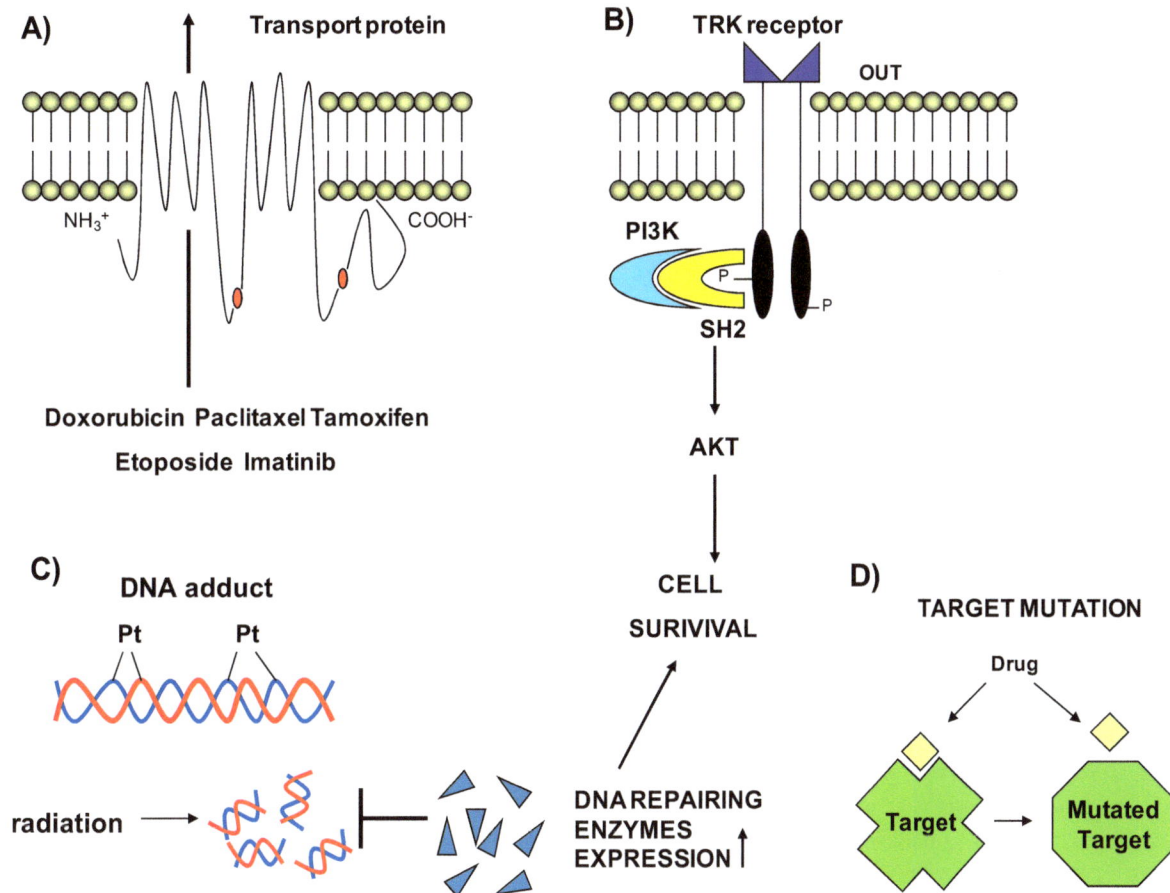

Figure 1: Mechanisms of drug resistance. Cancer cells may avoid drug toxicity by: *A)* Expression of cell membrane transporters (such as the ATP-binding cassette transporters) which drive antineoplastic drugs out of the cell decreasing their intracellular concentration and effectiveness or B) by acquirement of resistance to apoptosis either by enhanced activity of tyrosine kinase receptors that activate pro-survival pathways or C) by up-regulation of DNA repairing enzymes activity or expression or *D)* by mutation of drug targets.

Prostate cancer cells are typically androgen-dependent and androgen ablation is the standard systemic therapy for this disease. Androgen deprivation induces programmed cell death in normal, hyperplastic, preneoplastic, and malignant prostatic epithelial cells. Virtually all prostate cancer patients treated with androgen ablation respond but many of them eventually develop resistance, an ominous clinical state for which no consistently effective therapy exists. Amplification or mutation of the androgen receptor occurs in 20 to 30% of androgen ablation-resistant prostate cancers, suggesting that tumor cells become hypersensitive and respond to low levels of androgens or become promiscuous and can be stimulated by alternative ligands with structural homology to androgen. An alternative model for therapy resistance suggests that recruitment of non-steroid receptor signal transduction pathways can activate the androgen response in the setting of clinical androgen deprivation. Gene expression profiles for androgen ablation-resistant tumors reflected an apparent reactivation of the androgen-responsive program. These reflect the physiological changes that occur in treated tumors and may provide useful markers of response and targets for combination therapy [10].

Antibodies Resistance

CD20 may have kinase activity and function as a calcium channel. This may be an "ideal" antigen for targeted therapy, as it is not shed or internalized and does not circulate in the plasma as free protein, and various monoclonal antibodies have been raised against CD20, which exert differential effects on binding, and may have significant differential mechanisms of cytotoxicity. Unfortunately most of the responses to antibodies against CD20 are incomplete, and approximately 50% of patients may not respond to initial treatment. Antibody-mediated cellular cytotoxicity, mediated through ligation of the Fc portion of the monoclonal antibody to Fc receptors appears to be a major mechanism of action. Additionally, certain anti-CD20 monoclonal antibodies *in vitro* translocate CD20 into lipid rafts and activate the lytic complement. Treatment of tumor cells with antibodies that are capable of inducing a pro-apoptotic signal *via* their cell surface target structure may induce cellular responses against the tumor. Using cDNA microarrays in primary lymphoma specimens, it has been found that most of the gene expression pattern more similar to normal lymph nodes was from non-responders to anti-CD 20 therapies. Many of the overexpressed genes in this non-responder group were involved in cellular immune responses, including cytokine, complement and T cell receptor signaling. There are no data supporting that staining intensity of CD20 expression will predict the response to antibodies and, on the other hand, loss of CD20 expression is not generally considered to be an important resistance mechanism to this therapy. Polymorphisms that encode FcRIIIa with a valine instead of phenylalanine in amino acid position 158, result in higher affinity of IgG1 increasing antibody induced cellular toxicity [11] Friedberg, 2005]. Clinical studies in patients with non-Hodgkin lymphoma have suggested that serum anti-CD20 levels were higher in responding patients than in non-responders, but other results suggested that pharmacokinetics does not affect the response in patients with follicular lymphoma. Interestingly decreased responses to CD antibodies can be solved with prolonged schedules and higher doses [11].

CONCLUSIONS

Cancer cells display several effective mechanisms that overcome the effects of anti-neoplasic drugs. This response is a serious problem in the clinic because many patients run into failing treatments while the tumors grow or spread to other sites. Research identifying inhibitors of the ABC transporters or targeting specific mutants of growth or hormone receptors would help to solve this problem. In addition, it would be worthwhile to analyze gene expression profiles of patients before initiating a specific therapy. Taken together, investigations on mechanisms of drug resistance and more *personal* gene expression studies should help to identify potential responders to treatment and recommend more successful therapies to patients.

ACKNOWLEDGEMENTS

The preparation of this book is part of a group research project supported by Conacyt (Grant 82175-M to JC). We thank Cynthia Chow for revising the English language.

REFERENCES

[1]   Stavrovskaya AA and Stromskaya TP. Transport proteins of the ABC family and multidrug resistance of tumor cells. Biochemistry (Mosc) 2008; 73(5): 592-604.

[2]   Shain KH and Dalton WS. Cell adhesion is a key determinant in *de novo* multidrug resistance (MDR): new targets for the prevention of acquired MDR. Mol Cancer Ther 2001; 1(1): 69-78.

[3]   Liu Y, Peng H, and Zhang JT. Expression profiling of ABC transporters in a drug-resistant breast cancer cell line using AmpArray. Mol Pharmacol 2005; 68(2): 430-8.

[4]   Wang Q and Greene MI. Mechanisms of resistance to ErbB-targeted cancer therapeutics. J Clin Invest 2008; 18(7): 2389-92.

[5]   Guix M, Faber AC, Wang SE, *et al.* Acquired resistance to EGFR tyrosine kinase inhibitors in cancer cells is mediated by loss of IGF-binding proteins. J Clin Invest 2008; 118(7): 2609-19.

[6]   Osborne CK, Shou J, Massarweh S and Schiff R. Crosstalk between estrogen receptor and growth factor receptor pathways as a cause for endocrine therapy resistance in breast cancer. Clin Cancer Res 2005; 11: 865s-70s.

[7]   Antonescu CR, Besmer P, Guo T, *et al.* Acquired resistance to imatinib in gastrointestinal stromal tumor occurs through secondary gene mutation. Clin Cancer Res 2005; 11(11): 4182-90.

[8]   Katzenellenbogen BS. Antiestrogen resistance: mechanisms by which breast cancer cells undermine the effectiveness of endocrine therapy. J Nat Cancer Inst 1991; 83(20): 1434-5.

[9]   Agthoven TV, Sieuwerts AM, Meijer-van Gelder M, *et al.* Relevance of breast cancer antiestrogen resistance genes in human breast cancer progression and tamoxifen resistance. J Clin Oncol 2009; 27: 542-9.

[10] Holzbeierlein J, Lal P, LaTulippe E, *et al.* Gene expression analysis of human prostate carcinoma during hormonal therapy identifies androgen-responsive genes and mechanisms of therapy resistance. Am J Pathol 2004; 164(1): 217-27.

[11] Friedberg J. Unique toxicities and resistance mechanisms associated with monoclonal antibody therapy. Hematology 2005; 329-34.

CHAPTER 12

Antisense Oligodeoxyribonucleotides (AS-ODNs) for Cancer Gene Therapy: A Clinical Perspective

María Luisa Benítez-Hess and Luis Marat Alvarez-Salas*

Department of Genetics and Molecular Biology, Centro de Investigación y de Estudios Avanzados del I.P.N., Avenida Instituto Politécnico Nacional 2508, 7360 Mexico City, Mexico

Abstract: Gene therapy allows the specific control of disease-associated genes. It has been used to target specific genes on different types of cancer. A singular approach to regulate gene expression includes the administration of small synthetic Therapeutic Nucleic Acids (TNAs) which include Antisense Oligonucleotides (AS-ODNs). AS-ODNs utilize DNA sequence information from a disease gene to synthesize a molecule complementary to an accessible target mRNA. Although, many AS-ODNs have shown promising results targeting specific genes in different cancer types at a preclinical stage, only few of them have entered clinical trials. In this review, we will focus on the most successful AS-ODNs administered in clinical trials. The use of AS-ODNs on the clinical set up often produced unexpected results, suggesting that design and pre-clinical modifications are required to improve responsiveness to treatment. It is important to note that even though these molecules show advantage over conventional drugs for treating disease, the use of AS-ODNs as standard therapy for cancer is still far.

Keywords: Antisense, oligonucleotides, oligodeoxynucleotides, DNA, cancer, cancer therapy, gene therapy, clinical trial, therapeutic nucleic acids, therapeutic oligonucleotides.

INTRODUCTION

Cancer may be defined as the result of a complex network of accumulated and aberrant molecular interactions within a cell. When cellular homeostasis is affected, gene expression becomes abnormal and/or some atypical molecular interactions transform a normal cell into a tumor cell. Such are the products of mutated genes that result in gain of function (*i.e. ras, bcr-abl*) or normal receptors and signaling proteins in pathways that regulate apoptosis or the cell cycle and that are dysregulated by a mutation that results in the loss of protein function (*i.e. P53*) [1].

Actual therapies for most types of cancer include surgical resection, radiotherapy or chemotherapy. The last two inhibit tumor cell proliferation by the use of radiation or by administration of cytotoxic drugs affecting continuously proliferating cells. Although these therapies allow tumor size control and improve patient survival, in some instances there is no response and drug resistance and harmful side-effects are generally present. Over the last decade, more attention has been focused on therapeutic approaches that arise from a wider understanding of the molecular events controlling cellular life-span and proliferation, as well as the knowledge of the human genome.

The continuous discovery of molecular targets for cancer led to the development of innovative strategies, which include the use of Therapeutic Nucleic Acids (TNAs). These molecules are target-based drugs composed of small chemically synthesized nucleosides/nucleotides, DNA or RNA moieties that selectively interfere with metabolic pathways or the expression and functionality of proteins associated with malignant transformation. The use of nucleic acids as therapeutic agents dates back over 40 years with the initial usage of nucleoside analogues to fight disease. Since then, TNAs have found many uses for cancer detection and treatment. Such approaches are characterized by an increased specificity against malignant cells and reduced side-effect toxicity [2].

In the last 20 years, increasing efforts for the development of therapeutic oligonucleotides that block the flow of genetic information or stimulate immunity have resulted in the suppression of disease-associated phenotypes [3]. Approaches to therapeutic oligonucleotides include: 1) blocking of transcription by triplex-forming

*Address correspondence to Luis Marat Alvarez-Salas: Department of Genetics and Molecular Biology, Centro de Investigación y de Estudios Avanzados del I.P.N., Avenida Instituto Politécnico Nacional 2508, 7360 Mexico City, Mexico; E-mail: lalvarez@cinvestav.mx

oligodeoxyribonucleotides (TFOs); 2) stimulation of innate immune response by CpG-containing Oligonucleotides (CpG-ODNs); 3) translational arrest by Antisense Oligonucleotides (AS-ODNs), catalytic oligonucleotides (ribozymes and DNAzymes) or small interfering RNAs (siRNAs); and 4) inhibition of protein function by RNA aptamers [4]. In this review, we will focus on the clinical use of AS-ODNs as therapeutic moieties for different types of cancer.

Antisense Oligonucleotides (AS-ODNs)

Early demonstrations of antisense moieties for gene silencing used antisense RNA (AS-RNA) and showed very high target specificity with no unspecific (off-target) effects. The mechanism of action of AS-RNA relies in the formation of long (>100nt) and stable double-stranded RNA with the complementary target mRNA thus producing translational arrest (physical blockage of ribosome binding). However, most AS-RNA silencing approaches required intracellular expression and consequently were limited to cell culture applications. AS-RNA is usually sought for long-term gene suppression through the control of inducible promoters [5].

AS-ODNs utilize DNA sequence information from a disease gene to synthesize a molecule complementary to an accessible target mRNA. Like AS-RNAs, hybridization with the target RNA by Watson–Crick base pairing provides high specificity and affinity to produce translational arrest. In addition, due to their reduced length (usually 15-25nt), AS-ODNs can inhibit splicing, modulate polyA site selection or cause disruption of regulatory RNA structure (Fig. 1) [6]. The formation of DNA-RNA heteroduplexes has the extra advantage of activating cellular RNaseH causing cleavage of the target mRNA and thus increasing gene silencing potential [7].

AS-ODN Design Considerations

Target Accessibility

The specificity of AS-ODNs heavily relies on the fidelity of Watson-Crick hybridization [8]. However, the structural features of the target mRNA and intracellular mRNA–protein interactions constraints AS-ODN accessibility and consequently their effect [9, 10]. To avoid this limitation, some successful AS-ODNs are targeted to regions nearby the start codon or splicing donor/acceptor sites of a target mRNA as they are usually poorly structured to allow ribosome anchorage or accessibility for the splicing machinery [11].

Mapping antisense accessible regions within a target mRNA has been accomplished by using cell extracts, RNase digestion, ODN libraries and even ribozyme or DNAzyme libraries, resulting in very successful AS-ODNs [12-16]. Nevertheless, many effective AS-ODNs have been chosen by consideration of the thermodynamic or structural properties of the target RNA using computer algorithms [17-19]. This last approach still requires experimental confirmation by testing several AS-ODNs for adequate hybridization in a cellular environment [20, 21]. Therefore, a comprehensive study of the target mRNA sequence, structure and genomic stability must precede any experimental set-up for therapeutic AS-ODNs.

Cell Uptake

In general, oligonucleotides do not efficiently enter most cell types on *in vitro* applications. To achieve a useful level of cell uptake it is usually necessary to use transfection reagents [22], which may produce cytotoxicity levels unacceptable for therapeutic use [23, 24]. Although many transfection reagents are available, empirical testing is required to identify the best choice for transfecting a given cell type [25]. Various synthetic carriers including liposomes, polymeric nanoparticles and dendrimers have been extensively tested as AS-ODN delivery agents [26-28]. However, the particulate nature of these materials may limit their *in vivo* bio-distribution [29]. In addition to nanoparticle carriers, other approach has been to chemically conjugate AS-ODNs with various Cell-Penetrating Peptides (CPPs). Most CPPs are polycationic sequences with the ability to penetrate the cell membrane to the cytosol while carrying linked molecules such as AS-ODNs, peptides or even full proteins [30]. Although CPPs have obtained some success, the concentrations needed for biological effects are often higher than those usually considered for therapeutic AS-ODNs [31]. However, oligonucleotides efficiently enter cells *in vivo* through diverse administration routes [32]. AS-ODNs and other therapeutic oligonucleotides are usually internalized in cells through receptor-mediated endocytotic pathways [33].

Stability in Biofluids

As mentioned above, AS-ODNs can produce many effects including up-regulation, down-regulation or isoform shifting of a particular cancer-related gene. They can be administered as typical drugs, potentially allowing for precise control of gene expression. Because of their macromolecular nature, the stability and efficient delivery of AS-ODNs are often affected by the presence of nucleases in biological fluids. Thus, modification of oligonucleotide chemistry to improve antisense delivery and activity in biological fluids is an important factor to the success of AS-ODN therapeutics [34, 35].

Several nucleotide modifications have been introduced to increase AS-ODN stability in biofluids. To avoid changes in hybridization specificity, these changes include modifications in the phosphate backbone of nucleic acids and the ribose component of the nucleotide. First generation AS-ODNs consisted of sulfur-substituted DNA on the free oxygen molecules constituting a phosphodiester bond (phosphorothioate or PS linkages). Phosphorothioated ODNs (PS-ODNs) have sufficient resistance to nucleases while retaining the ability to form RNaseH substrates for efficient and highly specific silencing of the target RNA [36] (Fig. **1**). RNaseH activity would lead to destruction of the pre-mRNA in the nucleus before it could be spliced [37]. However, due to their strongly polyanionic nature PS-ODNs have proven less satisfactory regarding their affinity towards target sequences, specificity, cellular uptake, biodistribution and toxicity [36]. Nevertheless, PS-ODNs are the most extensively studied AS-ODNs in various models and have been tested in several human clinical trials [38].

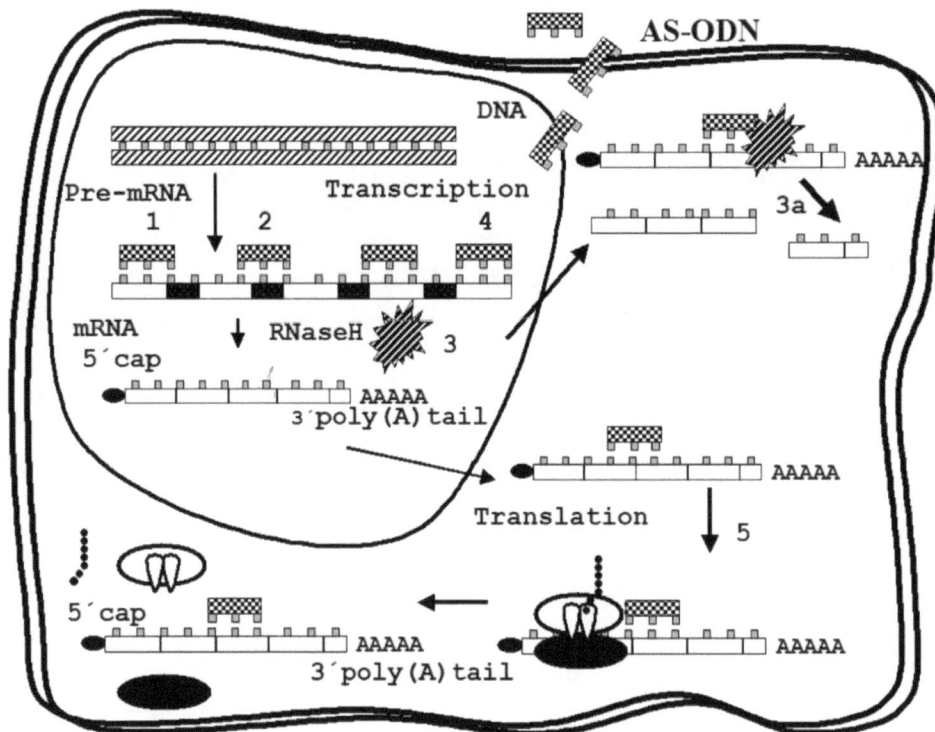

Figure 1: AS-ODNs mechanisms of action. 1) Blocking of capping; 2) Splicing inhibition of; 3) Induction of RNaseH on RNA/DNA heteroduplexes; 4) Polyadenylation inhibition; 5) Blocking of ribosome anchorage.

Sugar modifications such as 2'-*O*-methyl and 2'-methoxyethyl are relatively conservative changes that have been the main focus of research in recent years. They exhibit decreased toxicity, higher affinities for target sequences and very high resistance to nucleases compared with PS-ODNs [39, 40]. However, 2'-modified nucleotides cannot act as a substrate for RNaseH. There are only a few exceptions such as when using 2'-deoxy-2'-fluoro-arabinonucleic acids (2'-F-ANA), whose mixed hybrids with RNA were shown to be substrates for RNaseH [41, 42]. These so-called second generation AS-ODNs have increased biological activity, reduced off-target effects and increased *in vivo* stability, which makes oral administration feasible and have been used successfully from the bench to the clinic over the past several years [43]. Thus 2'-modified AS-ODNs are well suited to modulate gene expression by blocking splice sites and shifting alternative or aberrant splicing of targeted pre-mRNA (precursor to mRNA) [44]. They are also suitable for gene down-regulation by blocking ribosome anchorage to a target mRNA.

Newer generation AS-ODNs include Peptide Nucleic Acids (PNA) with the entire phosphate deoxyribose backbone replaced by uncharged *N*-(2-aminoethyl)-glycine linkages [45] and Phosphorodiamidate Morpholino Oligomers (PMOs) or 2′-methoxyethyl modified phosphorothioate oligonucleotides. PNAs have a non-charged backbone and thus hybridization is not affected by the intrastrand electrostatic repulsion enhancing affinity and rates of association and prevents binding to proteins that normally recognize polyanions, avoiding a major source of non-specific interactions that plagued PS-containing ODNs [46]. Additionally, PNAs do not appear to be substrates for nucleases or proteases [47].

PMOs are more water-soluble than PNAs and they too hybridize with RNA in a sequence-specific manner without inducing RNaseH degradation. PMO antisense molecules are steric blockers and inhibit gene expression by physically preventing binding or progression of splicing or translational machinery components [48]. PMOs dominate applications requiring exceptionally high specificity in complex systems [49]. Although other modifications are very promising for AS-ODN applications (*i.e.* LNAs), we shall limit to only those currently evaluated in cancer therapy clinical trials.

Immunostimulatory Issues

Other important consideration for the *in vivo* use of AS-ODNs is that oligonucleotides containing CpG motifs can stimulate the innate immune system [50]. While this stimulation may be advantageous for some therapies, it might also lead to misleading results. In fact, the activity observed with many therapeutic oligonucleotides (AS-ODNs, siRNA, *etc.*) in several animal models was, at least in part, due to innate immunity activation and not only to target mRNA degradation [51, 52]. The immunostimulatory effect of CpG motifs can be negated by using 4-methylcytosine and other cytosine derivatives within the AS-ODN sequence [53]. Nevertheless, including these modifications may induce toxic or off-target effects. Therefore, it is necessary to thoroughly evaluate AS-ODNs in immunocompetent animal models before clinical testing.

Clinical Trials for Anticancer AS-ODNs

Clinical trials for most AS-ODNs concentrate on several forms of degenerative diseases including cancer and seldom on viral inhibition. The first AS-ODNs under clinical trials used PS-ODNs targeted against cancer related genes such as apoptosis pathway proteins (*i.e. BCL-2*) [54], protein kinase C-α (*PKC-α*) [55], angiogenic factors [56, 57] and oncogenes (*c-raf, c-myb, c-myc*) [58-60]. Although powerful and specific *in vitro* gene silencing agents, most antisense PS-ODNs failed to survive phase I clinical trials due to severe side-effects [61]. Most common side-effects associated with PS-ODN include thrombocytopenia, elevation in hepatic transaminases, fever, rigors, complement activation and fatigue [54, 62]. These side-effects are not sequence-specific and probably related to the polyanionic nature of the PS-substituted backbone [63-66]. Nevertheless, some PS-ODNs showed promising therapeutical effects with less severe side-effects and progressed to phase II clinical trials.

There are several AS-ODNs developed for cancer treatments so we will briefly describe the type of cancer and describe the therapeutic target to which AS-ODNs are directed, as well we will relate clinical trials in which they have been tested. For each TNA, we will focus on the chemical composition, size of these TNAs (Table **1**). From the clinical trials will focus on the type of AS-ODN target, development stage and if there are applications to the Food and Drug Administration (FDA, Table **2**). In addition, we will mention the overall toxic effects reported for a particular AS-ODN, resuming all the trials reported (Table **3**).

Target: c-myc

The proto-oncogene *c-myc*, an important regulator of cell proliferation and differentiation, encodes a ubiquitously expressed nuclear phosphoprotein found mainly in heterodimeric complexes with the related *MAX* protein. The *MYC/MAX* complexes bind to DNA in a sequence-specific manner and activate transcription thereby inducing cell transformation and cell cycle progression.

Table 1: Main characteristics of AS-ODNs tested on clinical trials

AS-ODN	Modifications	Sequence	Size	Target
AVI-4126	Morpholino ring backbone	ACGTTGAGGGGCATCGTCGC	20nt	*c-myc* AUG start site
ISIS2503	Phosphorothioate linkages	GGGACTCCTCGCTACTGCCT	20nt	*Ha-ras* AUG start site
ISIS3521 (CGP64128A, ISIS 641A, LY900003, Aprinocarsen)	Phosphorothioate linkages	GTTCTCGCTGGTGAGTTTCA	20nt	3'-UTR of PKC-α mRNA
ISIS5132 (CGP 69846A)	Phosphorothioate linkages	TCCCGCCTGTGACATGCATT	20nt	3'-UTR of *RAF-1* mRNA
OGX-011 (ISIS112989)	2′-methoxyethyl nucleotides and phosphorothioate linkages	CAGCAGCAGAGTCTTCATCAT	21nt	Clusterin AUG start site
GTI-2040	Phosphorothioate linkages	GGCTAAATCGCTCCACCAAG	20nt	RNR2
Oblimersen (G3139, Genasense)	Phosphorothioate linkages	TCTCCCAGCGTGCGCCAT	18nt	First six codons of the *BCL-2* mRNA

Table 2: Summary of AS-ODNs tested in clinical trials

AS-ODN	Clinical trial	Type of Cancer
AVI-4126	Phase I	Solid tumors (Prostate and breast)
ISIS2503	Phase I	Advanced carcinoma
	Phase I	Colorectal cancer, non-small cell lung cancer, gastrointestinal tract cancers other than colorectal and pancreatic cancer, mesothelioma and leiomyosarcoma, breast cancer and a variety of other tumors
	Phase II	Advanced or metastatic pancreatic adenocarcinoma
ISIS3521 (CGP 64128A, ISIS641A, LY900003, Aprinocarsen)	Phase I	Ovarian, colon, pancreatic, or lung cancer. Other tumor histologies included granulose cell, gastric, esophageal, breast, and lymphoma
	Phase I	Advanced cancer lymphocytic lymphoma
	Phase I	Advanced cancer, Ovarian, colon, pancreatic, sarcoma, lung, gastric, esophageal, breast, melanoma, and lymphoma
	Phase II	Advanced ovarian carcinoma
	Phase I/II	Metastatic colorectal cancer
	Phase II	Non-Hodgkin's lymphoma
	Phase I/II	Non-small cell lung cancer
ISIS5132 (CGP 69846A)	Phase I	Refractory malignancies
	Phase I	Solid malignancies
	Phase I	Advanced cancer
	Phase II	Small-cell and non-small cell lung cancer.
ISIS5132 or ISIS3521	Phase II	Hormone-refractory prostate cancer
OGX-011 (ISIS 112989)	Phase I	Prostate cancer
	Phase I	Advanced cancer

GTI-2040	Phase I	Advanced solid tumor, or lymphoma
	Phase I/II	Renal cell carcinoma
Oblimersen (G3139, Genasense)	Phase I and II	Hormone-refractory prostate cancer
	Phase I	Advanced cancer
	Phase I	Hormone-refractory prostate cancer
	Phase I	Metastatic colorectal cancer
Oblimersen (G3139, Genasense)	Phase II	Recurrent B-cell non-Hodgkin's lymphoma
	Phase I	Solid tumors
	Phase I	Chronic lymphocytic leukemia
	Phase III FDA Application	Relapsed or refractory chronic lymphocytic leukemia
	Phase I	Leukemia
	Phase I and II	Acute myeloid leukemia
	Phase I	Non-Hodgkin's lymphoma
	Phase II	B-cell non-Hodgkin's lymphoma
	Phase II	Multiple myeloma
	Phase I, II, III FDA application	Advanced melanoma
	Phase I/II	Breast cancer
	Phase I and II	Small-cell lung cancer

Gains at chromosome 8q, where *c-myc* (8q24) is also located, are often associated to prostate cancer [67]. Additionally, *c-myc* consensus sites have been identified in the androgen receptor, and these seem to be involved in androgen-mediated up-regulation of androgen receptor mRNA. Androgen deprivation therapy has been observed to cause *c-myc* and androgen receptor gene amplifications associated with increased cell proliferation. Distinct changes in gene copy number before and after androgen ablation suggest possible involvement of the *c-myc* gene in the escape from androgen control, making *c-myc* a rational target for treatment of this disease. *C-myc* amplification is a feature of increasing grade and stage in prostate cancer and predicts adverse outcome in locally advanced disease [68].

Antisense *vs.* myc: AVI-4126

Phase I clinical trials for an antisense PS-ODN directed to *C-MYC* mRNA (AVI-4126) involved a single center, open label and dose-escalating application in healthy volunteers showing no toxicity or serious adverse events. *C-MYC* involvement in prostate cancer led to the clinical application in patients with advanced HRPC who have failed androgen ablation, thus defining the scope of AVI-4126-directed therapy for prostate cancer [69]. A second phase I study was conducted in patients undergoing resection surgery for prostate or breast tumors. Again, administration of the AS-ODN had no adverse events. Response to AVI-4126 therapy was tested in tumor samples and adjacent normal tissue from which the concentration and distribution of AVI-4126 was measured. Data revealed significant tissue accumulation of AVI-4126. Thus, AVI-4126 is a promising new agent that might be used alone or in combination with either hormonal or cytotoxic therapies [70].

Target: H-ras

Four human *ras* genes, *H-ras, N-ras* and the splice variants, *K-ras*A and *K-ras*B, have been implicated in the etiology and maintenance of the malignant phenotype. Human cancers demonstrate multiple abnormalities involving *ras* gene products directly or indirectly. These include activating mutations in at least one of the three *ras* genes at an early stage of tumor progression in 20–25% of all human tumors and overexpression of *ras* proteins, or overexpression of growth factors and their receptors whose downstream signaling is mediated by *RAS* pathways. *H-ras* itself has been implicated as an important growth promoter in pancreatic cell lines with mutations of *K-ras*. Because the *ras* signaling pathway has been implicated in a variety of tumors, it is reasonable to hypothesize that AS-ODNs directed to *RAS* mRNA may result in a more effective treatment for several cancers [71].

Table 3: Adverse effects reported on anticancer AS-ODNs gene therapy

AS-ODN	Adverse effects
AVI-4126	Acid indigestion, backaches, chest wall pain, fever blister in lip, headaches, herpetic lesion in mouth, leg cramps, nausea and neck pain
ISIS2503	Abdominal pain, anemia, anorexia, bilirubin, fatigue, fever, hematologic toxicity, nausea, neutropenia, sepsis from a liver abscess, thrombocytopenia and thrombosis
ISIS3521 (CGP 64128A ISIS 641A LY900003 Aprinocarsen)	Anemia, catheter-related events, chills, diarrhea, elevated aspartate aminotransferase or alanine aminotransferase (alt) concentration, Elevated serum levels of amylase and lipase, emesis, fatigue, fever, headache, mild hepatic toxicity, myalgia, myelosuppression, nausea, neutropenia, pancreatitis, rigors, thrombocytopenia and vomiting
ISIS5132 (ISIS3521)	Acute hemolytic anemia, acute renal failure, abnormal C3a levels, chills, dose-dependent complement activation, increased prothrombin and partial thromboplastin time, increased IL-1R-a levels, increased serum TNF-α levels, fatigue, fever, hypotension, mild anemia, mild leukopenia, nausea, sepsis, thrombocytopenia, vomiting, central venous catheter infections, fatigue, lethargy, nausea, thrombosis and thrombocytopenia
ISIS3521 or ISIS5132	Central venous catheter infections, fatigue, lethargy, nausea, thrombosis and thrombocytopenia
OGX-011 (ISIS112989)	Alopecia, anemia, anorexia, dehydration, diarrhea, dyspnea, elevation of liver enzymes, elevations in hepatic transaminase levels, fatigue, fever, leukopenia, mucositis, nausea, neutropenia, rigors, thrombocytopenia and vomiting
GTI-2040	Anorexia, complement activation, elevated hepatic transaminases and bilirubin levels, erythematous macular skin rash, fatigue, infections (non-neutropenic) with gram-negative pathogens, nausea and neutropenia
Oblimersen (G3139, Genasense)	Abdominal pain, alopecia, anemia, angioedema, anorexia, arthralgia, atrial fibrillation, back pain, catheter-related deep vein thrombosis, central venous catheter infection and bacteremia, cough, cytokine release reaction syndrome, diarrhea, drug-induced rash, duodenal obstruction, elevated serum transaminase levels, elevated hepatic transaminase levels, elevation of aspartate serum transferase, elevations in creatinine, hyperlacrimation, fatigue, febrile neutropenia, fever, fevers, hepatomegaly, hypokalemia, hypophosphatemia, hypotension, leukocytosis, leukopenia, lymphopenia, mucositis, myalgias, myelosuppression, nail bed changes and onchylosis, nausea, neutropenia, night sweats, palpitations, pemphigus, neutropenia, peripheral edema, peripheral neuropathy, polyuria, pulmonary embolism, pyrexia, rash, reduction in total leukocyte counts, rigors, sensory neuropathy, stomatitis, thrombocytopenia, urinary retention and vomiting

Antisense *vs.* ras: ISIS 2503

ISIS2503 is a PS-ODN targeting *H-RAS* mRNA. This AS-ODN has been tried in phase I and in phase II studies. Phase I trials on patients with diverse advanced solid tumors were treated with intravenous (i.v.) doses of ISIS2503 reporting non-consistent changes (decreases) on peripheral blood mononuclear cells (PBMCs) *H-RAS* mRNA levels. No patients achieved complete or partial responses (tumor size), although a few patients did have stabilization of disease for two months or longer [58].

A second phase I trial used ISIS2503 in combination with the anticancer drug gemcitabine (2',2'-difluorodeoxycytidine; a S-phase specific pyrimidine analogue), in patients with advanced solid tumors [71]. Co-administration of gemcitabine and ISIS2503 did not show any alteration on plasma disposition. Most patients treated with ISIS2503 showed prolonged disease stabilization. Therapeutic response was difficult to report because most of the patients discontinue the treatment before evaluation for tumor response. However, there was a single case in a breast cancer patient with a partial response presenting 80% decrease in subcutaneous metastasis and 50% reduction on liver metastases [71]. In phase II trials of ISIS2503-gemcitabine combined therapy was administrated to patients with metastatic or locally advanced pancreatic adenocarcinoma. Most patients had evidence of progressive disease and died during the 25-month follow-up. The overall 6-month survival after treatment percentage was 57.5%. However, the overall response rate was only 10.4%. Two additional patients experienced partial responses that were not confirmed on a subsequent scan [72]. From the phase II results, the combination of ISIS2503-gemcitabine produced an improvement in the patient survival of 6.7 months when compared with administration of gemcitabine alone (5.7 months) [73], and also the overall response rate increased from 5% with gemcitabine alone to 10% in combination with ISIS2503.

Target: Protein Kinase C (PKC)

PKC is an attractive target in cancer therapy. It is over-expressed in a variety of tumors, and several non-specific *PKC* inhibitors have demonstrated antitumor activity [74]. Experiments in keratinocytes have suggested that *PKC-α* is involved in mediating the transforming effects of oncogenic *ras* [75, 76]. AS-ODNs targeted against *PKC-α*, which have high specificity, can inhibit mRNA and protein expression as well as the growth of tumors *in vitro* and *in vivo*.

Antisense *vs.* PKC: ISIS3521

ISIS3521 antisense PS-ODN was administered in a phase I study on patients with different incurable malignancies, to characterize the safety profile and to determine the maximum tolerated dose of antisense. The maximum tolerated dose was 2.0 mg/kg/day. Pharmacokinetic measurements showed rapid plasma clearance and dose-dependent steady-state concentrations of ISIS3521. The primary metabolite seen in plasma was a shortened form of ISIS3521 by one nucleotide in the 3'-end. Evidence of tumor response lasting up to 11 months was observed in few patients with ovarian cancer. Interestingly, the ovarian tumor mass in these patients stabilized for several months before shrinking [64]. Phase II trials designed to determine the antitumor response, disease progression and toxicity of ISIS3521 in patients with advanced ovarian carcinoma showed no significant clinical activity [77].

A parallel study administered ISIS3521 three times weekly showed complete remissions in two patients with low-grade lymphoma [62]. Re-evaluation 3 months later revealed no clinical or radiologic evidence of relapse 12+ months after treatment. The other patient showed a recurrent lymphoma 4 months later. No further disease has been clinically evident, and no additional therapy has been administered for an additional 4+ months.

Another phase I trial was designed to determine the Maximum Tolerated Dose (MTD), toxicity profile, pharmacokinetics and antitumor activity of ISIS3521 in combination with 5-fluorouracil (5-FU, pyrimidine analog) and Leucovorin (LV) adjuvant (a mixture of 5-formyl derivatives from tetrahydrofolate) in patients with advanced cancer. The toxic symptoms reported are common in 5-FU therapy, and the number of patients with these toxicities did not appear to be greater than what might be expected from 5-FU/LV alone. Therefore, ISIS3521 is tolerable as a single-agent dose when given with 5-FU/LV and clinical improvement in antitumor activity was observed [78].

A phase I/II study of ISIS3521 in combination with cisplatin and gemcitabine in patients with advanced Non-Small Cell Lung Cancer (NSCLC) was conducted to assess the safety of the combination and to evaluate the antitumor activity of the triple drug combination in chemotherapy-naïve NSCLC patients. Results showed two patients with discernable antitumor activity. In addition, prolonged stabilization lasting 5 months was observed in two other patients. No pharmacokinetic interactions occurred with the combination. In the phase II portion, 36% of the patients showed response (one complete and 13 partial). The median time to treatment failure was 3.9 months, whereas the median time response to progression for the most of the patients was 4.4 months [79]. A separate phase II study of ISIS3521 in patients with previously treated low-grade non-Hodgkin's lymphoma resulted in partial response to the treatment. The overall median time to progression for all evaluable patients was 2.8 months. Clinically significant hematological toxicities were largely limited to thrombocytopenia [80].

Target: PKC-α AND RAF-1

Because of the diverse number of growth factor receptor tyrosine kinases associated with tumor growth, selective inhibition of the specific signal transduction pathways represents an attractive therapeutic target. The antiproliferative effects may be independent of the specific growth receptor family responsible for malignant growth [81, 82]. *RAF-1* is a 74kDa serine/threonine protein kinase that plays a broad role in oncogenic signaling connecting upstream growth factor-mediated tyrosine kinase stimulation with downstream activation of serine threonine kinases and the mitogenic signaling pathways. *RAF-1* is activated by phosphorylation after translocation to the plasma membrane by a mechanism that involves *RAS* in the mitogen-activated protein kinase pathway and hence is involved in oncogenic transformation and tumor cell proliferation [83].

PKC-α also has an important role in tumor growth and proliferation independent of *raf* interactions, and has been implicated in the transformation and growth of breast, colorectal, and prostate tumors [84-86]. The degree of *PKC-α* expression may also represent a biomarker of malignant transformation in the prostate with pathologic evidence; enhanced *PKC-α* expression is detectable in early prostate carcinoma specimens but not in adjacent benign prostatic epithelium [87]. *PKC-α* inhibition from a diverse array of strategies promotes apoptosis in androgen-independent prostate cell lines [88-91].

PKC-α and *RAF-1* are important elements of proliferative signal transduction pathways in both normal and malignant cells. Abrogation of either *RAF-1* or *PKC-α* function can both inhibit cellular proliferation and induce apoptosis in several experimental cancer models including prostate cancer cell lines. Both *RAF-1* and *PKC-α* protein expression can be potently inhibited *in vitro* by specific antisense oligonucleotides in a concentration-dependent and sequence-dependent manner. Furthermore, inhibition of *PKC-α* or *RAF-1* by antisense oligonucleotides has demonstrated broad antitumor activity in several human tumors tested *in vitro* and *in vivo* [20, 92, 93]. Therefore, inhibition of *PKC-α* and *RAF-1* appears to be a valid therapeutic strategy for androgen-independent prostate cancer [74].

Antisense *vs.* raf: ISIS5132

ISIS5132 AS-ODN comes from an extensive screening of more than 50 antisense-designed PS-ODNs targeted to human *c-raf* mRNA. ISIS5132 was identified as being the most potent inhibitor of *c-raf* gene expression both *in vitro* and *in vivo* C-RAF inhibition results in a dramatic alteration of downstream signaling events within the MAP kinase signaling pathway. Moreover, ISIS5132 displays potent antitumor activity against a broad spectrum of tumor types in mouse models and has progressed to phase I clinical trials.

In an effort to identify potential back-up compounds to ISIS5132, varieties of second-generation 2'-modifications have been evaluated for activity against *c-raf* in cell culture. A number of second-generation oligonucleotides with improved biophysical characteristics resulted in enhanced activity against *c-raf* in cell culture. Activity enhancement was most pronounced for 2'-O-methoxyethyl-modified oligonucleotides and this modification resulted in significantly improved antitumor activity *in vivo* [94].

A phase I trial with ISIS5132 in patients with refractory malignancies was designed to determine the maximum tolerated dose, toxicity profile, pharmacokinetics, and antitumor activity of the ISIS5132. Significant reductions in *RAF-1* mRNA expression in PBMCs were observed in most of the patients within 48 hours of initial ISIS5132 dosing. The median reduction was to 42%. These effects on *RAF-1* expression were seen at all dose levels and were not dose-dependent [95]. When ISIS5132 was administered to patients with solid malignancies, none of the patients achieved a complete response. The study was terminated before a true maximum tolerated dose level was reached, and toxicity was modest in all respects. Specifically, there was no relationship between ISIS5132 infusion and activation of the complement system [65]. Response to ISIS5132 in patients with advanced cancer showed specific target gene reduction in treated patients and that PBMCs are suitable tissues for biomarker studies in future trials. [96].

Two multicenter phase II trials were designed to determine if tumor responses can be achieved in progressive Small-Cell Lung Cancer (SCLC) or Non-Small Cell Lung Cancer (NSCLC) patients treated with ISIS5132 and to further characterize the safety of the compound. The study showed a 20% response rate with 95% confidence intervals for NSCLC and cannot draw any conclusions for SCLC patients as only a few were involved in the study [97].

Hormone Refractory Prostate Cancer (HRPC) represents an intrinsically chemoresistant malignancy. The absence of effective chemotherapy that prolongs life provides a strong clinical impetus for the evaluation of new therapeutic approaches for the treatment of this disease [98]. Phase II trials comparing two AS-ODNs (ISIS3521 and ISIS5132) targeting *PKC-α* and *RAF-1* was evaluated in patients with HRPC. The most common treatment-related toxicity observed with either AS-ODNs were mild to moderate fatigue and lethargy. The percentage of intact parental AS-ODN to total oligonucleotide detected remained stable throughout the infusion period. The absence of tumor regressions produced the termination of the study and may indicate the limited importance of *RAF-1* and *PKC-α* in HRPC patients [98].

The standard treatment for metastatic colorectal cancer has been 5'-Fluorouracil, folinic acid (adjuvant) and CPT-11 (Irinotecan hydrochloride, a semi-synthetic derivative of the topoisomerase I inhibitor plant alkaloid camptothecin). Given the limited survival advantage and the toxicity of the treatment, there is a need to identify more active or less toxic agents. A Phase II trial comparing ISIS3521 and ISIS5132 was evaluated in patients with colorectal cancer.

Few patients receiving ISIS3521or ISIS5132 had stable disease; thus neither AS-ODN induced objective responses in untreated colorectal cancer patients [99].

Target: Clusterin

Recent investigations demonstrated that tumor resistance to therapy could arise from the increased activity of antiapoptotic pathways by up-regulation of antiapoptotic genes. Among these genes, clusterin (testosterone-repressed prostate message-2, apolipoprotein J or sulfated glucoprotein-2) plays functionally relevant roles in the acquisition of therapy-resistant prostate cancer, and thus is considered a potential therapeutic target. The clusterin gene locates at 8p21-p12 and has been linked to numerous physiologic and pathologic processes [100]. Clusterin binds to a wide variety of biological ligands and to be regulated by the transcription factor, Heat Shock Factor-1 (HSF-1), suggesting that clusterin functions like a heat shock protein to chaperone and stabilize conformations of proteins during periods of cell stress. In humans clusterin exists as both an intracellular truncated 55kDa form and a 75-80kDa extracellular heterodimeric secreted glycoprotein [101, 102]. The ability of clusterin to inhibit apoptosis has been shown to act through inhibition of activated *BAX*, a proapoptotic Bcl-2 family member [103]. In cancer, clusterin has been defined as an antiapoptotic protein that is activated after therapeutic stress [104, 105].

Antisense *vs.* Clusterin: OGX-011 (ISIS112989)

OGX-011 is an antisense PS-ODN complementary to clusterin mRNA [106]. The first phase I study with OGX-011 used a new adjuvant design to identify effective biological dosing [107]. Patients with localized prostate cancer and high-risk symptoms were enrolled on a dose escalation study and treated with OGX-011 for 1 month followed by prostatectomy. With this design an effective biological dose was established for OGX-011 based on its ability to suppress clusterin mRNA by >90%. Being a chaperone, the development of OGX-011 was conceptually applied to combined therapy with other anticancer drugs. Several cancers that over-express clusterin are also Docetaxel-sensitive; therefore, OGX-011-Docetaxel combination was evaluated in a phase I trial in patients with advanced cancer. Dose-limiting toxicity was not observed at any of the dose levels evaluated, and adverse events were limited (Table **3**). QRT-PCR analysis demonstrated a statistically significant dose-dependent decrease in clusterin RNA expression. To determine whether suppression of clusterin levels by OGX-011 treatment was associated with increased apoptosis, the apoptotic index was evaluated in prostatectomy specimens resulting in significantly higher apoptotic index in OGX-11 treated subjects. The presence of OGX-011 in plasma and prostate tissue was detected approximately 2-3 hours and concentration of OGX-011 in prostate tissue increased with dose [107]. Phase II trials of OGX-011 in combination with Docetaxel resulted of this trial show that OGX-011 was well tolerated and had a predictable plasma pharmacokinetic profile. More importantly, concentrations of OGX-011 could be achieved in prostate tissue that resulted in dose-dependent decreases in clusterin expression and an associated increase of the apoptotic index. Non-hematological toxicities were minimal [108]. Randomized Phase III trials are currently in the planning stages [109].

Target: Ribonucleotide Reductase (RNR)

The human Ribonucleotide Reductase (RNR) catalyzes the synthesis of 2'-deoxyribonucleotides from the corresponding ribonucleoside 5'-diphosphates. RNR consists of two subunits R1 and R2: Expression of both the R1 and R2 genes is required for enzymatic activity. R1 is a 160kDa dimer that contains at least two different effector-binding sites, and R2 is a 78kDa dimer that contains a non-heme iron that participates in catalysis by forming an unusual free radical on the aromatic ring of a tyrosine residue. Interestingly, R1 and R2 are encoded by different genes located on separate chromosomes, and the mRNAs for the two proteins are differentially expressed throughout the cell cycle. The mRNA levels for the R2 subunit is highest during late G1/early S phase when DNA replication occurs [110].

Antisense *vs.* RNR2: GTI-2040

The *RNR2* mRNA sequence targeted by GTI-2040 is identical in rat, monkey, mouse, and human. Given the sequence conservation, GTI-2040 efficacy and toxicity can be evaluated in a number of animal models [111, 112]. *RNR2* over-expression increases the drug resistant properties of cancer cells, whereas *RNR2* expression in antisense orientation leads to the reversal of drug resistance and results in decreased proliferation of tumor cells [113, 114]. Thus, specific inhibition of RNR2 expression is involved in an antiproliferative effect and may have antineoplastic benefits [114].

GTI-2040 produces a significant decrease of *RNR2* mRNA levels in several tumor cell lines resulting in a sequence-specific and dose-dependent antitumor activity. In murine models, GTI-2040 appeared to be active against a wide range of cancer types producing a significant decrease in tumor growth and end-point weight. Interestingly, GTI-2040 has exceptional efficacy against renal carcinomas (A498 and Caki-1) showing a dramatic growth inhibition of Caki-1 and A498 renal tumors and has higher antitumor efficacy compared with other *RNR2*-based therapeutic compounds such as 5-FU, gemcitabine and vinblastine. The observed antitumor activity of GTI-2040 is not attributable to CpG-mediated immune stimulation but combination of GTI-2040-mediated *RNR2* down-regulation and immune stimulation may be tested for an enhanced antitumor efficacy [112].

A phase I trial with continuous i.v. infusion of GTI-2040 in patients with advanced solid tumors or lymphoma indicated no complete or partial objective tumor responses. Few patients experienced disease stabilization for a period between 2 and 6 months. Constitutional toxicities consisting of fatigue and anorexia were the most common toxicities [115]. Results from this study recommended a higher dose of GTI-2040 with dose limiting toxicities being the fatigue and transient elevation of serum hepatic transaminases. Based on these considerations, a phase I/II trial combining GTI-2040 and oral administration of Capecitabine was tested in patients with advanced renal carcinoma. In the initial phase I portion of the protocol none of the first three patients experienced dose limiting toxicity. For the phase II portion, results from the total patients show that only one had a decrease greater than 30% in baseline lesion measurements but also developed new lesions and was thus characterized as progressive disease. Therefore, the combination of GTI-2040 and Capecitabine was not recommended for further evaluation in renal cancer [115, 116].

Target: BCL-2

The *BCL-2* family includes both proapoptotic and antiapoptotic proteins that regulate caspase-9 and -3 activation after a diverse array of apoptotic stimuli including DNA damage, chemo/hormonal therapy and irradiation [117]. After an apoptotic stimulus, *BAX* (the prototypic proapoptotic protein) undergoes homodimerization and localizes in the outer mitochondrial membrane, resulting in loss of mitochondrial membrane integrity, release of cytochrome c, activation of caspase-9, and initiation of caspase-mediated cell death. *BCL-2* inhibits apoptosis through competitive dimerization with *BAX*, thus preventing homodimerization and loss of mitochondrial membrane integrity [118, 119]. Overexpression of *BCL-2* protein has been demonstrated in tumors from patients with malignant melanoma, non-Hodgkin's lymphoma, and carcinomas of the prostate (hormone-refractory), colon, small cell and non-small cell lung, and breast and several leukemias [120-125].

Antisense *vs.* bcl-2: Oblimersen (Genasense, G3139)

Oblimersen is an antisense PS-ODNs targeted to the *BCL-2* mRNA causing a specific down-regulation of *BCL-2* expression, which leads to increased apoptosis and has been thoroughly tested in several clinical settings alone or in combination for a number of malignancies. It has been suggested that immunoactivation, rather than antisense activity, is primarily responsible for the therapeutic efficacy of Oblimersen as it showed significant immunostimulatory activities probably due to the presence of two CpG motifs in the sequence [126, 127]. Randomized clinical trials have been reported evaluating the efficacy and tolerability of Oblimersen in lung cancer, chronic lymphocytic leukemia, multiple myeloma, and malignant melanoma. In addition, nonrandomized trials evaluated Oblimersen in combination with different classes of chemotherapy agents and monoclonal antibodies in gastric, colon, breast, hepatocellular, prostate, and Merkel cell carcinoma; non-Hodgkin's lymphoma; acute myeloid leukemia; chronic myelogenous leukemia and multiple myeloma [128].

Oblimersen in HRPC

Phase I trials designed to determine Oblimersen safety in patients with HRPC reported a decline in *BCL-2* levels during treatment, but no major antitumor responses were observed. Fatigue and elevated transaminase levels were the only adverse events likely related to treatment [129]. Later phase I trials using Oblimersen in combination with Mitoxantrone (the standard chemotherapy for patients with HRPC) showed that Oblimersen was well tolerated. Two patients had >50% reductions in prostate-specific antigen [130].

Another phase I trial using a combination of Oblimersen and Docetaxel in patients with HRPC showed common PS-ODN toxicity effects (Table **3**). *BCL-2* showed decrements in PBMCs. Seven of these 12 patients had significant reduction in prostate-specific antigen lasting at least 4 weeks and the majority of the tumor specimens from treated patients exhibited weak *BCL-2* expression. The absence of severe toxicities evidence and the inhibition of *BCL-2* in

PBMCs and tumor tissue, and antitumor activity in HRPC patients granted further clinical evaluation of this combination. Phase II trials using the same combination showed prostate-specific antigen responses was reported on 52% of the patients, whereas 33% of the patients with bidimensionally measurable disease had objective responses. From the overall treatment, 69% of the patients had net decrements in normalized *BCL-2* levels. The main toxicities of the combination Oblimersen-Docetaxel are shown on Table **3** [131, 132].

Oblimersen in Colorectal Cancer

A combination therapy of Oblimersen and Irinotecan was tested in a phase I trial in patients with metastatic colorectal cancer. Results showed that the combination is feasible in pretreated patients with advanced colorectal cancer. Reduction in levels of *BCL-2* protein in PBMCs was documented following treatment. Only one patient had a partial response for 10 months. Another patient having previous exposure to Irinotecan had persistent stable disease for 10 months [133].

Paclitaxel induces prolonged mitotic arrest, resulting in hyperphosphorylation of *BCL-2* [134]. Phase I trials in patients with advanced solid tumors using Oblimersen in combination with Carboplatin and Paclitaxel showed that there was a small partial response. *BCL-2* expression was reduced by Oblimersen treatment in PBMCs. However, there was no change in detectable *BAX* expression in PBMCs as well as in biopsy specimens after Oblimersen administration nor alteration of the pharmacokinetics of Paclitaxel or Carboplatin [135].

Oblimersen in Chronic Lymphocytic Leukemia

Oblimersen was also evaluated on phase I, II and III clinical trials in patients with advanced chronic lymphocytic leukemia (relapsed or refractory to treatment with fludarabine). Phase I studies determined the maximum-tolerated dose, efficacy, safety, and pharmacokinetics of Oblimersen in stable or responding patients. During the phase II portion of the study, 8% of the patients showed partial responses. Other evidence of antitumor activity included: reduction in splenomegaly, disappearance of hepatomegaly, reduction of lymph node size and reduction in circulating lymphocyte counts [136]. Phase III trials designed to evaluate Oblimersen effect in comparison with other chemotherapeutic drugs (Fludarabine plus cyclophosphamide) in patients with relapsed or refractory chronic lymphocytic leukemia showed complete or nodular partial response in 17% of the patients in G3139 group compared with 7% of the patients in the chemotherapy group. A small number of patients had a treatment-related adverse event with an outcome of death (Table **3**). Causes of death were generally similar except for tumor lysis/cytokine release syndrome in two patients with underlying cardiac disease [137]. In 2006, the FDA agreed that the study did not demonstrate "substantial" evidence of effectiveness thus negating wide-spread use of Oblimersen.

Oblimersen in Non-Hodgkin's Lymphoma

BCL-2 is over-expressed in most low-grade non-Hodgkin's lymphoma cases and approximately 50% of high-grade non-Hodgkin's lymphoma cases. It has been demonstrated that the eradication of lymphoma in an animal model can be achieved by a 14-day subcutaneous infusion of Oblimersen [138]. These observations provided the rationale for a phase I trial of Oblimersen non-Hodgkin's lymphoma patients. Treatment resulted in toxicity reports (Table **3**) [54]. A phase II trial with Oblimersen in combination with rituximab in patients with recurrent B-cell non-Hodgkin's lymphoma, reported a 23% of complete responses and 19% of partial responses. Patients with follicular lymphoma achieved a 40% and 20% respective response. Overall, the combination was well tolerated and myelosuppression was the main hematological toxicity in this study. The combination of rituximab and G3139 was effective in patients with rituximab-refractory disease, suggesting that G3139 could overcome mechanisms of rituximab-resistance [139].

Oblimersen in Myeloid Leukemia

Patients with acute myeloid leukemia or acute lymphoblastic leukemia received Oblimersen and chemotherapy treatment (FLAG) on a phase I trial. Results demonstrated that Oblimersen can be administered safely with FLAG chemotherapy. The specific role of Oblimersen in inducing 45% overall disease response could not be discriminated from the antileukemic activity of FLAG. Thus, the results of this trial provide justification for future investigation of Oblimersen in acute leukemia [125]. Another phase I trial with patients with acute myeloid leukemia, received a standard multicourse chemotherapeutic program that included anthracyclines and Oblimersen treatment. The combination therapy demonstrated to be feasible and safe with a toxicity profile similar to that expected with chemotherapy alone. Of the treated patients, 48% achieved complete remission; in addition, 10% of the patients achieved incomplete remission. Among the patients assessable for both clinical response and *BCL-2* protein levels, the median level of *BCL-2* normalized to total proteins were decreased compared with baseline levels [140].

A phase I trial using Oblimersen and Gemtuzumab Ozogamicin (GO; humanized anti-CD33 monoclonal antibody conjugated to Calicheamicin) in patients with acute myeloid leukemia. The 20% of the patients alive achieved major response and survived >6 months. Serious adverse events for the Oblimersen/GO combinations were qualitatively similar to those reported for GO alone requiring wider randomized trial to assess effect [141]. Using this study as a platform, a phase III randomized trial in untreated acute myeloid leukemia patients aged more than 60 years was designed to definitively assess the contribution of Oblimersen to the chemotherapeutical activity. However, patient recruitment for this trial was stopped because early analysis indicated that the experimental treatment would not significantly improve overall survival

Oblimersen in Multiple Myeloma

Multiple myeloma remains an incurable malignancy. Despite responses to conventional and high-dose chemotherapy, deregulation of signaling pathways and impairment of apoptosis contribute to resistance to chemotherapy and radiotherapy. A phase I trial was designed to evaluate Oblimersen in combination with dexamethasone and thalidomide, showed that 73%of the patients had documented responses. The only predictive variable for response was an early and statistically significant increase in polyclonal immunoglobulin M for responders. This polyclonal IgM activation suggested that alternative pathways that do not involve stimulation of the B-cell receptor are involved. One possibility is that Oblimersen may stimulate the innate immune system to secrete polyclonal IgM. Clinical response did not correlate with *BCL-2* expression in contrast to RT-PCR analysis. The biological data derived from this study suggested that Oblimersen is active against its target *BCL-2* mRNA, at least in some patients, showing decrease in *BCL-2* mRNA by RT-PCR analysis in patients with partial response. Although several reversible toxic effects were reported (Table **3**), the combination of Oblimersen with thalidomide and dexamethasone is feasible and effective in refractory and relapsed multiple myeloma [142].

Oblimersen in Malignant Melanoma

Melanoma is a localized disease frequently curable by surgical excision. However, metastatic melanoma is inherently resistant to most systemic treatments, and survival of patients with advanced disease has not improved in more than 30 years. Drug resistance in melanoma has been partially attributed to overexpression of the *bcl-2* proto-oncogene. AS-ODNs targeted against *BCL-2* mRNA decreased *BCL-2* protein concentrations, increased tumor-cell apoptosis, and led to tumor responses in a mouse xenotransplantation model when combined with systemic Dacarbazine.

Phase I, II and III clinical studies were designed to investigate the effect of Oblimersen in combination with Dacarbazine in patients with advanced malignant melanoma expressing *BCL-2*. Phase I/II trials showed a 40% decrease in *BCL-2* protein in serial tumor biopsy samples measured by Western Blot and increased tumor-cell apoptosis, which was greatly increased after Dacarbazine treatment. The combination regimen was well tolerated and six patients had anti-tumor response. Results of a dose-ranging study suggested that Oblimersen might improve response to Dacarbazine and overall survival in patients with advanced melanoma without increasing toxicity [143]. In phase III trials, the overall response was 13.5% for patients receiving the combination and 7.5% for patients only receiving Dacarbazine. The proportion of patients with durable responses (≥ 6 months) was significantly higher in the combination group as well as the proportion of patients who discontinued treatment because of treatment-related adverse events. It was seen that the combination significantly improved multiple clinical outcomes in patients with advanced melanoma [144]. However, FDA concerns on Oblimersen performance status, tumor-related symptoms and toxicity undermined the approval of wide-spread use of Oblimersen alone or in combination for malignant melanoma.

Oblimersen in Breast Cancer

Approximately 40% to 80% of invasive breast carcinomas express *BCL-2*. Although *BCL-2* may be a weak prognostic indicator for breast cancer, studies have shown that *BCL-2* expression can be associated with chemotherapy resistance [145-147]. Preclinical models have established that *BCL-2* down-regulation leads to increased apoptosis and improved response to chemotherapy *in vivo* [148]. A phase I/II study with localized and inoperable advanced breast cancer was designed to evaluate administration of Oblimersen in combination with bolus Doxorubicin and Docetaxel. Phase I results showed that there was no pathologic complete responses in treated patients. Pharmacodynamic studies showed limited *BCL-2* down-regulation in primary tumors, probably related to issues with insufficient drug delivery to the intact tumor. Oblimersen in combination with doxorubicin and Docetaxel was well tolerated. The response rates for the phase II portion of the trial showed that most patients treated had a confirmed partial response, showing a limited down-regulation of *BCL-2* protein or mRNA in the primary breast cancers sampled after Oblimersen administration. However, no patients achieved a complete pathologic response within the breast and draining axillary lymph nodes and show that there was no additional efficacy with the combination suggesting that the combination therapy may, in fact, be worse than chemotherapy alone [149]. This worsening of clinical outcome has been shown in other solid tumor types, such as small cell lung cancer, where a randomized phase II trial revealed a statistically significant worse overall survival for patients receiving Oblimersen in combination with carboplatin and etoposide [150].

Oblimersen in Small-Cell Lung Cancer (SCLC)

SCLC represents approximately 15% of all lung tumors. The majority of patients have extensive-stage disease at the time of diagnosis. An antisense oligonucleotide directed against the *BCL-2* mRNA increased the efficacy of cisplatin and etoposide against human SCLC lines in tissue culture and as murine xenografts [151]. A phase I trial with the administration of G3139 (3 mg/kg/day) and paclitaxel (175 mg/m2) in patients with SCLC showed that few patients had clinical or objective disease progression within a month of evaluation [152]. Another combination was tested in a phase I trial involving the administration of Oblimersen and carboplatin and etoposide showing no statistical significance in changing *BCL-2* levels [153].

A Phase II trial designed to evaluate toxicity and efficacy of the combination of Oblimersen, carboplatin and etoposide for the treatment of chemotherapy-naïve extensive-stage SCLC showed an overall response rate of 61% for combination therapy and 60% for chemotherapy. The 1-year survival rate for combination therapy is far less than the pre-specified 51% cutoff percentage for a trial success. This was associated with a median survival of 8.6 months for combined therapy and 10.6 months for chemotherapy. Although the survival comparison between treatments was not a prospectively planned study end-point, the hazard ratio for death suggests that the addition of Oblimersen to standard therapy for this disease may have had a negative impact on survival. Emerging data from several groups suggest that this lack of efficacy may be due to insufficient suppression of *BCL-2 in vivo*. Additional evaluation of this agent in SCLC is not warranted [150].

CONCLUDING REMARKS

Contrary to the rationale of antisense use, most AS-ODNs that have reached clinical trials failed to convincingly show therapeutic effect without significant and sometimes unexpected toxic effects. Many clinical issues arose from the previously unknown off-target and immunostimulatory effects derived from chemical moieties frequently used to stabilize AS-ODNs. Determination of response or partial response has been difficult because there is no initial parameter to evaluate. Most AS-ODNs clinical trials lack a preclinical genetic characterization of the expression of a particular gene directly in the tumor. More importantly, AS-ODNs lacked sufficient and objective evaluation before entering clinical trials. Several aspects were not considered: metabolism or degradation of the molecule during administration, effective AS-ODN concentration at the target site and target validation in patients to be treated with the AS-ODN molecule. Thus, determination of whether a particular gene of interest is over-expressed or not in tumors and the basal target mRNA level become main points for patient criteria accrual. Only a handful of AS-ODNs against clinically validated cancer genes have shown success in preclinical reports, such as human papillomavirus genes in cervical cancer [154, 155]. However, the recent availability of prophylactic measures has been favored towards prevention rather than treatment of cervical cancer.

Nevertheless, AS-ODNs lead the way for more powerful technologies such as siRNAs and DNAzymes and the lessons learned from AS-ODN clinical application should provide better clinical protocols and selection criteria. We propose that to enter clinical trials AS-ODNs should undergo more preclinical testing under the following guidelines:

1) AS-ODNs should be considered as specific cytostatic molecules within the target tumor while their metabolites may be considered as potentially unspecific cytotoxic molecules. Thus, AS-ODN integrity should be conserved during long periods of time to minimize toxic effects.

2)   Determination of the basal level of expression of the target gene. Variations in normal subjects as well as in tumor-treated patients must be included as a part of the criteria for clinical testing. This involves molecular characterization of the target to determine basal level of the messenger prior to treatment.

3)   Because the chemical nature of the AS-ODN is of great importance to determine toxicity and other effects related to the complete molecule, pharmacokinetics and pharmacodynamics studies in immunocompetent animal models must precede clinical testing. Thus, effects related to the bioavailability of the complete AS-ODN molecule at the site of action and toxic effects will be minimized.

4)   Patient selection by comparing target mRNA levels to organize groups to receive treatment.

5)   Result evaluation of AS-ODN therapy after each treatment cycle should be at a molecular level by sampling PBMCs and by fine needle aspiration of the tumor, or, if possible, sequential tumor biopsies when treatment has finished. Tumor progression or proportion of patients should be evaluated with evidence of partial or total responses at a defined time point after the start of therapy.

REFERENCES

[1]   Hanahan D, Weinberg RA. The hallmarks of cancer. Cell 2000; 100: 57-70.

[2]   Leonetti C, Zupi G. Targeting different signaling pathways with antisense oligonucleotides combination for cancer therapy. Curr Pharm Des 2007; 13: 463-70.

[3]   Bennett CF. Efficiency of antisense oligonucleotide drug discovery. Antisense Nucleic Acid Drug Dev 2002; 12: 215-24.

[4]   Alvarez-Salas LM. Nucleic acids as therapeutic agents. Curr Top Med Chem 2008; 8: 1379-404.

[5]   Sazani P, Vacek MM, Kole R. Short-term and long-term modulation of gene expression by antisense therapeutics. Curr Opin Biotechnol 2002; 13: 468-72.

[6]   Crooke RM. Antisense oligonucleotides as therapeutics for hyperlipidaemias. Expert Opin Biol Ther 2005; 5: 907-17.

[7]   Bonham MA, Brown S, Boyd AL, *et al.* An assessment of the antisense properties of RNase H-competent and steric-blocking oligomers. Nucleic Acids Res 1995; 23: 1197-203.

[8]   Alvarez-Salas LM, Benitez-Hess ML, DiPaolo JA. Advances in the development of ribozymes and antisense oligodeoxynucleotides as antiviral agents for human papillomaviruses. Antivir Ther 2003; 8: 265-78.

[9]   Vickers TA, Wyatt JR, Freier SM. Effects of RNA secondary structure on cellular antisense activity. Nucleic Acids Res 2000; 28: 1340-7.

[10] Pan WH, Devlin HF, Kelley C, *et al.* A selection system for identifying accessible sites in target RNAs. RNA 2001; 7: 610-21.

[11] Bacon TA, Wickstrom E. Walking along human c-myc mRNA with antisense oligodeoxynucleotides: maximum efficacy at the 5' cap region. Oncogene Res 1991; 6: 13-9.

[12] Ho SP, Britton DH, Stone BA, Behrens DL, *et al.* Potent antisense oligonucleotides to the human multidrug resistance-1 mRNA are rationally selected by mapping RNA-accessible sites with oligonucleotide libraries. Nucleic Acids Res 1996; 24: 1901-7.

[13] Venturini F, Braspenning J, Homann M, *et al.* Kinetic selection of HPV 16 E6 /E7-directed antisense nucleic acids: anti-proliferative effects on HPV 16-transformed cells. Nucleic Acids Res 1999; 27: 1585-92.

[14] Cairns MJ, Hopkins TM, Witherington C, *et al.* Target site selection for an RNA-cleaving catalytic DNA. Nat Biotechnol 1999; 17: 480-6.

[15] Scherr M, Reed M, Huang CF, *et al.* Oligonucleotide Scanning of Native mRNAs in Extracts Predicts Intracellular Ribozyme Efficiency: Ribozyme-Mediated Reduction of the Murine DNA Methyltransferase. Mol Ther 2000; 2: 26-38.

[16] Lloyd BH, Giles RV, Spiller DG, *et al.* Determination of optimal sites of antisense oligonucleotide cleavage within TNFalpha mRNA. Nucleic Acids Res 2001; 29: 3664-73.

[17] Sczakiel G, Homann M, Rittner K. Computer-aided search for effective antisense RNA target sequences of the human immunodeficiency virus type 1. Antisense Res Dev 1993; 3: 45-52.

[18] Wraight CJ,.White PJ. Antisense oligonucleotides in cutaneous therapy. Pharmacol Ther 2001; 90: 89-104.

[19] Ding Y,.Lawrence CE. Statistical prediction of single-stranded regions in RNA secondary structure and application to predicting effective antisense target sites and beyond. Nucleic Acids Res 2001; 29: 1034-46.

[20] Monia BP, Johnston JF, Geiger T, *et al.* Antitumor activity of a phosphorothioate antisense oligodeoxynucleotide targeted against *C-raf* kinase. Nat Med 1996; 2: 668-75.

[21]   Dean NM, McKay R, Condon TP, *et al.* Inhibition of protein kinase C-a expression in human A549 cells by antisense oligonucleotides inhibits induction of intercellular adhesion molecule 1 (ICAM-1) mRNA by phorbol esters. J Biol Chem 1994; 269: 16416-24.

[22]   Conrad AH, Behlke MA, Jaffredo T, *et al.* Optimal lipofection reagent varies with the molecular modifications of the DNA. Antisense Nucleic Acid Drug Dev 1998; 8: 427-34.

[23]   Lv H, Zhang S, Wang B, *et al.* Toxicity of cationic lipids and cationic polymers in gene delivery. J Control Release 2006; 114: 100-9.

[24]   Akhtar S, Benter I. Toxicogenomics of non-viral drug delivery systems for RNAi: Potential impact on siRNA-mediated gene silencing activity and specificity. Adv Drug Deliv Rev 2007; 117: 3623-32.

[25]   Braasch DA,.Corey DR. Novel antisense and Peptide nucleic Acid strategies for controlling gene expression. Biochemistry 2002; 41: 4503-10.

[26]   Oishi M, Hayama T, Akiyama Y, *et al.* Supramolecular assemblies for the cytoplasmic delivery of antisense oligodeoxynucleotide: polyion complex (PIC) micelles based on poly(ethylene glycol)-SS-oligodeoxynucleotide conjugate. Biomacromolecules 2005; 6: 2449-54.

[27]   Yoo H, Juliano RL. Enhanced delivery of antisense oligonucleotides with fluorophore-conjugated PAMAM dendrimers. Nucleic Acids Res 2000; 28: 4225-31.

[28]   Fattal E, Couvreur P, Dubernet C. "Smart" delivery of antisense oligonucleotides by anionic pH-sensitive liposomes. Adv Drug Deliv Rev 2004; 56: 931-46.

[29]   Juliano R. Challenges to macromolecular drug delivery. Biochem Soc Trans 2007; 35: 41-3.

[30]   Jarver P, Langel K, El-Andaloussi S, *et al.* Applications of cell-penetrating peptides in regulation of gene expression. Biochem Soc Trans 2007; 35: 770-4.

[31]   Alam MR, Dixit V, Kang H, *et al.* Intracellular delivery of an anionic antisense oligonucleotide *via* receptor-mediated endocytosis. Nucleic Acids Res 2008; 36: 2764-76.

[32]   Agrawal S, Kandimalla ER. Antisense and/or immunostimulatory oligonucleotide therapeutics. Curr Cancer Drug Targets 2001; 1: 197-209.

[33]   Juliano R, Alam MR, Dixit V, *et al.* Mechanisms and strategies for effective delivery of antisense and siRNA oligonucleotides. Nucleic Acids Res 2008; 36: 4158-71.

[34]   Micklefield J. Backbone modification of nucleic acids: synthesis, structure and therapeutic applications. Curr Med Chem 2001; 8: 1157-79.

[35]   Uhlmann E, Ryte A, Peyman A. Studies on the mechanism of stabilization of partially phosphorothioated oligonucleotides against nucleolytic degradation. Antisense Nucleic Acid Drug Dev 1997; 7: 345-50.

[36]   Agrawal S,.Zhang R. Pharmacokinetics of oligonucleotides. Ciba Found Symp 1997; 209: 60-75.

[37]   Wagner RW, Matteucci MD, Lewis JG, *et al.* Antisense gene inhibition by oligonucleotides containing C-5 propyne pyrimidines. Science 1993; 260: 1510-3.

[38]   Gleave ME,.Monia BP. Antisense therapy for cancer. Nat Rev Cancer 2005; 5: 468-79.

[39]   Mercatante D,.Kole R. Modification of alternative splicing pathways as a potential approach to chemotherapy. Pharmacol Ther 2000; 85: 237-43.

[40]   Crooke ST. Progress in antisense technology. Annu Rev Med 2004; 55: 61-95.

[41]   Wilds CJ,.Damha MJ. Duplex recognition by oligonucleotides containing 2'-deoxy-2'-fluoro-D-arabinose and 2'-deoxy-2'-fluoro-D-ribose. Intermolecular 2'-OH-phosphate contacts versus sugar puckering in the stabilization of triple-helical complexes. Bioconjug Chem 1999; 10: 299-305.

[42]   Noronha AM, Wilds CJ, Lok CN, *et al.* Synthesis and biophysical properties of arabinonucleic acids (ANA): circular dichroic spectra, melting temperatures, and ribonuclease H susceptibility of ANA.RNA hybrid duplexes. Biochemistry 2000; 39: 7050-62.

[43]   Agrawal S, Zhao Q. Mixed backbone oligonucleotides: improvement in oligonucleotide-induced toxicity *in vivo*. Antisense Nucleic Acid Drug Dev 1998; 8: 135-9.

[44]   Sierakowska H, Gorman L, Kang SH, *et al.* Antisense oligonucleotides and RNAs as modulators of pre-mRNA splicing. Methods Enzymol 2000; 313: 506-21.

[45]   Hyrup B,.Nielsen PE. Peptide nucleic acids (PNA): synthesis, properties and potential applications. Bioorg Med Chem 1996; 4: 5-23.

[46]   Demidov VV, Potaman VN, Frank-Kamenetskii MD, *et al.* Stability of peptide nucleic acids in human serum and cellular extracts. Biochem Pharmacol 1994; 48: 1310-3.

[47]   Hamilton SE, Simmons CG, Kathiriya IS, *et al.* Cellular delivery of peptide nucleic acids and inhibition of human telomerase. Chem Biol 1999; 6: 343-51.

[48] Amantana A, Iversen PL. Pharmacokinetics and biodistribution of phosphorodiamidate morpholino antisense oligomers. Curr Opin Pharmacol 2005; 5: 550-5.

[49] Karkare S, Bhatnagar D. Promising nucleic acid analogs and mimics: characteristic features and applications of PNA, LNA, and morpholino. Appl Microbiol Biotechnol 2006; 71: 575-86.

[50] Liu HM, Newbrough SE, Bhatia SK, *et al.* Immunostimulatory CpG oligodeoxynucleotides enhance the immune response to vaccine strategies involving granulocyte-macrophage colony- stimulating factor. Blood 1998; 92: 3730-6.

[51] Zhao Q, Temsamani J, Iadarola PL, *et al.* Effect of different chemically modified oligodeoxynucleotides on immune stimulation. Biochem Pharmacol 1996; 51: 173-82.

[52] Weiner GJ, Liu HM, Wooldridge JE, *et al.* Immunostimulatory oligodeoxynucleotides containing the CpG motif are effective as immune adjuvants in tumor antigen immunization. Proc Natl Acad Sci USA 1997; 94: 10833-7.

[53] Braasch DA, Liu Y, Corey DR. Antisense inhibition of gene expression in cells by oligonucleotides incorporating locked nucleic acids: effect of mRNA target sequence and chimera design. Nucleic Acids Res 2002; 30: 5160-7.

[54] Waters JS, Webb A, Cunningham D, *et al.* Phase I clinical and pharmacokinetic study of bcl-2 antisense oligonucleotide therapy in patients with non-Hodgkin's lymphoma. J Clin Oncol 2000; 18: 1812-23.

[55] Roychowdhury D,.Lahn M. Antisense therapy directed to protein kinase C-alpha (affinitak, LY900003/ISIS 3521): Potential role in breast cancer. Semin Oncol 2003; 30: 30-3.

[56] Pavco PA, Bouhana KS, Gallegos AM, *et al* Antitumor and antimetastatic activity of ribozymes targeting the messenger RNA of vascular endothelial growth factor receptors. Clin Cancer Res 2000; 6: 2094-103.

[57] Morrissey DV, Lee PA, Johnson DA, *et al.* Characterization of nuclease-resistant ribozymes directed against hepatitis B virus RNA. J Viral.Hepat 2002; 9: 411-8.

[58] Cunningham CC, Holmlund JT, Geary RS, *et al.* A Phase I trial of H-ras antisense oligonucleotide ISIS 2503 administered as a continuous intravenous infusion in patients with advanced carcinoma. Cancer 2001; 92: 1265-71.

[59] Luger SM, O'Brien SG, Ratajczak J, *et al.* Oligodeoxynucleotide-mediated inhibition of c-myb gene expression in autografted bone marrow: a pilot study. Blood 2002; 99: 1150-8.

[60] Link BK, Ballas ZK, Weisdorf D, *et al.* Oligodeoxynucleotide CpG 7909 delivered as intravenous infusion demonstrates immunologic modulation in patients with previously treated non-Hodgkin lymphoma. J Immunother 2006; 29: 558-68.

[61] Chan JH, Lim S, Wong WS. Antisense oligonucleotides: from design to therapeutic application. Clin Exp Pharmacol Physiol 2006; 33: 533-40.

[62] Nemunaitis J, Holmlund JT, Kraynak M, *et al.* Phase I evaluation of ISIS 3521, an antisense oligodeoxynucleotide to protein kinase C-alpha, in patients with advanced cancer. J Clin Oncol 1999; 17: 3586-95.

[63] Shaw DR, Rustagi PK, Kandimalla ER, *et al.* Effects of synthetic oligonucleotides on human complement and coagulation. Biochem Pharmacol 1997; 53: 1123-32.

[64] Yuen AR, Halsey J, Fisher GA, *et al.* Phase I study of an antisense oligonucleotide to protein kinase C-alpha (ISIS 3521/CGP 64128A) in patients with cancer. Clin Cancer Res 1999; 5: 3357-63.

[65] Cunningham CC, Holmlund JT, Schiller JH, *et al.* A phase I trial of *c-Raf* kinase antisense oligonucleotide ISIS 5132 administered as a continuous intravenous infusion in patients with advanced cancer. Clin Cancer Res 2000; 6: 1626-31.

[66] Rudin CM, Holmlund J, Fleming GF, *et al.* Phase I Trial of ISIS 5132, an antisense oligonucleotide inhibitor of *c-raf*-1, administered by 24-hour weekly infusion to patients with advanced cancer. Clin Cancer Res 2001; 7: 1214-20.

[67] Sato K, Qian J, Slezak JM *et al.* Clinical significance of alterations of chromosome 8 in high-grade, advanced, nonmetastatic prostate carcinoma. J Natl Cancer Inst 1999; 91: 1574-80.

[68] Quinn DI, Henshall SM, Sutherland RL. Molecular markers of prostate cancer outcome. Eur J Cancer 2005; 41: 858-87.

[69] Iversen PL, Arora V, Acker AJ, *et al.* Efficacy of antisense morpholino oligomer targeted to c-myc in prostate cancer xenograft murine model and a Phase I safety study in humans. Clin Cancer Res 2003; 9: 2510-9.

[70] Devi GR, Beer TM, Corless CL, *et al. In vivo* bioavailability and pharmacokinetics of a c-MYC antisense phosphorodiamidate morpholino oligomer, AVI-4126, in solid tumors. Clin Cancer Res 2005; 11: 3930-8.

[71] Adjei AA, Dy GK, Erlichman C, *et al.* A phase I trial of ISIS 2503, an antisense inhibitor of H-ras, in combination with gemcitabine in patients with advanced cancer. Clin Cancer Res 2003; 9: 115-23.

[72] Alberts SR, Schroeder M, Erlichman C, *et al.* Gemcitabine and ISIS-2503 for patients with locally advanced or metastatic pancreatic adenocarcinoma: a North Central Cancer Treatment Group phase II trial. J Clin Oncol 2004; 22: 4944-50.

[73] Burris HA, Moore MJ, Andersen J, *et al.* Improvements in survival and clinical benefit with gemcitabine as first-line therapy for patients with advanced pancreas cancer: a randomized trial. J Clin Oncol 1997; 15: 2403-13.

[74] Basu A. The potential of protein kinase C as a target for anticancer treatment. Pharmacol Ther 1993; 59: 257-80.

[75] Dlugosz AA, Cheng C, Williams EK, *et al.* Alterations in murine keratinocyte differentiation induced by activated rasHa genes are mediated by protein kinase C-alpha. Cancer Res1994; 54: 6413-20.

[76]   Ways DK, Kukoly CA, deVente J, *et al.* MCF-7 breast cancer cells transfected with protein kinase C-alpha exhibit altered expression of other protein kinase C isoforms and display a more aggressive neoplastic phenotype. J Clin Invest 1995; 95: 1906-15.

[77]   Advani R, Peethambaram P, Lum BL, *et al.* A Phase II trial of aprinocarsen, an antisense oligonucleotide inhibitor of protein kinase C alpha, administered as a 21-day infusion to patients with advanced ovarian carcinoma. Cancer 2004; 100: 321-6.

[78]   Mani S, Rudin CM, Kunkel K, *et al.* Phase I clinical and pharmacokinetic study of protein kinase C-alpha antisense oligonucleotide ISIS 3521 administered in combination with 5-fluorouracil and leucovorin in patients with advanced cancer. Clin Cancer Res 2002; 8: 1042-8.

[79]   Villalona-Calero MA, Ritch P, Figueroa JA, *et al.* A phase I/II study of LY900003, an antisense inhibitor of protein kinase C-alpha, in combination with cisplatin and gemcitabine in patients with advanced non-small cell lung cancer. Clin Cancer Res 2004; 10: 6086-93.

[80]   Rao S, Watkins D, Cunningham D, *et al.* Phase II study of ISIS 3521, an antisense oligodeoxynucleotide to protein kinase C alpha, in patients with previously treated low-grade non-Hodgkin's lymphoma. Ann Oncol 2004; 15: 1413-8.

[81]   Margolis B, Skolnik EY. Activation of Ras by receptor tyrosine kinases. J Am Soc Nephrol 1994; 5: 1288-99.

[82]   Schonwasser DC, Marais RM, Marshall CJ, *et al.* Activation of the mitogen-activated protein kinase/extracellular signal-regulated kinase pathway by conventional, novel, and atypical protein kinase C isotypes. Mol Cell Biol 1998; 18: 790-8.

[83]   Tanaka Y, Honda T, Matsuura K, *et al. In vitro* selection and characterization of DNA aptamers specific for phospholamban. J Pharmacol ExpTher 2009;

[84]   O'Brian C, Vogel VG, Singletary SE, *et al.* Elevated protein kinase C expression in human breast tumor biopsies relative to normal breast tissue. Cancer Res 1989; 49: 3215-7.

[85]   Kopp R, Noelke B, Sauter G, Schildberg FW, Paumgartner G, Pfeiffer A. Altered protein kinase C activity in biopsies of human colonic adenomas and carcinomas. Cancer Res 1991; 51: 205-10.

[86]   Liu B, Maher RJ, Hannun YA, *et al.* 12(S)-HETE enhancement of prostate tumor cell invasion: selective role of PKC alpha. J Natl Cancer Inst 1994; 86: 1145-51.

[87]   Cornford P, Evans J, Dodson A, *et al.* Protein kinase C isoenzyme patterns characteristically modulated in early prostate cancer. Am J Pathol 1999; 154: 137-44.

[88]   Henttu P, Vihko P. The protein kinase C activator, phorbol ester, elicits disparate functional responses in androgen-sensitive and androgen-independent human prostatic cancer cells. Biochem Biophys Res Commun 1998; 244: 167-71.

[89]   Olsen CM, Marky LA. Energetic and hydration contributions of the removal of methyl groups from thymine to form uracil in G-quadruplexes. J Phys Chem B 2009; 113: 9-11.

[90]   Laufer SD, Recke AL, Veldhoen S, *et al.* Noncovalent Peptide-Mediated Delivery of Chemically Modified Steric Block Oligonucleotides Promotes Splice Correction: Quantitative Analysis of Uptake and Biological Effect. Oligonucleotides 2009; 19: 63-80.

[91]   Lonnberg H. Solid-Phase Synthesis of Oligonucleotide Conjugates Useful for Delivery and Targeting of Potential Nucleic Acid Therapeutics. Bioconjug Chem 2009; 20: 1065-94.

[92]   Dean NM, McKay R. Inhibition of protein kinase C-α expression in mice after systemic administration of phosphorothioate antisense oligodeoxynucleotides. Proc Natl Acad Sci USA 1994; 91: 11762-6.

[93]   Monia BP, Sasmor H, Johnston JF, *et al.* Sequence-specific antitumor activity of a phosphorothioate oligodeoxyribonucleotide targeted to human *C-raf* kinase supports an antisense mechanism of action *in vivo*. Proc Natl Acad Sci USA 1996; 93: 15481-4.

[94]   Abes S, Ivanova GD, Abes R. *et al.* Peptide-based delivery of steric-block PNA oligonucleotides. Methods Mol Biol 2009; 480: 85-99.

[95]   Stevenson JP, Yao KS, Gallagher M, *et al.* Phase I Clinical/Pharmacokinetic and Pharmacodynamic Trial of the *c-raf*-1 Antisense Oligonucleotide ISIS 5132 (CGP 69846A). J Clin Oncol 1999; 17: 2227.

[96]   O'Dwyer PJ, Stevenson JP, Gallagher M, *et al. c-raf*-1 depletion and tumor responses in patients treated with the *c-raf*-1 antisense oligodeoxynucleotide ISIS 5132 (CGP 69846A). Clin Cancer Res 1999; 5: 3977-82.

[97]   Coudert B, Anthoney A, Fiedler W, *et al.* Phase II trial with ISIS 5132 in patients with small-cell (SCLC) and non-small cell (NSCLC) lung cancer. A European Organization for Research and Treatment of Cancer (EORTC) Early Clinical Studies Group report. Eur J Cancer 2001; 37: 2194-8.

[98]   Tolcher AW, Reyno L, Venner PM, *et al.* A randomized phase II and pharmacokinetic study of the antisense oligonucleotides ISIS 3521 and ISIS 5132 in patients with hormone-refractory prostate cancer. Clin Cancer Res 2002; 8: 2530-5.

[99]   Cripps MC, Figueredo AT, Oza AM, *et al.* Phase II randomized study of ISIS 3521 and ISIS 5132 in patients with locally advanced or metastatic colorectal cancer: a National Cancer Institute of Canada clinical trials group study. Clin Cancer Res 2002; 8: 2188-92.

[100] Jones SE,. Jomary C. Clusterin. Int J Biochem Cell Biol 2002; 34: 427-31.

[101] Humphreys DT, Carver JA, Easterbrook-Smith SB, *et al.* Clusterin has chaperone-like activity similar to that of small heat shock proteins. J Biol Chem 1999; 274: 6875-81.

[102] Michel D, Chatelain G, North S, *et al.* Stress-induced transcription of the clusterin/apoJ gene. Biochem J 1997; 328: 45-50.

[103] Zhang H, Kim JK, Edwards CA, *et al.* Clusterin inhibits apoptosis by interacting with activated BAX. Nat Cell Biol 2005; 7: 909-15.

[104] Zellweger T, Chi K, Miyake H, *et al.* Enhanced radiation sensitivity in prostate cancer by inhibition of the cell survival protein clusterin. Clin Cancer Res 2002; 8: 3276-84.

[105] Miyake H, Hara S, Arakawa S, *et al.* Over expression of clusterin is an independent prognostic factor for nonpapillary renal cell carcinoma. J Urol 2002; 167: 703-6.

[106] Zellweger T, Miyake H, Cooper S, *et al.* Antitumor activity of antisense clusterin oligonucleotides is improved *in vitro* and *in vivo* by incorporation of 2'-O-(2-methoxy)ethyl chemistry. J Pharmacol Exp Ther 2001; 298: 934-40.

[107] Chi KN, Eisenhauer E, Fazli L, *et al.* A phase I pharmacokinetic and pharmacodynamic study of OGX-011, a 2'-methoxyethyl antisense oligonucleotide to clusterin, in patients with localized prostate cancer. J Natl Cancer Inst 2005; 97: 1287-96.

[108] Chi KN, Siu LL, Hirte H, *et al.* A phase I study of OGX-011, a 2'-methoxyethyl phosphorothioate antisense to clusterin, in combination with docetaxel in patients with advanced cancer. Clin Cancer Res 2008; 14: 833-9.

[109] Chi KN, Zoubeidi A, Gleave ME. Custirsen (OGX-011): a second-generation antisense inhibitor of clusterin for the treatment of cancer. Expert Opin Investig Drugs 2008; 17: 1955-62.

[110] Engstrom Y, Eriksson S, Jildevik I, *et al.* Cell cycle-dependent expression of mammalian ribonucleotide reductase. Differential regulation of the two subunits. J Biol Chem 1985; 260: 9114-6.

[111] Fan H, Villegas C, Wright JA. Ribonucleotide reductase R2 component is a novel malignancy determinant that cooperates with activated oncogenes to determine transformation and malignant potential. Proc Natl Acad Sci USA 1996; 93: 14036-40.

[112] Vassilakos A, Lee Y, Viau S, *et al.* GTI-2040 displays cooperative anti-tumor activity when combined with interferon alpha against human renal carcinoma xenografts. Int J Oncol 2009; 34: 33-42.

[113] Huang A, Fan H, Taylor WR, *et al.* Ribonucleotide reductase R2 gene expression and changes in drug sensitivity and genome stability. Cancer Res 1997; 57: 4876-81.

[114] Chen S, Zhou B, He F, Yen Y. Inhibition of human cancer cell growth by inducible expression of human ribonucleotide reductase antisense cDNA. Antisense.Nucleic.Acid.Drug Dev 2000; 10: 111-6.

[115] Desai AA, Schilsky RL, Young A, *et al.* A phase I study of antisense oligonucleotide GTI-2040 given by continuous intravenous infusion in patients with advanced solid tumors. Ann Oncol 2005; 16: 958-65.

[116] Stadler WM, Desai AA, Quinn DI, *et al.* A Phase I/II study of GTI-2040 and capecitabine in patients with renal cell carcinoma. Cancer Chemother Pharmacol 2008; 61: 689-94.

[117] Tsujimoto Y, Ikegaki N, Croce CM. Characterization of the protein product of bcl-2, the gene involved in human follicular lymphoma. Oncogene 1987; 2: 3-7.

[118] Zha H, Aime-Sempe C, Sato T, *et al.* Proapoptotic protein Bax heterodimerizes with Bcl-2 and homodimerizes with Bax *via* a novel domain (BH3) distinct from BH1 and BH2. J Biol Chem 1996; 271: 7440-4.

[119] Tanaka S, Saito K, Reed JC. Structure-function analysis of the Bcl-2 oncoprotein. Addition of a heterologous transmembrane domain to portions of the Bcl-2 beta protein restores function as a regulator of cell survival. J Biol Chem 1993; 268: 10920-6.

[120] McDonnell TJ, Troncoso P, Brisbay SM, *et al.* Expression of the protooncogene bcl-2 in the prostate and its association with emergence of androgen-independent prostate cancer. Cancer Res 1992; 52: 6940-4.

[121] Grover R,.Wilson GD. Bcl-2 expression in malignant melanoma and its prognostic significance. Eur J Surg Oncol 1996; 22: 347-9.

[122] Gascoyne RD, Adomat SA, Krajewski S, *et al.* Prognostic significance of Bcl-2 protein expression and Bcl-2 gene rearrangement in diffuse aggressive non-Hodgkin's lymphoma. Blood 1997; 90: 244-51.

[123] Bhatavdekar JM, Patel DD, Ghosh N, *et al.* Coexpression of Bcl-2, c-Myc, and p53 oncoproteins as prognostic discriminants in patients with colorectal carcinoma. Dis Colon Rectum 1997; 40: 785-90.

[124] Carbognani P, Tincani G, Crafa P, *et al.* Biological markers in non-small cell lung cancer. Retrospective study of 10 year follow-up after surgery. J Cardiovasc Surg 2002; 43: 545-8.

[125] Marcucci G, Byrd JC, Dai G, *et al.* Phase 1 and pharmacodynamic studies of G3139, a Bcl-2 antisense oligonucleotide, in combination with chemotherapy in refractory or relapsed acute leukemia. Blood 2003; 101: 425-32.

[126] Krieg AM, Guga P, Stec W. P-chirality-dependent immune activation by phosphorothioate CpG oligodeoxynucleotides. Oligonucleotides 2003; 13: 491-9.

[127] Pan X, Chen L, Liu S, *et al.* Antitumor activity of G3139 lipid nanoparticles (LNPs). Mol Pharm 2009; 6: 211-20.

[128] Herbst RS,.Frankel SR. Oblimersen sodium (Genasense bcl-2 antisense oligonucleotide): a rational therapeutic to enhance apoptosis in therapy of lung cancer. Clin Cancer Res 2004; 10: 4245s-8s.

[129] Morris MJ, Tong WP, Cordon-Cardo C, *et al.* Phase I trial of BCL-2 antisense oligonucleotide (G3139) administered by continuous intravenous infusion in patients with advanced cancer. Clin Cancer Res 2002; 8: 679-83.

[130] Chi KN, Gleave ME, Klasa R, *et al.* A phase I dose-finding study of combined treatment with an antisense Bcl-2 oligonucleotide (Genasense) and mitoxantrone in patients with metastatic hormone-refractory prostate cancer. Clin Cancer Res 2001; 7: 3920-7.

[131] Tolcher AW, Kuhn J, Schwartz G, *et al.* A Phase I pharmacokinetic and biological correlative study of oblimersen sodium (genasense, g3139), an antisense oligonucleotide to the bcl-2 mRNA, and of docetaxel in patients with hormone-refractory prostate cancer. Clin Cancer Res 2004; 10: 5048-57.

[132] Tolcher AW, Chi K, Kuhn J, *et al.* A phase II, pharmacokinetic, and biological correlative study of oblimersen sodium and docetaxel in patients with hormone-refractory prostate cancer. Clin Cancer Res 2005; 11: 3854-61.

[133] Mita MM, Ochoa L, Rowinsky EK, *et al.* A phase I, pharmacokinetic and biologic correlative study of oblimersen sodium (Genasense, G3139) and irinotecan in patients with metastatic colorectal cancer. Ann Oncol 2006; 17: 313-21.

[134] Scatena CD, Stewart ZA, Mays D, *et al.* Mitotic phosphorylation of Bcl-2 during normal cell cycle progression and Taxol-induced growth arrest. J Biol Chem 1998; 273: 30777-84.

[135] Liu G, Kolesar J, McNeel DG, *et al.* A phase I pharmacokinetic and pharmacodynamic correlative study of the antisense Bcl-2 oligonucleotide g3139, in combination with carboplatin and paclitaxel, in patients with advanced solid tumors. Clin Cancer Res 2008; 14: 2732-9.

[136] O'Brien SM, Cunningham CC, Golenkov *et al.* Phase I to II multicenter study of oblimersen sodium, a Bcl-2 antisense oligonucleotide, in patients with advanced chronic lymphocytic leukemia. J Clin Oncol 2005; 23: 7697-702.

[137] O'Brien S, Moore JO, Boyd TE, *et al.* Randomized phase III trial of fludarabine plus cyclophosphamide with or without oblimersen sodium (Bcl-2 antisense) in patients with relapsed or refractory chronic lymphocytic leukemia. J Clin Oncol 2007; 25: 1114-20.

[138] Cotter FE, Johnson P, Hall P, *et al*, Morgan G. Antisense oligonucleotides suppress B-cell lymphoma growth in a SCID-hu mouse model. Oncogene 1994; 9: 3049-55.

[139] Pro B, Leber B, Smith M, *et al.* Phase II multicenter study of oblimersen sodium, a Bcl-2 antisense oligonucleotide, in combination with rituximab in patients with recurrent B-cell non-Hodgkin lymphoma. Br J Haematol 2008; 143: 355-60.

[140] Marcucci G, Stock W, Dai G, *et al.* Phase I study of oblimersen sodium, an antisense to Bcl-2, in untreated older patients with acute myeloid leukemia: pharmacokinetics, pharmacodynamics, and clinical activity. J Clin Oncol 2005; 23: 3404-11.

[141] Moore J, Sciter K, Kolitz J, *et al.* A Phase II study of Bcl-2 antisense (oblimersen sodium) combined with gemtuzumab ozogamicin in older patients with acute myeloid leukemia in first relapse. Leuk Res 2006; 30: 777-83.

[142] Badros AZ, Goloubeva O, Rapoport AP, *et al.* Phase II study of G3139, a Bcl-2 antisense oligonucleotide, in combination with dexamethasone and thalidomide in relapsed multiple myeloma patients. J Clin Oncol 2005; 23: 4089-99.

[143] Jansen B, Wacheck V, Heere-Ress E, *et al.* Chemosensitisation of malignant melanoma by BCL2 antisense therapy. Lancet 2000; 356: 1728-33.

[144] Bedikian AY, Millward M, Pehamberger H, *et al.* Bcl-2 antisense (oblimersen sodium) plus dacarbazine in patients with advanced melanoma: the Oblimersen Melanoma Study Group. J Clin Oncol 2006; 24: 4738-45.

[145] Hellemans P, van Dam PA, Weyler J, *et al.* Prognostic value of bcl-2 expression in invasive breast cancer. Br J Cancer 1995; 72: 354-60.

[146] Joensuu H, Pylkkanen L, Toikkanen S. Bcl-2 protein expression and long-term survival in breast cancer. Am J Pathol 1994; 145: 1191-8.

[147] Silvestrini R, Veneroni S, Daidone MG, *et al.* The Bcl-2 protein: a prognostic indicator strongly related to p53 protein in lymph node-negative breast cancer patients. J Natl Cancer Inst 1994; 86: 499-504.

[148] Chi KC, Wallis AE, Lee CH, *et al.* Effects of Bcl-2 modulation with G3139 antisense oligonucleotide on human breast cancer cells are independent of inherent Bcl-2 protein expression. Breast Cancer Res Treat 2000; 63: 199-212.

[149] Moulder SL, Symmans WF, Booser DJ, *et al.* Phase I/II study of G3139 (Bcl-2 antisense oligonucleotide) in combination with doxorubicin and docetaxel in breast cancer. Clin Cancer Res 2008; 14: 7909-16.

[150] Rudin CM, Salgia R, Wang X, *et al.* Randomized phase II Study of carboplatin and etoposide with or without the bcl-2 antisense oligonucleotide oblimersen for extensive-stage small-cell lung cancer: CALGB 30103. J Clin Oncol 2008; 26: 870-6.

[151] Zangemeister-Wittke U, Schenker T, Luedke GH, *et al.* Synergistic cytotoxicity of bcl-2 antisense oligodeoxynucleotides and etoposide, doxorubicin and cisplatin on small-cell lung cancer cell lines. Br J Cancer 1998; 78: 1035-42.

[152] Rudin CM, Otterson GA, Mauer AM, *et al.* A pilot trial of G3139, a bcl-2 antisense oligonucleotide, and paclitaxel in patients with chemorefractory small-cell lung cancer. Ann Oncol 2002; 13: 539-45.

[153] Rudin CM, Kozloff M, Hoffman PC, *et al.* Phase I study of G3139, a bcl-2 antisense oligonucleotide, combined with carboplatin and etoposide in patients with small-cell lung cancer. J Clin Oncol 2004; 22: 1110-7.

[154] Alvarez-Salas LM, Arpawong TE, DiPaolo JA. Growth inhibition of cervical tumor cells by antisense oligodeoxynucleotides directed to the human papillomavirus type 16 E6 gene. Antisense Nucleic Acid Drug Dev 1999; 9: 441-50.

[155] Marquez-Gutierrez MA, Benitez-Hess ML, DiPaolo JA, *et al.* Effect of combined antisense oligodeoxynucleotides directed against the human papillomavirus type 16 on cervical carcinoma cells. Arch Med Res 2007; 38: 730-8.

CHAPTER 13

Directions of Future Cancer Research

Javier Camacho

Department of Pharmacology, Centro de Investigación y de Estudios Avanzados del Instituto Politécnico Nacional, Avenida Instituto Politécnico Nacional 2508, México D. F. 07360, Mexico

Abstract: Basic oncology concepts as well as recent discoveries in cancer research have been described throughout this book. This final chapter aims to present some suggested directions in future cancer research based on both the information provided in this book and on the current high throughput technology available today. Several ideas arise, from prevention and epidemiological studies to gene expression and proteomic in a personalized-based manner. Definitely, interaction of the diverse cancer experts in the world should lead to a better understanding of this disease. Multidisciplinary cancer research should also lead to discovery of more accurate methods to diagnose the disease at early stages and provide more efficient anti-cancer therapies, to the benefit of cancer patients.

Keywords: Epidemiological studies, pharmaco-epidemiology, cancer prevention, early markers, drug resistance, personalized therapy, clinical trials, mutations, etiological factors.

INTRODUCTION

Cancer research produces thousands of new articles per month in the scientific field. Despite the tremendous production and the hundreds of clinical trials for cancer patients that are currently running, the disease remains a major cause of death worldwide with a high mortality-to-incidence ratio [1].

Major efforts have been made in all of the areas of cancer research and billions of dollars have been spent in developing new drug designs, *in vitro* and *in vivo* assays, clinical trials, *etc.* Nevertheless, in spite of such huge investment and decades of investigation, most of the new anti-cancer drugs have failed to pass the different phases of clinical trials [2] and unfortunately after many years of research the goal of treating cancer patients has not been reached.

In addition, many attempts to introduce new cancer markers have also failed in part because these new markers may appear as a result of local inflammation or because hormonal status modifies its expression. Cancer research is needed in different fields from finding early markers to new drug design, more personalized diagnose and therapy, *etc.* Following, some directions in specific cancer research topics will be discussed.

Epidemiology

Epidemiological studies have been extremely helpful in identifying certain cancer-associated factors, for example viral infection, environmental exposure to carcinogens, family history of cancer or smoking [3]. Other types of epidemiology-related studies associate the occurrence of some single polymorphisms in nucleotides in different populations. Several reports also show that some dietary habits may decrease cancer incidence. However, it is also common to find controversies between epidemiological studies. While such controversies may be due to real differences between populations, it is also conceivable that an international network could be formed in order to make epidemiological studies as homogeneous as possible. This way, more specific parameters can be measured and the same variables taken into account.

Pharmaco-epidemiology is another important area in which international networks may help to identify potential chemo-protective or chemotherapeutic agents. Many countries have very well organized databases that could be used

---

*****Address correspondence to Javier Camacho:** Department of Pharmacology, Centro de Investigación y de Estudios Avanzados del Instituto Politécnico Nacional, Avenida Instituto Politécnico Nacional 2508, México D. F. 07360, Mexico; E-mail: fcamacho@cinvestav.mx

to help identify whether patients using certain drugs for other diseases not related to cancer may have different risk in developing certain cancer types. Unfortunately, in this case the same problem arises. While some reports indicate a cancer protective effect of using certain drugs for some patients, other reports do not find an effect or may even find a negative association.

It would be very beneficial both to encourage all of the countries to create pharmacological databases and also to form international networks inviting pharmacologists to perform these kinds of studies as a whole group. This may have a high impact on cancer research because if currently used drugs are found to be associated with cancer incidence –at least for some types of cancers – then new drugs that have already succeeded in clinical trials may potentially be included for cancer therapy saving time, money, and lives.

Early Detection

A variety of tumors can be successfully treated if detected at early stages. However, in many cases tumors are diagnosed at advanced malignant stages or when the primary tumor has already spread to other organs and at which point most of the therapies fail.

Several investigations have been designed in order to find new cancer biomarkers. Unfortunately, because cancer is a multi-factorial disease, participation of potential cancer biomarkers in different phenomena may mask the real utility of such markers. Inflammation is one such process in which many potential cancer biomarkers are also increased, leading to many false positive results. Hormones and metabolic stages may also enhance the expression of some potential cancer biomarkers, leading to a confusing situation in cancer detection. More recently new potential markers including some ion channels have been proposed as early tumor markers. Diagnostic kits grouping different potential cancer markers should increase specificity and sensitivity of diagnostic methods.

In some types of tumors, early detection as a result of frequent screening has led for example to a decrease of cervical cancer incidence in some countries. In other words, increased frequent screening in patients exposed to some cancer risk factors might also help to decrease cancer mortality.

Non-invasive molecular tests including blood-based analysis, would be very helpful in the detection of cancer at an early stage [4].

Cancer Models

Another problem related to cancer as a multi-factorial disease is that most cancer types require many years to develop. This makes it difficult to obtain animal models that accurately simulate what occurs in humans.

In many models only one cancer-associated factor is studied. However, some studies have shown the combined effect of different cancer-risk factors. These kinds of experiments could lead to more representative cancer models in which different early markers and therapeutic targets may be found.

Studies looking for biomarkers and therapeutic targets in animal models recreating more closely human tumor development, together with the development of kits identifying several cancer biomarkers, should improve early diagnosis. Early detection would allow treatment of patients at stages where current therapies are efficient.

Drug Design and Clinical Trials

As hundreds of proteins have a role in tumor cell proliferation, it is difficult to find drugs targeting so many pathways. Many drugs are designed to target very specific proteins. In some cases, this may be extremely successful. However, for most types of cancer drugs targeting several targets are needed. How can this be accomplished? A possible solution lies in targeting proteins having a *master* role in cell cycle, proliferation or apoptosis. The protein p53, named *the guardian of the genome* some years ago, is an example of such potential targets.

Drug resistance is another major problem in drug design. As several players have been identified, discovery of inhibitors of multi-drug resistance proteins should help to improve chemotherapy [5].

A very interesting field of research in drug design comes along with pharmaco-epidemiology studies. Every day new roles for old drugs are found. This is the case for example for some anti-histamine or some calcium channel blockers which now are known to also inhibit cell proliferation. Therefore, pharmaco-epidemiological studies identifying old drugs protecting against cancer might be used to design new anti-cancer drugs. This way these new drugs might target different proteins and serve for different diseases. This would come together for more accurate cancer models in which new therapeutic targets are identified.

Traditional clinical trials can limit the real potential effect of new drugs. Some clinical trials are performed initially with patients who have not responded to previous treatments. Cancer cells may have developed drug resistance by different mechanisms and the new drugs may not have the same effect as if they have been tested at earlier stages. Following very rigorous ethical rules, new drugs may be tested at earlier stages in combination with standard drugs. Despite this is possible for many drugs, clinical trials policies could be more open to facilitate cancer drug testing to the benefit of cancer patients.

In this direction, old drugs currently used for other diseases but proven to have anti-proliferative effects *in vitro* or *in vivo* may be taken into the clinic.

"Personalized" Diagnosis and Therapy

High-throughput technologies are becoming more easily available to the clinic. Many elegant studies have identified gene expression signatures for many tumors. In this way, some tumors might be classified based on gene and protein expression. Not only is classification possible but also such gene and protein expression of the specific tumor might help to identify responders from non-responders to specific therapies. This approach could possibly be very helpful in the near future for cancer diagnose and therapy [6].

Unfortunately, many of these strategies do not include the identification of mutated genes/proteins or even the presence of polymorphisms. Because mutations or polymorphism may determine the response to a specific therapy, an extended version of such gene and protein expression strategies are required. In addition, training programs to process the samples and analyze very large amounts of gene and protein expression data are needed if this kind of diagnosis-prognosis method is intended to reach the clinic. Further, the cost of these high-throughput studies would be at the moment very high if expected to be used for thousands of patients.

Inclusion of detection of gene mutations, modified proteins and single polymorphisms, together with technological advances lowering the costs of the studies, will no doubt help to improve cancer diagnosis, prognosis and therapy in a more personalized- based manner.

Cancer Prevention

It is not uncommon to hear of people who despite having followed a healthy lifestyle develop cancer, while others living an unhealthy lifestyle with *"bad"* habits do not.

This is because genetic background also plays a major role in pre-disposing some patients to developing cancer, which might be taken as a reason for closer screening of some patients. Epidemiological and molecular studies should help in identifying such risk patients and prevent them from developing cancer [7].

Many factors have been associated with cancer including viruses, obesity, carcinogen exposure, lifestyle, *etc.* More accurate *in vitro* and *in vivo* models together with samples from risk patients should help to identify more early cancer markers.

Epidemiological studies have also proposed several natural products (for instance anti-oxidants) as cancer chemo-protectors. Strong and consistent evidence has been found associating physical activity with reduced cancer risk [8]. In addition, pharmacological manipulation has also gained interest for cancer prevention. For instance, aspirin use has been suggested to prevent colorectal cancer [9]. Definitely, a healthy life-style in concert with closer screening detecting potential cancer biomarkers should help to prevent cancer in many patients.

CONCLUSIONS

Billions of dollars have been invested in cancer research, and thousands of new cancer research articles representing the work of thousands of scientists arise throughout the world. Nevertheless, cancer is still an increasing and major health problem.

New technologies, however, are also arising and scientists are working together globally to fight against cancer. Without a doubt, the interactions among epidemiologists, cell and molecular biologists, oncologists, engineers, *etc.* will be important in helping to find a solution to this terrible disease.

Specifically, discovery of new early markers and more general drugs targeting master proteins together with the identification of natural agents that help prevent cancer should all help to decrease mortality from this disease.

ACKNOWLEDGEMENTS

The preparation of this book is part of a group research project supported by Conacyt (Grant 82175-M to JC). I thank Cynthia Chow for revising the English language.

REFERENCES

[1] Kamangar, F, Dores GM, Anderson WF. Patterns of cancer incidence, mortality, and prevalence across five continents: defining priorities to reduce cancer disparities in different geographic regions of the world. J Clin Oncol 2006; 24: 2137-50.

[2] Roberts TG, Goulart BH, Squitieri L, *et al.* Trends in the risk and benefits to patients with cancer participating in phase 1 clinical trials. JAMA 2004; 292: 2130-40.

[3] Hemminki K, Lorenzo Bermejo J, Försti A. The balance between heritable and environmental aetiology of human disease. Nat Rev Genet 2006; 7(12): 958-65.

[4] Hanash SM, Baik CS, Kallioniemi O. Emerging molecualr biomarkers—blood-based strategies to detect and monitor cancer. Nat Rev Clin Oncol 2011; 8(3): 142-50.

[5] Stavrovskaya AA and Stromskaya TP. Transport proteins of the ABC family and multidrug resistance of tumor cells. Biochemistry (Mosc) 2008; 73(5): 592-604.

[6] Wistuba II, Gelovani JG, Jacoby JJ, *et al.* Methodological and practical challenges for personalized cancer therapies. Nat Rev Clin Oncol 2011; 8(3): 142-50.

[7] Song M, Lee KM, Kang D. Breast cancer prevention based on gene-environment interaction. Mol Carcinog 2011; 50: 280-90.

[8] Friedenreich CM, Neilson HK, Lynch BM. State of epidemiological evidence on physical activity and cancer prevention. Eur J Cancer 2010; 46: 2593-604.

[9] Rothwell PM, Fowkes FG, Belch JF, *et al.* Effect of daily aspirin on long-term risk of death due to cancer: analysis of individual patients data from randomized trials. Lancet 2011; 377: 31-41.

Author Index

Author	(Chapter Number)
Alvarez-Salas Luis Marat	XII
Angulo Carla	I
Benítez-Hess María Luisa	XII
Bravo-Gómez María Elena	X
Cabrera Muñoz Lourdes	IX
Camacho Javier	IIC, XI
Cortés Enoc Mariano	IIE
De Vizcaya-Ruiz Andrea	IIA
Dueñas-González Alfonso	IV
García-Cuellar Claudia	IV
Gariglio Patricio	IIE, III
Gutiérrez Ranier	IIB
Gutiérrez Jorge	IIE
Hernández-Montes Jorge	VII
Hernández-Zavala Araceli	IIA
Hinojosa Luz María	IIC
Huerta Miriam	I
López-Bayghen Esther	I
Márquez-Rosado Lucrecia	V, VI
Meléndez Zajgla Jorge	VIII
Monroy-García Alberto	VII
Mora-García María de Lourdes	VII
Morales-Vásquez Flavia	IIC
Muriel Pablo	IID
Ortiz Cindy Sharon	XI
Pérez-Carreon Julio Isael	VIII
Ponce Verónica	IX
Restrepo Iván	XI
Rivera Guevara Claudia	X
Rodríguez-Rasgado Jesús Adrián	IIC
Ruiz-Azuara Lena	X
Vázquez José Juan	IIE

Subject Index

A

ABC transporters	VIII, 11; XI, 1
Adiponectin	IIB, 2
Aflatoxins	VIII, 4
Air pollution	IIA, 6
Angiogenesis	V, 6; VI, 1,3
Antibodies	VII, 10; IX, 1; XI 2
Antigen	VII, 1; IX, 1
Antisense oligonucleotides	XII, 1
Apoptosis	I, 1,7; IIE, 8; III, 4; V, 1
Aromatase	IIC, 1
Arsenic	IIA, 6
Autophagy	I, 1,7;

B

Bcl	I, 9; III, 4; V, 1; XI 2; XII, 11
Benzene	IIA, 5
Biomarkers	IX, 1; XIII, 2
Body mass index	IIB, 1
Breast cancer	IIC, 1; XI, 3; XII, 13

C

Cancer models	VIII 1, XIII, 2
Cancer stem cells	VIII, 9
Carcinogens	IIA, 1; VIII, 2
Casiopeínas	X, 1
Caspases	I, 8;
Causes of cancer	IIA, IIB, IIC, IID, IIE
Cell cycle	I, 1;
Cell lines	VIII, 9
Cervical cancer	IIE, 1;
Chemical carcinogenesis	VIII, 2
Chemotherapy	X, 1; XI 1
Chromatin	IV, 2
Cirrhosis	IID, 2
Clinical trials	X, 7; XII, 4; XIII 2
Cyclin-dependent kinases	I, 1,2;
Cyclins	I, 1; V, 2
Cytochrome P450	IIA, 3; VIII, 2

D

Dendritic cells	VII, 1
DNA-adducts	IIA, 2; VIII, 2; XI, 4
DDT	IIA, 4
Death receptor	I, 8;
Drug design and development	X, 1; XIII 1
Drug resistance	XI, 1

E

Environment   IIA, 1;

Epidermal growth factor   III, 5; V, 1; IX, 1; XI 2

Epigenetics   IV, 1

Estrogens   IIA, 6; IIB, 3; IIC,1; IID, 1; IIE,1; XI, 3

Extravasation   VI, 1

F

Focal adhesion kinase   V, 7

G

Gene knockdown   VIII, 9

Genotoxicity   IIA, 1; VIII, 2; VIII, 8

H

Hepatitis virus   IID, 1; VIII, 2

Hepatocellular carcinoma   IID, 1; VIII, 5

HER2   III, 3; IX, 1; XI 2

Histones   IV, 1

Histone deacetylases   IV, 2

Human Papilloma Virus   IIE, 1; VIII, 2

I

Immune system   VII, 1

Inflammation   VII, 1

Immunotherapy   VII, 6

Initiation   VIII, 4

Insulin-like growth factor   IIB, 1; XI, 3

Invasion   VI, 1

Intravasation   VI, 1

J

JAK-STAT   V, 1

K

Kinases   I, 1; V, 1; XI 2

L

Leptin   IIB, 1

Leukemia   IX, 1; XI, 3; XII, 12

Libraries   X, 3; XII, 1

Lung cancer   IIA, 1; IIB,1; XII, 14

M

MAP kinase   III, 3; V, 1; XI, 3

Metals   IIA, 6; X, 10
Methylation   IIA, 5; IV, 1
Metastasis   VI, 1
Migration   VI, 1
Mitosis Promoting Factor   I, 2;
Molecular diagnosis and prognosis   IX, 1
Multidrug resistance   VIII, 11; XI, 1
Myc   III, 2; VIII, 8; XII, 4

N

NFκB   V, 1
Nitrosamines   VIII, 4
Nitrosoureas   VIII, 4; XI, 2

O

Obesity   IIB, 1
Oncogenes   III, 1; V, 1

P

Pap smear   IX, 1
p53   IIA, 2; III, 1; V, 1; VIII, 8
Pesticides   IIA, 1;
Particulate matter   IIA, 6
Pharmacophore   X, 2
Phorbol esters   VIII, 4
Phosphatases   I, 3;
PI3 kinase   I, 4; IIB, 2; III, 3; V, 1; XI 2
PKC   XII, 9
Polycyclic aromatic hydrocarbons   IIA, 2; VIII, 2
Pre-clinical studies   VIII, 1; X, 2
Promotion   VIII, 4
Prostate specific antigen   IX, 1
PTEN   V, 1

R

Radiation   IIA, 1;
Ras   IIA, 2; III, 3; V, 1; VIII, 4; XII, 1
Reactive Oxygen Species   IIA, 6; VII, 1
Retinoblastoma   III, 7; VIII, 8
Retinoids   IIE, 1
Ribozymes   XII, 1

S

siRNA   VIII, 9; XII, 2
Sarcomas   IX, 4
Src   V, 8; XII, 1
Structure-activity relationships   X, 6

T

Tamoxifen   IIC, 1; XI, 3

Tobacco smoking   IIA, 1,2; IIE, 2
Transforming growth factor   III, 5
Tumor Necrosis Factor   I, 8; VII, 9
Tumor suppressor genes   III, 1

U

Ubiquitin   I, 2,6;

V

Vascular endothelial growth factor   V, 2
Vinca alkaloids   X, 2

W

Wnt   III, 11;

www.ingramcontent.com/pod-product-compliance
Lightning Source LLC
Chambersburg PA
CBHW050834220326
41598CB00006B/363